Neurobiology
of
Primary
Dementia

Association for Research in
Nervous and Mental Disease

Neurobiology
of
Primary
Dementia

EDITED BY
Marshal F. Folstein, M.D.

With the assistance of Stephen Gilman

*Association for Research in
Nervous and Mental Disease*

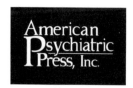

American
Psychiatric
Press, Inc.

Washington, DC
London, England

Copyright © 1998 Association for Research in Nervous and Mental Disease
ALL RIGHTS RESERVED
Manufactured in the United States of America on acid-free paper
First Edition
01 00 99 98   4 3 2 1

American Psychiatric Press, Inc.
1400 K Street, N.W., Washington, DC 20005
www.appi.org

Library of Congress Cataloging-in-Publication Data
Neurobiology of primary dementia / edited by Marshal F. Folstein.
    p. cm.
   Includes bibliographical references and index.
   ISBN 0-88048-915-4 (alk. paper)
   1. Senile dementia—Pathophysiology.   2. Alzheimer's disease—
Pathophysiology.   3. Neurobiology.   I. Folstein, Marshal F.
II. Association for Research in Nervous and Mental Disease.
   [DNLM: 1. Dementia.   2. Brain—physiopathology.   WM 220 N491
1998]
IN PROCESS
616.8′3107—dc21
DNLM/DLC
for Library of Congress   97-27523
                                                   CIP

British Library Cataloguing in Publication Data
A CIP record is available from the British Library.

Contents

Contributors

Robert H. Binstock, Ph.D.
Professor of Aging, Health, and Society, Case Western Reserve
University School of Medicine

Thomas D. Bird, M.D.
University of Washington Medical School, VA Medical Centers,
Seattle and Tacoma, Washington

David R. Borchelt, Ph.D.
Department of Pathology and the Neuropathology Laboratory,
The Johns Hopkins University School of Medicine

Michael R. Chun, M.D.
Gertrude H. Sergievsky Center, Department of Neurology, School
of Public Health

Stephen J. DeArmond, M.D., Ph.D.
Departments of Neuropathology (Neuropathology Unit) and
Neurology University of California, San Francisco

David W. Desmond, Ph.D.
Department of Neurology, Columbia University, College of
Physicians and Surgeons, New York

Marshal F. Folstein, M.D.
Chairman and Professor, Department of Psychiatry, New England
Medical Center, Tufts University School of Medicine

Susan E. Folstein, M.D.
Professor of Psychiatry, Tufts University School of Medicine,
Director of Child & Adolescent Psychiatry, New England Medical
Center

Samuel E. Gandy, M.D., Ph.D.
Department of Neurology and Neuroscience, Cornell University
Medical College

Albert Heyman, M.D.
Department of Medicine (Neurology), Duke University School of
Medicine

Barry D. Jordan, M.D.
Assistant Attending Neurologist, Sports Neurology Program,
Hospital for Special Surgery

Thomas H. Lampe, M.D.
University of Washington Medical School, VA Medical Centers,
Seattle and Tacoma, Washington

Lee J. Martin, Ph.D.
Department of Pathology and the Neuropathology Laboratory,
The Johns Hopkins University School of Medicine

Richard Mayeux, M.D., M.S.E.
Gertrude H. Sergievsky Center, Departments of Neurology,
Psychiatry, Center for Alzheimer's Disease Research in the City
of New York, and Division of Epidemiology

Thomas H. Murray, Ph.D.
Center for Biomedical Ethics, Case Western Reserve University
School of Medicine

Sergio Paradiso, M.D.
Department of Psychiatry, University of Iowa College of Medicine

Donald L. Price, M.D.
Departments of Pathology, Neurology, Neuroscience, and the
Neuropathology Laboratory, The Johns Hopkins University
School of Medicine, Department of Neurology, Cornell University
Medical College, New York

Richard W. Price, M.D.
Professor of Neurology, University of California, San Francisco,
Chief of Neurology Service, San Francisco General Hospital

Stanley I. Rapoport, M.D.
Chief, Laboratory of Neurosciences, National Institute on Aging,
National Institutes of Health

Murray A. Raskind, M.D.
VA Puget Sound Health Care System, Mental Health Programs,
Department of Psychiatry and Behavioral Sciences

Norman Relkin, M.D., Ph.D.
Assistant Professor of Neurology and Neuroscience, New York
Hospital—Cornell University Medical Center

Robert G. Robinson, M.D.
Department of Psychiatry, University of Iowa College of Medicine

Gerard D. Schellenberg, Ph.D.
University of Washington Medical School, VA Medical Centers,
Seattle and Tacoma, Washington

Peter Schofield, M.B.B.S., F.R.A.C.P., M.S.E.
Gertrude H. Sergievsky Center, Department of Neurology, School
of Public Health

Dennis J. Selkoe, M.D.
Professor of Neurology and Neuroscience, Center for Neurologic
Diseases, Brigham and Women's Hospital, Department of
Neurology, Harvard Medical School

Sangram S. Sisodia, Ph.D.
Departments of Pathology, Neuroscience, and the Neuropathology Laboratory, The Johns Hopkins University School of Medicine

Yaakov Stern, Ph.D.
Gertrude H. Sergievsky Center, Departments of Neurology, Psychiatry, and the Center for Alzheimer's Disease Research in the City of New York

Thomas K. Tatemichi, M.D. (deceased)
Gertrude H. Sergievsky Center, Department of Neurology, Columbia University, College of Physicians and Surgeons

Leon J. Thal, M.D.
Department of Neurosciences, University of California, San Diego, Department of Neurology, SDVAMC

Gopal Thinakaran, Ph.D.
Department of Pathology and Neuropathology Laboratory, The Johns Hopkins University School of Medicine

Ellen M. Wijsman, Ph.D.
University of Washington Medical School, VA Medical Centers, Seattle and Tacoma, Washington

Preface

Neurobiology of Primary Dementia, the 74th publication of the Association for Research in Nervous and Mental Disease (ARNMD), is a report of a conference on primary dementia held December 2–3, 1994. The primary dementias are ideal examples of the kinds of topics discussed in the reports of this society because the investigation and treatment of primary dementias bring together neurologists, psychiatrists, psychologists, and other scientists interested in mental disorders caused by brain diseases.

In the 80 years since the defining pathological description of Alzheimer's disease, research methods progressed from clinical pathological correlations and family history studies to an exploration of cellular neurochemistry and genomic pathology suggesting new treatments. These new studies are represented in this volume.

The topics of the book include epidemiology of Alzheimer's dementia by Mayeux, indicating the continuum of causality from gene expression to symptom expression, a process that occurs over decades with multiple mechanisms and thus multiple opportunities for intervention and prevention; genetic studies; the chemistry of amyloid production and processing, head trauma as a risk factor for Alzheimer's disease and other dementias; imaging studies revealing the pathology during life; potential laboratory diagnostic tests through analysis of genes and gene products; drug treatments under investigation; patient management; principles of genetic counseling; and ethics of dementia care in the changing socioeconomic health care environment. Other diseases causing dementia are represented by chapters on AIDS dementia, prions, and vascular disease as a cause of depression and dementia.

We are in the midst of one of those infrequent turning points in science when advances arise from theory and technique that are accessible only to cutting-edge investigators and laboratories. Every day, new discoveries are published. Some of the technical details of work of just a few years ago when this conference was held are already out of date. But for those students specializing in other areas or just beginning to work on dementia, this volume provides a useful primer of ideas from experts leading the field and points to the direction for research in the next millennium.

MARSHAL F. FOLSTEIN, M.D.

CHAPTER

1

The Epidemiology of Dementia Among the Elderly: Experience in a Community-Based Registry

Michael R. Chun, M.D., Peter Schofield, M.B.B.S., F.R.A.C.P., M.S.E., Yaakov Stern, Ph.D., Thomas K. Tatemichi, M.D.[†], and Richard Mayeux, M.D., M.S.E.

Introduction

Although Alzheimer's disease (AD) represents the most frequent cause of dementia, it is clearly not the only cause. Dementia may occur as a manifestation of cerebrovascular disease and other de-

Support for this paper came from the following federal grants: AG07232, AG10963, AG08702, and from the Charles S. Robertson Memorial Gift for Alzheimer's Disease Research from the Banbury Fund.

We thank the faculty of the Center for Geriatrics who developed the concept

[†]Deceased.

generative and metabolic diseases that occur during life with similar profound and debilitating consequences. The prevalence and incidence of diseases causing dementia, other than AD, vary depending on the type of population depicted. For example, in most hospital- and clinic-based series, AD accounts for more than half of the diagnosed patients with dementia (Sacktor and Mayeux 1994). A heterogeneous group of disorders accounts for the remaining causes of dementia. Population-based studies have generally reported a higher frequency of AD and lower frequency of other types of dementia (Copeland et al. 1992; Cummings and Benson 1992; Fratiglioni et al. 1991; Kokemen et al. 1988; Skoog et al. 1993), though AD can coexist with other causes of dementia in the elderly. For example, over a 15-year period in Rochester, Minnesota, AD alone accounted for 65% of the identified causes of dementia (Kokemen et al. 1992), but this number increased to 72% when concomitant conditions were included. Investigations in Liverpool, England (Copeland et al. 1992), and Stockholm, Sweden (Fratiglioni et al. 1991), suggest similar proportions. We have seen a similar trend among individuals aged 65 years and older in an urban New York community; dementias other than AD accounted for approximately 21% of the dementia cases (Sacktor and Mayeux 1994). Important differences in the types of dementia have also been found in a Swedish investigation (Skoog et al. 1993) of patients over age 85, where 44% were noted to have AD, yet another 47% had AD dementia associated with cerebrovascular disease. Among Asian populations the proportions of vascular dementia may also be higher.

There is little doubt that nomenclature and definitions explain much of the differences in rates of AD, vascular dementia, and other forms of dementia in some of these studies. Had these studies

of the registry: Barry Gurland, M.D., Rafael Lantigua, M.D., and David Wilder, Ph.D.; and the faculty of the Gertrude H. Sergievsky Center who participated in the studies within the registry: Ned Sacktor, M.D., Karen Marder, M.D., Karen Bell, M.D., George Dooneief, M.D., Mary Sano, Ph.D., and Ming-Xin Tang, Ph.D. We also thank Nicole Schupf, Ph.D., Dr.P.H., for her critical review of parts of this manuscript.

(Copeland et al. 1992; Fratiglioni et al. 1991; Kokemen et al. 1988) included mixed dementia in the proportion of dementia attributed to AD, the reported prevalence rates for AD would have been slightly higher and that for other forms of dementia much lower. Nonetheless, the proportion of dementias related to diseases other than AD is surprisingly high and remains constant with increasing age. Reviews of a large number of studies indicate that dementias other than AD apparently account for a third or more of the causes of dementia overall (Cummings and Benson 1992; Sacktor and Mayeux 1994). Though clinically diverse and distinct in etiology, this group of disorders falls into two major categories: dementias associated with cerebrovascular diseases and dementias associated with degenerative diseases of the basal ganglia.

A Service-Based Dementia Registry

We have chosen to discuss the epidemiology from the perspective of a service-based disease registry. The registry does not provide true prevalence or incidence rates. Rather, we considered that with the imminent restructuring of the health care system in the United States, health care service providers such as visiting nurse services, home health aids, and nursing homes will become a referral source for many neurologic problems such as dementia. An understanding of the frequencies and causes of dementia and cognitive impairment in elderly people who use these services will become increasingly important. The registry also differs from clinic- or hospital-based studies because all individuals who use health-related services at any level were eligible. Thus, a service-based registry provides an estimate of all or nearly all patients seeking medical attention or public or private assistance for their illnesses. Moreover, a registry provides an advantage because most previous studies of cognitive decline in the elderly have been performed on inpatient populations (Erkinjuntti et al. 1986; Freemon 1976; Marsden and Harrison 1972; Smith and Kiloh 1981) or have focused on dementia rather than cognitive impairment (Broe et al.

1976; Jorm et al. 1988; Macer et al. 1991; Williamson et al. 1964). The registry described here reflects the probable caseload to be anticipated by neurologists and other physicians who care for older patients with dementia.

In the creation of a registry in an urban community for persons over age 65, we were able to identify most individuals with suspected memory problems and characterize the severity and causes of those memory problems. Severity was established by using a neuropsychological paradigm to separate subjects into four categories: those with dementia and those with moderate, mild, or no cognitive impairment. We describe the profiles of these groups and consider how such a registry might be used. We also review a few of the major known antecedents for the most common forms of dementia.

The development of the registry and the prospective investigation of AD and related dementias began in 1988 and was limited to a portion of the Washington Heights community of northern Manhattan (from 155th Street to 181st Street and from Harlem River Drive to Riverside Drive). According to the 1990 census, approximately 9,000 people over the age of 65 resided in this area. A network of community-based service providers including visiting nurse services, home health care agencies, nursing homes, senior centers, and housing and other community agencies (e.g., Meals-on-Wheels, Seniors Helping Seniors, Homebound Elderly) was used to identify individuals with possible memory problems. We also monitored admission and discharge lists from Columbia Presbyterian Medical Center (and affiliated hospitals) and contacted the private medical practitioners and health maintenance organizations (HMOs) in the community. Because many individuals used one or more of the services, ascertainment relied on a capture-recapture method to provide an exhaustive survey of cases.

For ethnic group classification, we used the format suggested by the 1990 United States Census Bureau (Census of Population and Housing 1990). The 1990 census allows for the identification of Hispanics as a cultural group, with further designation of African-American, Caucasian, or other. We separated subjects into four ethnic groups according to self-report: African-American, Hispanic,

Caucasian, and other, based on direct interview with the subjects or their family members.

Once identified, subjects were screened with a standardized questionnaire (Gurland et al. 1984) and initially classified into three groups: no impairment, borderline impairment, and possible dementia. A sample of each group received a detailed examination consisting of two sessions, as illustrated in Figure 1–1. We focused on subjects whose scores indicated possible impairment, but 40% of those with no impairment on screening were also evaluated.

In the first part of the evaluation, a physician obtained a standardized history, recorded all medications, and performed a neurological and general physical examination. A neurologist completed three measures of activities of daily living: the Blessed Dementia Index (Blessed et al. 1968), the Schwab and England Activities of Daily Living (Schwab and England 1969), and the Barthel Index (Mahoney and Barthel 1965). He or she then estimated whether cognitive impairment or dementia was present and if so the etiology. A modified Clinical Dementia Rating (CDR) (Hughes et al. 1982) was assigned to reflect severity of dementia.

The second part of the evaluation comprised a complete neuropsychological assessment and a set of screening items for depression (the Hamilton Rating Scale for Depression [Hamilton

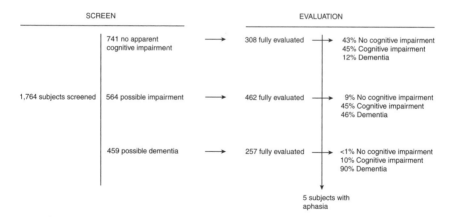

Figure 1–1. Screening and evaluation of subjects for a service-based dementia registry.

1960]), psychosis, and alcohol abuse (Structured Clinical Interview for DSM-III-R Diagnosis [SCID] screen [Spitzer and Williams 1986]), all conducted in English or Spanish (subject's preference). The evaluation contained tests of memory (short and long term, verbal and nonverbal), orientation, abstract reasoning, language (naming, verbal fluency, comprehension, and repetition), and construction (copying and matching). A neuropsychological paradigm using cutoff scores necessary but not sufficient for the diagnosis of dementia has been described previously (Stern et al. 1992). Briefly, subjects met the neuropsychological criteria for dementia if they performed below the cutoff scores on at least two of three memory tests and two other nonmemory areas.

A team of physicians and neuropsychologists then reviewed the results of these evaluations at a diagnostic consensus conference. Any available ancillary information, including medical charts and computed tomography (CT) or magnetic resonance imaging (MRI) scan reports, was reviewed. The diagnosis of dementia required evidence of dementia, based on the neuropsychological paradigm, and evidence of impairment in social or occupational function, based on the formal functional assessments and elicited history. Criteria of the National Institute of Neurological and Communicative Disorders and Stroke–Alzheimer's Disease and Related Disorders Association (McKhann et al. 1984) were used for the diagnosis of probable or possible AD.

Subjects without dementia were assigned to one of three categories based on their neuropsychological test performance. Subjects in the first category—*moderate cognitive impairment*—usually met the CDR criteria for questionable dementia. Subjects had scores that approached paradigm criteria for dementia, or subjects met criteria but had no functional impairment. Subjects in the second category—*mild cognitive impairment*—had more than one test score below cutoffs but were not close to paradigm criteria. These subjects were not as impaired as those in category one but were still clearly abnormal. Subjects in the third category—*no cognitive impairment*—had no more than one low test score and the test results were classified as not having any apparent clinical significance; that is, their scores were close to or within normal range.

Results Over the First 4 Years

A total of 1,764 individuals were initially identified and screened (see Figure 1–1). Sources of subjects were home health care agencies (38.5%), regional medical facilities (30.0%), local nursing homes (10.8%), volunteers: self-referrals and friend or relative referrals (11.5%), senior centers and housing (5.9%), other community agencies (2.3%) and other (<1%). The overall refusal rate from referral sources was about 20%. Screening scores estimated that 741 (42%) subjects had no impairment, 564 (32%) had possible impairment, and 459 (26%) had possible dementia. Obviously, the frequency of possible cognitive impairment and dementia was higher than would be observed in a typical population sample because of the source of subjects. The objective of the registry was to identify all individuals in a geographic area who used medical services because of dementia or cognitive decline.

A total of 1,027 subjects underwent a full evaluation by physicians and neuropsychologists. Reasons why screened subjects were not evaluated included refusals (17%), inability to locate subject (6%), death (7%), deferral (63%; 90% of these subjects had no impairment on screening), and other (7%). The demographics of evaluated subjects are provided in Table 1–1. After evaluation, 514 (50%) met the criteria for dementia, 146 (14%) were found to have moderate impairment, 199 (19%) had mild impairment, and the remaining 168 (16%) subjects were classified as having no clinically

Table 1–1. Demographics of 1,027 fully evaluated subjects by ethnic group

Race	N	Age[a]	Education[b]
Caucasian	157	83.1 (8.6)	10.9 (3.9)
African-American	363	79.5 (8.2)	8.3 (3.5)
Hispanic	480	77.1 (7.7)	5.6 (4.2)
Other	27	83.4 (8.0)	8.6 (4.8)

[a]Mean age at time of evaluation (standard deviation).
[b]Mean highest grade of education (standard deviation).

significant cognitive deficit (Table 1–2). The records of nine persons were incomplete, preventing classification. Five individuals were unclassifiable because of a left hemispheric stroke that caused aphasia (their data are not included in the 1,027). Mean age was significantly different among all groups. However, there were no significant gender or ethnic differences among these groups. Distributions of severity of cognitive impairment of subjects from different referral sources are given in Table 1–3.

Of those with dementia, 45% had probable AD, an additional

Table 1–2. Demographics of evaluated subjects and severity of impairment

Severity of impairment	N	Age[a]	Caucasian[b] (%)	African-American[b] (%)	Hispanic[b] (%)
Dementia	514	82.1 (8.0)	57	57	46
Moderate cognitive impairment	146	78.4 (7.6)	11	14	14
Mild impairment	199	76.2 (7.4)	15	14	21
No impairment	168	73.3 (6.8)	17	14	18
Total	1,027[c]		100	100	100

[a]Mean age at time of evaluation (standard deviation).
[b]Percentage of subjects of a given ethnicity in each category.
[c]Includes five patients with aphasia.

Table 1–3. Sources of evaluated subjects and severity of impairment

	Source of subjects (%)		
Severity of impairment	Nursing homes	Home health care agencies	Regional medical facilities
Dementia	86	53	56
Moderate cognitive impairment	5	18	11
Mild impairment	5	18	14
No impairment	4	11	19
Total	100	100	100

17% had probable or possible AD with stroke, and 6% had Parkinson's disease with dementia (Table 1–4). Dementia due only to vascular causes accounted for 7% (36/514). In about 7% of subjects the dementia syndrome was only related to one or more strokes. Metabolic and toxic dementias accounted for less than 1% each.

There were some minor differences among causes of dementia within ethnic groups. Among Caucasians with dementia, 12% had Parkinson's disease with dementia compared with 4%–5% of African-Americans and Hispanics. Stroke-related dementia was found in 12% of Hispanics, compared with only 2%–3% in Caucasians and African-Americans. These differences may simply reflect the use of such services by individuals with these conditions rather than differences in the actual rate of diseases.

Table 1–4.   Causes of dementia

Diagnosis	N (%)	Ethnic group (%)		
		Caucasian[a] (N = 84)	African-American[a] (N = 201)	Hispanic[a] (N = 214)
Probable Alzheimer's disease	230 (44.7)	46	46	42
Alzheimer's disease with stroke	88 (17.1)	12	20	17
Alzheimer's disease with other concomitant dementia	51 (9.9)	13	10	7
Other dementia	45 (8.8)	7	10	8
Stroke-related dementia	36 (7.0)	2	3	12[b]
Dementia, cause unknown	29 (5.6)	5	4	6
Parkinson's disease with dementia	29 (5.6)	12[b]	4	5
Toxic dementia (including alcohol)	4 (<1)	2	1	0
Metabolic dementia	2 (<1)	0	0	1
Total	514	100	100	100

[a]Percentage of subjects of a given ethnicity for each diagnosis.
[b]Significant difference compared to other ethnic groups (P < .05).

In those subjects with cognitive impairment, an obvious contributing factor was noted in 46 subjects: stroke (14), alcohol abuse
(8), depression (8), effects of medications (4), head trauma (3),
Parkinson's disease (2), brain tumors (2), schizophrenia (1), mental retardation (1), hypothyroidism (1), anoxia (1), and normal-
pressure hydrocephalus (1). Classification of subjects by screen
versus evaluation is indicated in Table 1–5. Among all evaluated
subjects, 90% of those with possible impairment by screening score
turned out to have at least mild impairment after evaluation. In
contrast, only 55% of those with a no-impairment screening score
were found to have some degree of impairment. In terms of distinguishing subjects with mild cognitive impairment or worse from
those with no impairment, the screen had a sensitivity of 80.0%, a
specificity of 75.1%, and a positive predictive value of 94.0%.

From the evaluated subjects, we can estimate the amount of
impairment in the total group because screening questionnaire performance reflected the degree of cognitive impairment found on
full evaluation. In extrapolating screening scores to the original
1,764 subjects, 1,100 (62%) subjects are estimated to have had at
least mild cognitive impairment, of whom 625 (35%) had dementia.
Because these estimates are most relevant in the context of our
sources of subjects, the frequency of cognitive impairment and dementia estimated from this type of registry probably reflects that
found in people using services such as home health care agencies
and nursing homes. Although estimates of prevalence are obtained
using different sampling techniques, characteristics of the registry
are useful in examining this subpopulation.

Table 1–5. Classification of subjects by screen versus evaluation

Classification from screening questionnaire	Classification from full evaluation			
	Dementia (%)	Cognitive impairment (%)	Normal (%)	
No impairment	12	43	45	100%
Borderline impairment	47	43	10	100%
Possible dementia	93	7	<1	100%

Discussion

As expected (Census of Population and Housing 1990; Macer et al. 1991; Thal et al. 1988), probable and possible AD were the most frequent causes of dementia, present in 77%, followed by vascular disease, present in 24%. Because the prevalence of AD, Parkinson's disease, and vascular disease was high in this age group, and dementias due to more than one cause were expected, we used overlap categories such as AD plus stroke and Parkinson's disease with dementia. Although the association between Parkinson's disease and Caucasians has been described (Marttila and Rinne 1981), the association between stroke-related dementia and Hispanics has not. Clearly, the incidence of stroke-related dementia in Hispanics deserves further investigation in the population-based study that is currently under way in the same community.

The Common Dementias

Regardless of how or where dementia has been examined, three forms are consistently cited as the most frequent: AD, dementia with cerebrovascular disease, and dementia in patients with Parkinson's disease. Here we briefly review the epidemiology of these three conditions.

Alzheimer's disease.   The frequency of AD has been well studied over the last few years. It is well-known that the prevalence or proportion of cases in the population rises steeply with age; estimates of as high as 40% in subjects age 80 years or older have been reported (Evans et al. 1989). The prevalence of AD appears to be comparable in all ethnic groups in the United States once educational differences are taken into account (Gurland et al. 1995). Incidence rates (or the rate of newly acquired disease) in the United States and Europe are also exceedingly high (Hebert et al. 1995), as indicated in Figure 1–2. Despite differences in diagnostic

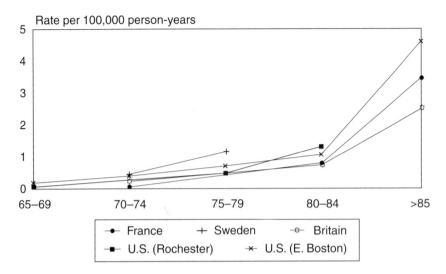

Figure 1–2. Age-specific incidence rates for Alzheimer's disease in the United States and Europe during the last 30 years.
Source. Based on data from Table 4, Breteler et al. 1992 and Hebert et al. 1995.

criteria, there is a striking consistency that indicates a steady increase in risk of AD with age.

Though AD occurs as a rare autosomal dominant disease among individuals ages 35 to 50, in the majority of cases AD is sporadic and occurs later in life. A few of these early-onset heritable forms of familial AD have been genetically linked to chromosome 21 and a series of mutations in the amyloid precursor protein (Chartier-Harlin et al. 1991; Citron et al. 1992; Goate et al. 1991; Murrell et al. 1991; Naruse et al. 1991; St. George-Hyslop et al. 1987, 1990). More recently, a gene on chromosome 14 that accounts for more than 70% of familial cases was discovered (Sherrington et al. 1995). In the same year, Schellenberg et al. (Levy-Lahad et al. 1995a,b) identified a gene on chromosome 1 responsible for early-onset AD in the Volga German families.

Late-onset familial AD has been linked to a region of chromosome 19 (Pericak-Vance et al. 1991), and more recently it has been associated with the ε4 allele of apolipoprotein-E (APOE-ε4) (Brogaonkar et al. 1993; Corder et al. 1993, 1994; Maestre et al. 1995; Mayeux et al. 1993b; Payami et al. 1993; Poirier et al. 1993; Saunders et al. 1993a,b; Strittmatter et al. 1993). If the APOE protein has a direct role in increasing the risk of AD, then a large proportion of the population, between 4% and 30% depending on the ethnic group, may be at risk by virtue of carrying at least one APOE-ε4 allele. The association may not be as robust among African-Americans and Hispanics, which suggests that there may be genetic or environmental modifiers (Maestre et al. 1995) or linkage disequilibrium. Other potential genetic risks include shared susceptibility to Down's syndrome (Schupf et al. 1994) and Parkinson's disease (van Duijn et al. 1991).

Only a few environmental risk factors have been consistently associated with AD. Traumatic head injury (Mayeux et al. 1993a; Mortimer et al. 1991), which may increase the risk of AD in conjunction with APOE-ε4 (Mayeux et al. 1995b), has been associated with AD. Illiteracy and reduced years of formal education have also been associated with AD (Evans et al. 1993; Stern et al. 1994). It is not clear whether this represents an issue related to detection or whether it is related to the concept of increased *cognitive reserve* as suggested by Katzman (Zhang et al. 1990) and Stern et al. (1994). Cigarette smoking has been purported to act as a protective factor (Broe et al. 1990; Graves et al. 1990, 1991; Herbert et al. 1992; Letenneur et al. 1994). Biological evidence that smoking facilitates nicotinic receptor function could mean that smoking delays some of the signs of AD.

Cerebrovascular dementia.   Although stroke and dementia are frequently found in the same person (Tatemichi et al. 1990, 1992a), it is often uncertain whether stroke is directly causal, contributory, or coincidental (Brust 1983; Scheinberg 1988; Tatemichi 1990). Two proposed sets of diagnostic criteria by Chui et al. (1992) and Román et al. (1993) constitute a significant advance but should not be considered definitive, because important gaps in knowledge still exist (Drachman 1993). In our registry, vascular dementias were divided into AD plus stroke and stroke-related dementia. The difference between these two categories is meant to reflect different processes of decline. Persons diagnosed with AD plus stroke were felt to have signs or symptoms of a stroke but still showed a gradual cognitive decline consistent with AD and not temporally related to the stroke. Individuals with stroke-related dementia were not felt to show such decline but had onset of dementia temporally related to one or more strokes. The distinction is retrospective and often difficult; when the two categories are combined, the association we noted between stroke-related dementia and Hispanics diminished.

Vascular dementia has been defined as a clinical syndrome of acquired intellectual impairment resulting from cerebrovascular disease. This definition properly includes both hemorrhagic and ischemic cerebrovascular disease (Brust 1988; Loeb 1988; Román et al. 1993), though most often ischemic damage is the predominant cause (Chui 1989; Chui et al. 1992; Scheinberg 1988). The presence of cerebrovascular disease can be inferred by a history compatible with stroke, which may occur in about 50% of patients with vascular dementia (Mayer-Gross et al. 1969) or even more frequently (Erkinjuntti et al. 1988). Among those who lack a history, stroke may be clinically obvious, with persisting focal neurological signs on examination. Silent strokes (Desmond et al. 1993), cerebral infarction with transient signs (Bogousslavsky and Regli 1984; Perrone et al. 1979; Waxman and Toole 1983), strokes in strategic areas not associated with hemiplegia or hemisensory loss (Tatemichi et al. 1992b), and others may result in cumulative damage to the cerebral white matter, leading to progressive but not apoplectic cognitive (or physical) impairment, as in Binswanger's disease. In any of these circumstances brain imaging is critical, as recognized by both diagnostic criteria (Chui et al. 1992; Román et al. 1993). There are no definitive brain CT or MRI criteria for vascular dementia, but the absence of any imaging evidence of cerebrovascular disease strongly refutes vascular etiology.

The ischemic score (IS) proposed in 1975 by Hachinski and colleagues (1975) was intended as a clinical method to distinguish vascular from degenerative dementia. Among the four pathological validation studies that provide detailed information on the IS (Erkinjuntti et al. 1988; Fischer et al. 1991; Molsa et al. 1985; Rosen et al. 1979), the one clinical feature found to discriminate significantly between multi-infarct dementia (MID) and AD in all studies was a history of prior stroke. One conclusion from this analysis is that the most discriminating elements of the IS merely identify evidence for recent or remote stroke (Loeb and Gandolfo 1983).

Katzman et al. (1988) summarized nine studies with a total of 784 patients, confirming the impression gained from pathological series: AD was six times as common as vascular dementia (65.9% versus 10.8%), although brain imaging was not used to verify diagnoses in most cases. We agree with Chui (1989) that clinical dementia series are likely to underestimate the contribution of cerebrovascular disease. Prevalence estimates for vascular dementia in hospital-based series vary from 12% to 30%. Tatemichi et al. (1990) estimated the prevalence and incidence of dementia following ischemic stroke using information from the Stroke Data Bank cohort; among 726 testable patients older than 60 years, with acute ischemic stroke, 15.9% were found to have dementia at stroke onset. Among the 610 patients who initially were without dementia, the incidence of dementia occurring in the 2-year follow-up was strongly related to age, increasing from 5.5% for a patient aged 60 years to 10.5% for a 90-year-old. In a consecutive series of 251 stroke patients over 60 years (mean age 71.9 years) admitted to Columbia-Presbyterian Medical Center 3 months after acute brain infarction and a group of 249 stroke-free control subjects (mean age 70.8 years) recruited from a similar neighborhood (Gurland et al. 1995), dementia was diagnosed or was present in 26.8% of stroke patients and 3.2% of the control. Three interesting studies, from Newcastle (for severe cases) (Kay et al. 1964), Appigiano (Rocca et al. 1990), and Gothenburg (Skoog et al. 1993), all reported a higher proportion of vascular dementia than AD. However, the latter two studies included mixed dementia cases in the vascular dementia group. Thus, vascular dementia accounts for 10%–20% of the total causes of dementia in most hospital and community studies.

Hypertension, atrial fibrillation, congestive heart failure, coronary heart disease, carotid bruit, diabetes, cigarette smoking, hyperlipidemia, peripheral vascular disease, transient ischemic attack, and stroke have all been cited as potential precursors of vascular dementia (Cummings 1987; Hachinski et al. 1989). Stroke can complicate preexisting AD, with no contributory role to the dementia syndrome. It has been proposed that the vascular disease potentiating the clinical effects of AD may be more subtle than the obvious focal stroke that usually brings a patient to clinical attention; rather, white matter ischemic changes that are common in clinically (Diaz et al. 1991) and pathologically diagnosed patients with AD (Brun and Englund 1986) may contribute to dementia in patients with subclinical AD when either alone is insufficient, or they may accelerate the progressive course in patients with clinically apparent AD. The high prevalence of amyloid angiopathy in patients with AD (Glenner et al. 1981; Mandybur 1975) has led to the suggestion that this microangiopathy bears a pathogenetic relationship to the white matter demyelination and incomplete infarctions in AD (Gray et al. 1985), similar to that proposed for the role of arteriosclerotic changes in the development of Binswanger's disease (Hachinski 1990). APOE-ε4 allele may also be associated with dementia in patients with stroke (Slooter et al. 1997).

Parkinson's disease with dementia.   The prevalence of Parkinson's disease with or without dementia increases with age (Mayeux et al. 1992, 1995a). For example, the prevalence of Parkinson's disease at age 80 is approximately 1%, and a significant proportion of that group of individuals have dementia as an important manifestation. In previous studies it has been established that dementia in Parkinson's disease increases more than threefold if the onset of the motor signs of Parkinson's disease is after rather than before age 70 and that the cumulative incidence of dementia reaches 65% by age 85 (Mayeux et al. 1990). The risk of dementia among patients with Parkinson's disease exceeds, by twofold, that expected for individuals of the same age without Parkinson's disease (Marder et al. 1995).

Risk factors for dementia in patients with Parkinson's disease include advanced age, severe motor manifestations, the presence of depression or psychosis, and hypomimia (Marder et al. 1995; Stern et al. 1993). A family history of dementia is more frequent among patients with Parkinson's disease and dementia than among those without dementia (Marder et al. 1990). A similar indication of shared susceptibility has been observed by Hofman et al. (1989), who reported higher-than-normal incidence of Parkinson's disease among family members of patients with AD. However, this relationship needs further investigation. There is no evidence that Parkinson's disease with or without dementia shares established genetic risk factors with AD in terms of polymorphisms of apolipoprotein-ε4 (Marder et al. 1994).

Cognitive Impairment in the Absence of Dementia

We found that there were no ethnic differences among groups with varying levels of cognitive impairment in the absence of dementia among individuals in the registry. However, there was an association between advancing age and the level of impairment. Age was still the strongest predictor of AD (Breteler et al. 1992), and the older, moderately impaired subjects were at higher risk for progressing to dementia, regardless of its cause. Patients with a CDR of 0.5—similar to our moderately impaired group—progressed to a more advanced stage of dementia or had AD at autopsy (Morris et al. 1991; Rubin et al. 1989). The risk for dementia in the younger, mildly impaired subjects is less clear.

More emphasis was directed in the registry toward determining etiologies for patients with dementia than for those with cognitive impairment alone. However, it appears that stroke, depression, medication effects, and alcohol were some of the more frequently identified contributors in the cognitively impaired. Although some reports (Larson et al. 1985; Maletta et al. 1982; Smith and Kiloh 1981) have suggested a significant role of depression in dementia (pseudodementia), in the registry depression was infrequently associated with cognitive impairment and was not related to dementia. This result may reflect the selection process: since most of our subjects came from home health agencies, hospitals, and nursing homes, subjects with depression sufficient to cause dementia may have been identified and treated before they entered our study.

Additional investigations for patients in the registry were limited because of inaccessible laboratory and brain imaging data in some cases. The results from previous laboratory investigations were obtained when possible. However, a previous study of 200 outpatients with suspected dementia (of whom 24% had laboratory tests before study enrollment) indicated that brain imaging did not lead to any treatment changes or contribute to the diagnosis of dementia by the consensus group (Larson et al. 1985). Additionally, Thal et al. (1988) found in a selected population that data such as CT scans, EEGs, and serum studies aided the diagnosis in only 6% of the cases. It is likely that our population was less selected than these two groups, and in a small percentage of cases the diagnosis could be aided by laboratory tests. However, there would be no effect on the frequency of dementia, cognitive impairment, and nonimpairment because this was determined by neuropsychological performance and functional status.

It was clear from our experience in the registry that a significant number of individuals with cognitive impairment in the absence of dementia sought or used health-related services, which suggests that this group may have serious morbidity. Many go on to develop dementia, as would be expected. Thus, intervention at this stage would be of great benefit. However, in a subgroup of subjects progression to dementia does not occur. Certainly further investigation of this group is indicated.

Conclusions

We have reviewed the epidemiology of the most common forms of dementia and have described the frequency and some characteristics of dementia and cognitive impairment in an ethnically diverse registry of individuals who use community-based health care services. The experience in a community-based registry indicates that the burden of impairment among the elderly population is evident and impressive.

In 1990 major health care goals for the United States were specified in the Department of Health and Human Services document "Healthy People 2000" (1990). For the elderly, the directive is to improve function in people age 65 and older. More specifically, a

20% reduction in the number of people requiring assistance for personal care activities by the year 2000 has been mandated. We believe that this goal can be realized only by identifying the magnitude and etiologies of various forms of dementia and cognitive impairment in the elderly.

References

Blessed G, Tomlinson BE, Roth M: The association between quantitative measures of dementia and of senile changes in the cerebral gray matter of elderly subjects. Br J Psychol 225:797–811, 1968

Bogousslavsky J, Regli F: Cerebral infarction with transient signs (CITS): do TIAs correspond to small deep infarcts in internal carotid occlusion? Stroke 15:536–539, 1984

Breteler MMG, Claus JJ, van Duijn CM, et al: Epidemiology of Alzheimer's disease. Epidemiol Rev 14:59–82, 1992

Broe GA, Akhtar AJ, Andrews GR, et al: Neurological disorders in the elderly at home. J Neurol Neurosurg Psychiatry 36:362–366, 1976

Broe GA, Henderson AS, Creasey H, et al: A case-control study of Alzheimer's disease in Australia. Neurology 40:1698–1707, 1990

Brogaonkar DS, Schmidit LC, Martin SE, et al: Linkage of late-onset Alzheimer's disease with apolipoprotein-E type 4 on chromosome 19. Lancet 342:625, 1993

Brun A, Englund E: A white matter disorder in dementia of the Alzheimer type: a pathoanatomical study. Ann Neurol 19:253–262, 1986

Brust JCM: Dementia and cerebrovascular disease, in The Dementias. Edited by Mayeux R, Rosen WG. New York, Raven, 1983, pp 131–147

Brust JCM: Vascular dementia is overdiagnosed. Arch Neurol 45:799–801, 1988

Census of Population and Housing, 1990: Summary tape file 1. Technical documentation prepared by Bureau of Census. Washington, DC, Bureau of Census, 1991

Chartier-Harlin M-C, Crawford F, Houlden H, et al: Early-onset Alzheimer's disease caused by mutations at codon 717 of the beta-amyloid precursor protein gene. Nature 353:844–846, 1991

Chui HC: Dementia: a review emphasizing clinicopathologic correlation and brain-behavior relationships. Arch Neurol; 46:806–814, 1989

Chui HC, Victoroff JI, Margolin D, et al: Criteria for the diagnosis of ischemic vascular dementia proposed by the state of California Alzheimer's Disease Diagnostic and Treatment Centers. Neurology 42:473–480, 1992

Citron M, Oltersdorf T, Haass C, et al: Mutation of the beta-amyloid precursor protein in familial Alzheimer's disease increases beta-protein production. Nature 360:672–674, 1992

Copeland JR, Davidson IA, Dewey ME, et al: Alzheimer's disease, other dementias, depression, and pseudodementia: prevalence, incidence, and three-year outcome in Liverpool. Br J Psychiatry 161:230–239, 1992

Corder EH, Saunders AM, Strittmatter WJ, et al: Gene dose of apolipoprotein-E type 4 allele and the risk of Alzheimer's disease in late onset families. Science 261:921–923, 1993

Corder EH, Saunders AM, Risch NJ, et al: Apolipoprotein-E type 2 allele decreases the risk for late onset Alzheimer's disease. Nat Genet 7: 180–184, 1994

Cummings JL: Multi-infarct dementia. Psychosomatics 28:117–126, 1987

Cummings JL, Benson DF: Dementia. A Clinical Approach. 2nd Edition. Boston, Butterworth-Heinemann, 1992

Desmond DW, Tatemichi TK, Figueroa M, Stern Y: Stroke-related cognitive dysfunction persists after physical recovery (abstract). J Clin Exp Neuropsychol 15:99, 1993

Diaz JF, Merskey H, Hachinski VC, et al: Improved recognition of leukoaraiosis and cognitive impairment in Alzheimer's disease. Arch Neurol 48:1022–1025, 1991

Drachman DA: New criteria for the diagnosis of vascular dementia: do we know enough yet? Neurology 43:246–249, 1993

Erkinjuntti T, Wikström J, Palo J, Autio L: Dementia among medical inpatients: evaluation of 2000 consecutive admissions. Arch Intern Med 146:1923–1926, 1986

Erkinjuntti T, Haltia M, Palo J, et al: Accuracy of the clinical diagnosis of vascular dementia: a prospective clinical and post-mortem neuropathological study. J Neurol Neurosurg Psychiatry 1037–1044, 1988

Evans DA, Funkenstein HH, Albert MS, et al: Prevalence of Alzheimer's disease in a community population of older persons higher than previously reported. JAMA 262:2551–2556, 1989

Evans DA, Beckett LA, Albert MS, et al: Level of education and change in cognitive function in a community population of older persons. Ann Epidemiol 3:71–77, 1993

Fischer P, Jellinger K, Gatterer G, Danielczyk W: Prospective neuropathological validation of Hachinski's Ischemic Score in dementia. J Neurol Neurosurg Psychiatry 54:580–583, 1991

Fratiglioni L, Grut M, Forsell Y, et al: Prevalence of Alzheimer's disease and other dementias in an elderly urban population: relationship with age, sex, and education. Neurology 41:1886–1892, 1991

Freemon FR: Evaluation of patients with progressive intellectual deterioration. Arch Neurol 33:658–659, 1976

Glenner GG, Henry JM, Fujihara S: Congophilic angiopathy in the pathogenesis of Alzheimer's degeneration. Ann Pathol 1:105–108, 1981

Goate A, Chartier-Harlin M-C, Mullan M, et al: Segregation of a missense mutation in the amyloid precursor protein gene with familial Alzheimer's disease. Nature 349:704–706, 1991

Graves AB, White E, Koepsell TD, et al: A case-control study of Alzheimer's disease. Ann Neurol 28:766–774, 1990

Graves AB, van Duijn CM, Chandra V, et al: Alcohol and tobacco consumption as risk factors for Alzheimer's disease: a collaborative reanalysis of case-control studies. Int J Epidemiol 20(suppl 2):S48-S57, 1991

Gray F, Dubas F, Roullet E, Escourolle R: Leukoencephalopathy in diffuse hemorrhagic cerebral amyloid angiopathy. Ann Neurol 18:54–59, 1985

Gurland B, Golden RR, Teresi JA, Challop J: The SHORT-CARE: an efficient instrument for the assessment of depression, dementia and disability. J Gerontol 39:166–169, 1984

Gurland B, Wilder D, Cross P, et al: Relative rates of dementia by multiple case definitions, over two prevalence periods, in three cultural groups. Am J Geriatric Psych 3:6–12, 1995

Hachinski VC: The decline and resurgence of vascular dementia. Can Med Assoc J 142:107–111, 1990

Hachinski VC, Iliff LD, Zilhka E, et al: Cerebral blood flow in dementia. Arch Neurol 32:632–637, 1975

Hachinski VC, Mirsen TR, Merskey H: Changing concepts of vascular dementia, in Cerebrovascular Diseases. Edited by Ginsberg MD, Dietrich WD. New York, Raven, 1989, pp 181–191

Hamilton M: A rating scale for depression. J Neurol Neurosurg Psychiatry 23:56–62, 1960

Herbert LE, Scherr PA, Beckett LA, et al: Relation of smoking and alcohol consumption to incident of Alzheimer's disease. Am J Epidemiol 135:347–355, 1992

Hebert LE, Scherr PA, Beckett LA, et al: Age-specific incidence of Alzheimer's disease in a community population. JAMA 273:1354–1359, 1995

Hofman A, Schulte W, Tanja TA, et al: History of dementia and Parkinson's disease in 1st-degree relative of patients with Alzheimer's disease. Neurology 39:1589–1592, 1989

Hughes CP, Berg L, Danziger WL, et al: A new clinical scale for the staging of dementia. Br J Psychiatry 140:566–572, 1982

Jorm AF, Korten AE, Jacomb PA: Projected increases in the number of dementia cases for 29 developed countries: application of a new method for making projections. Acta Psychiatr Scand 78:493–500, 1988

Katzman R, Lasker B, Bernstein N: Advances in the diagnosis of dementia: accuracy of diagnosis and consequences of misdiagnosis of disorders causing dementia, in Aging and the Brain. Edited by Terry RD. New York, Raven, 1988, pp 17–62

Kay DWK, Beamish P, Roth M: Old age mental disorders in Newcastle upon Tyne, I: a study of prevalence. Br J Psychiatry 110:146–158, 1964

Kokemen E, Chandra V, Schoenberg BS: Trends in incidence of dementing illness in Rochester, Minnesota in three quinquennial periods, 1960–1974. Neurology 38:975–980, 1988

Larson EB, Reifler BV, Sumi SM, et al: Diagnostic evaluation of 200 elderly outpatients with suspected dementia. J Gerontol A Biol Sci Med Sci 40(5):827–842, 1985

Letenneur L, Dartigues J, Commenges D, et al: Tobacco consumption and cognitive impairment in elderly people: a population-based study. Ann Epidemiol 4:449–454, 1994

Levy-Lahad E, Wasco W, Poorkaj P, et al: Candidate gene for the chromosome 1 familial Alzheimer's disease locus. Science 269:973–977, 1995a

Levy-Lahad E, Wijsman EM, Nemens E, et al: A familial Alzheimer's disease locus on chromosome 1. Science 269:970–973, 1995b

Loeb C: Clinical criteria for the diagnosis of vascular dementia. Eur Neurol 28:87–92, 1988

Loeb C, Gandolfo C: Diagnostic evaluation of degenerative and vascular dementia. Stroke 14:399–401, 1983

Macer CA, Davis DR, Brandes DA, Still CN: A report on dementia in South Carolina, 1988–1990. J S C Med Assoc 87:531–535, 1991

Maestre G, Ottman R, Stern Y, et al: Apolipoprotein-E and Alzheimer's disease: ethnic variation in genotypic risks. Ann Neurol 37:254–259, 1995

Mahoney FI, Barthel DW: Functional evaluation: the Barthel Index. Md Med J 14:61–65, 1965

Maletta GJ, Pirozzolo FJ, Thompson G, Mortimer J: Organic mental disorders in a geriatric outpatient population. Am J Psychiatry 139:521–523, 1982

Mandybur TI: The incidence of cerebral amyloid angiopathy in Alzheimer's disease. Neurology 25:120–126, 1975

Marder K, Flood P, Cote L, Mayeux R: A pilot study of risk factors for dementia in Parkinson's disease. Mov Disord 5:156–161, 1990

Marder K, Maestre G, Cote LJ, et al: The apolipoprotein-4 allele in Parkinson's disease with and without dementia. Neurology 44:1330–1331, 1994

Marder K, Tang M-X, Cote L, et al: Predictors of dementia in community-dwelling elderly patients with Parkinson's disease. Arch Neurol 52:695–701, 1995

Marsden CD, Harrison MJG: Outcome of investigation of patients with presenile dementia. BMJ 2:249–252, 1972

Marttila RJ, Rinne UK: Epidemiology of Parkinson's disease: an overview. J Neural Transm 51:135–148, 1981

Mayer-Gross W, Slater E, Roth M: Clinical Psychiatry, 3rd Edition. London, Bailliere, Tindall, Carssell, 1969

Mayeux R, Chen J, Mirabello E, et al: An estimate of the incidence of dementia in patients with idiopathic Parkinson's disease. Neurology 40:1513–1517, 1990

Mayeux R, Denaro J, Hemenegildo N, et al: A population-based investigation of Parkinson's disease with and without dementia: relationship to age and gender. Arch Neurol 49:492–497, 1992

Mayeux R, Ottman R, Tang M-X, et al: Genetic susceptibility and head injury as risk factors for Alzheimer's disease among community-dwelling elderly persons and their first-degree relatives. Ann Neurol 33:494–501, 1993a

Mayeux R, Stern Y, Ottman R, et al: The apolipoprotein ε4 allele in patients with Alzheimer's disease. Ann Neurol 34:752–754, 1993b

Mayeux R, Marder K, Cote LJ, et al: The frequency of idiopathic Parkinson's disease among middle-aged and elderly black, Hispanic, and white men and women in northern Manhattan (1988–1993). Am J Epidemiol 142:820–827, 1995a

Mayeux R, Ottman R, Maestre G, et al: Synergistic effects of traumatic head injury and apolipoprotein-ε4 in patients with Alzheimer's disease. Neurology 45:555–557, 1995b

McKhann G, Drachman D, Folstein M, et al: Clinical diagnosis of Alzheimer's disease: report of the NINCDS-ADRDA work group under the auspices of Department of Health and Human Services task force on Alzheimer's disease. Neurology 34:939–944, 1984

Molsa PK, Paljarvi L, Rinne JD, et al: Validity of clinical diagnosis in vascular dementia: a prospective clinico-pathological study. J Neurol Neurosurg Psychiatry 48:1085–1090, 1985

Morris JC, McKeel DWW, Storandt M, et al: Very mild Alzheimer's disease: informant-based clinical, psychometric, and pathologic distinction from normal aging. Neurology 41:469–478, 1991

Mortimer JA, van Duijn CM, Chandra V, et al: Head trauma as a risk factor for Alzheimer's disease: a collaborative re-analysis of case-control studies. Int J Epidemiol 20(suppl 2):S28–S35, 1991

Murrell J, Farlow M, Ghetti B, Benson MD: A mutation in the amyloid protein associated with hereditary Alzheimer's disease. Science 254: 97–99, 1991

Naruse S, Igarashi S, Kobayashi H, et al: Mis-sense mutation Val-to-Ile in exon 17 of amyloid precursor protein gene in Japanese familial Alzheimer's disease. Lancet 337:1342–1343, 1991

Payami H, Kaye J, Heston LL, et al: Apolipoprotein-E genotype and Alzheimer's disease (letter). Lancet 342:738, 1993

Pericak-Vance MA, Bebout JL, Gaskell PC, et al: Linkage studies in familial Alzheimer disease: evidence for chromosome 19 linkage. Am J Hum Genet 48:1034–1050, 1991

Perrone P, Candelise L, Scotti G, et al: CT evaluation in patients with transient ischemic attack: correlation between clinical and angiographic findings. Eur Neurol 18:217–221, 1979

Poirier J, Davignon J, Bouthillier D, et al: Apolipoprotein E polymorphism and Alzheimer's disease. Lancet 342:697–699, 1993

Rocca WA, Bonaiuto S, Lippi A, et al: Prevalence of clinically diagnosed Alzheimer's disease and other dementing disorders: a door-to-door survey in Appignano, Macerata Province, Italy. Neurology 40:626–631, 1990

Román CG, Tatemichi TK, Erkinjuntti T, et al: Vascular dementia: diagnostic criteria for research studies. Report of the NINDS-AIREN International Work Group. Neurology 43:250–260, 1993

Rosen WG, Terry RD, Fuld P, et al: Pathological verification of ischemic score in differentiation of dementias. Ann Neurol 7:486–488, 1979

Rubin EH, Morris JC, Grant EA, Vendegna T: Very mild senile dementia of the Alzheimer type, I: clinical assessment. Arch Neurol 46:379–382, 1989

Sacktor N, Mayeux R: Dementia and delirium, in Merritt's Textbook of Neurology, 9th Edition. Edited by Rowland LP. Baltimore, MD, Williams & Wilkins, 1994, pp 1–8

Saunders AM, Strittmatter WJ, Pericak-Vance MA, et al: Apolipoprotein-E ε4 allele distribtions in late-onset Alzheimer's disease and in other amyloid-forming diseases. Lancet 342:710–711, 1993a

Saunders AM, Strittmatter WJ, Schmechel D, et al: Association of apolipoprotein-E allele ε4 with late-onset familial and sporadic Alzheimer's disease. Neurology 43:1467–1472, 1993b

Scheinberg P: Dementia due to vascular disease—a multifactorial disorder. Stroke 19:1291–1299, 1988

Schupf N, Dapell D, Lee J, et al: Increased risk for Alzheimer's disease in mothers of adults with Down syndrome. Lancet 344:353–356, 1994

Schwab JF, England AD: Projection technique for evaluating surgery in Parkinson's disease, in Third Symposium on Parkinson's Disease. Edited by Gillinhan FS, Donaldson MN. Edinburgh, E & S Livingstone, 1969, pp 152–157

Sherrington R, Rogaev EL, Liang Y: Cloning of a gene bearing mis-sense mutations in early-onset familial Alzheimer's disease. Nature 375:754–760, 1995

Skoog I, Nilsson L, Palmertz B, et al: A population-based study of dementia in 85-year-olds. N Engl J Med 328:153–158, 1993

Slooter AJC, Tang M-X, van Duijn C, et al: Apolipoprotein E4 increases the risk of dementia within patients with stroke: a population-based investigation. JAMA 277:818–821, 1997

Smith JS, Kiloh LG: The investigation of dementia: results in 200 consecutive admissions. Lancet 1:824–827, 1981

Spitzer RL, Williams JBW: Structured Clinical Interview for DSM III-R-Hamilton Version. New York, New York State Psychiatric Institute, 1986

Stern Y, Andrews H, Pittman J, et al: Diagnosis of dementia in a heterogeneous population: development of a neuropsychological paradigm-based diagnosis of dementia and quantified correction for the effects of education. Arch Neurol 49:453–460, 1992

Stern Y, Marder K, Tang MX, et al: Antecedent clinical features associated with dementia in Parkinson's disease. Neurology 46:1690–1693, 1993

Stern Y, Gurland B, Tatemichi TK, et al: Influence of education and occupation on the incidence of dementia. JAMA 271:1004–1010, 1994

St. George-Hyslop PH, Tanzi RE, Polinsky RJ, et al: The genetic defect causing familial Alzheimer's disease maps on chromosome 21. Science 235:885–890, 1987

St. George-Hyslop PH, Haines JL, Farrer LA, et al: Genetic linkage studies suggest Alzheimer's disease is not a single homogeneous disorder. Nature 347:194–196, 1990

Strittmatter WJ, Saunders AM, Schmechel D, et al: Apolipoprotein-E: high affinity binding to beta-amyloid and increased frequency of type 4 allele in late-onset familial Alzheimer's disease. Proc Natl Acad Sci U S A 90:1977–1981, 1993

Tatemichi TK: How acute brain failure becomes chronic: a view of the mechanisms and syndromes of dementia related to stroke. Neurology 40:1652–1659, 1990

Tatemichi TK, Foulkes MA, Mohr JP, et al: Dementia in stroke survivors in the Stroke Data Bank cohort: prevalence, incidence, risk factors and computed tomographic findings. Stroke 21:858–866, 1990

Tatemichi TK, Desmond DW, Mayeux R, et al: Dementia after stroke: baseline frequency, risks, and clinical features in a hospitalized cohort. Neurology 42:1185–1193, 1992a

Tatemichi TK, Desmond DW, Prohovnik I, et al: Confusion and memory loss from capsular genu infarction: a thalamocortical disconnection syndrome. Neurology 42:1966–1979, 1992b

Thal LJ, Grundman M, Klauber MR: Dementia: characteristics of a referral population and factors associated with progression. Neurology 38:1083–1090, 1988

U.S. Department of Health and Human Services, Public Health Service: Healthy people 2000 (DHHS Publ No PHS-91-50213). Washington, DC, U.S. Government Printing Office, 1990

van Duijn CM, Clayton D, Chandra V, et al: Familial aggregation of Alzheimer's disease and related disorders: a collaborative reanalysis of case-control studies. Int J Epidemiol 20(suppl 2):S13–S20, 1991

Waxman SG, Toole JF: Temporal profile resembling TIA in the setting of cerebral infarction. Stroke 14:433–437, 1983

Williamson J, Stokoe IH, Gray S, et al: Old people at home: their unreported needs. Lancet 2:1117–1120, 1964

Zhang MY, Katzman R, Salmon D, et al: The prevalence of dementia and Alzheimer's disease in Shanghai, China: impact of age, gender and education. Ann Neurol 27:428–437, 1990

2

Familial Alzheimer's Disease: Genetic Studies

Thomas D. Bird, M.D., Thomas H. Lampe, M.D.,
Ellen M. Wijsman, Ph.D., and
Gerard D. Schellenberg, Ph.D.

Introduction

The two best-documented risk factors for developing Alzheimer's disease (AD) are increasing age and a family history of the disease. The contribution of family history has been consistently recognized by careful epidemiologic studies, including those done in Sweden more than 30 years ago (Larson et al. 1963; Sjogren et al. 1952; Van Duijn et al. 1991). In addition, many families with a high incidence of AD over multiple generations have been described since the original report of Schottky in 1932 and summarized by Cook et al. in 1979. (AD in such large multiplex kindreds is commonly referred to as familial AD, or FAD.) These observations established that there must be important genetic influences in AD, but the precise nature of these factors remained obscure for many decades.

One approach to identifying these genetic influences has been *linkage analysis*. This strategy analyzes large kindreds with multiple generations of AD likely to represent an autosomal dominant single-gene inheritance pattern. The inheritance of the clinical disease is followed through the family in conjunction with a variety of polymorphic DNA markers. If the disease and a specific marker segregate together in the family, then they are said to be linked. This linkage provides evidence that the gene influencing AD resides on the same chromosome as the genetic marker. The gene or genes are then identified by positional cloning technology, and new insights are gained into the pathogenesis and potential treatment of AD. These techniques are being successfully applied to AD as we describe in the following sections.

Chromosome 21 and Amyloid Precursor Protein

Another clue to genetic factors in AD has been its relation to Down's syndrome. At first anecdotally and later systematically, it was recognized that middle-aged adults with trisomy 21 have an extraordinarily high frequency of the neuropathologic hallmarks of AD. This observation strongly suggested a contribution of genetic material on chromosome 21 to the development of AD. This theory seemed to be confirmed by initial linkage studies of a few large FAD kindreds that suggested linkage of the disease to markers on chromosome 21 (St. George-Hyslop et al. 1987). The amyloid precursor protein (APP) gene in the mid portion of the long arm of chromosome 21 became a candidate gene (Figure 2–1). APP is the precursor of Aβ amyloid that accumulates in the neuritic plaques of patients with AD. Mutations in the APP gene leading to cerebral hemorrhagic amyloid angiopathy of the Dutch type were a stimulus to search for APP gene mutations in AD (Levy et al. 1990). Such mutations were discovered in two FAD families by Goate et al. (1991). Several different mutations in the APP gene have now been demonstrated to be associated with FAD (St. George-Hyslop 1993). The most common mutation is a substitution of isoleucine for valine at codon position 717. Clinical and pathologic details of several

Chromosome 21

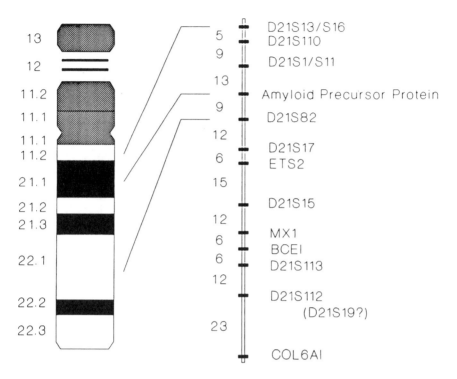

Figure 2–1. Chromosome 21 indicating the position of the amyloid precursor protein (APP) gene. Point mutations within this gene are responsible for early-onset FAD in several families.

of these APP mutation families are available (Karlinsky et al. 1992; Mullan et al. 1993b).

These events represent a major advance in our understanding of the pathogenesis of AD. APP gene mutations represent the first cause of AD to be discovered and directly implicate changes in APP in the metabolic cascade of events leading to dementia. Furthermore, DNA analysis of a single blood sample can be used (if so desired) in specific families with APP mutations as a diagnostic test for having inherited the critical predisposing factor for the disease (Lannfelt et al. 1995).

Chromosome 19

Although the discovery of APP gene mutations represents a landmark in the understanding of AD, it is clear that this solves only one piece of a very complex puzzle. Further genetic linkage studies showed that many FAD kindreds with both early and late onset did not show linkage to any markers on chromosome 21 (Schellenberg et al. 1988, 1991a,b). This difference was noted especially in families with late-onset disease. Furthermore, exhaustive searches of large populations with both familial and sporadic AD have determined that worldwide only a dozen or so AD families have APP mutations. Thus there must certainly be other genetic factors.

Schellenberg et al. had noted an association of FAD with an allele of APO C2 whose locus was known to be on chromosome 19 (Schellenberg et al. 1987, 1992a) (Figure 2–2). Pericak-Vance and colleagues produced suggestive evidence for linkage of late-onset FAD to markers on the long arm of chromosome 19 (Pericak-Vance et al. 1991). More recently, Strittmatter et al. (1993) and Corder et al. (1993) have shown a dramatic association between the APOE 4 allele on chromosome 19 and risk for AD. This association has been amply confirmed and appears to hold true for late-onset, early-onset, and sporadic cases of AD. APOE may be directly involved in the pathogenesis of AD, or there may be other genetic factors near APOE that are also involved. In any event, a gene or genes on chromosome 19 are clearly also involved in the development of AD (Roses 1994). These genes may primarily influence age at onset and may interact with additional, as yet unidentified, inherited and environmental factors.

Chromosome 14

Schellenberg at al. (1988, 1991b) reported that not all early-onset FAD kindreds showed linkage to markers on chromosome 21, and this was confirmed in a larger collection of families (St. George-

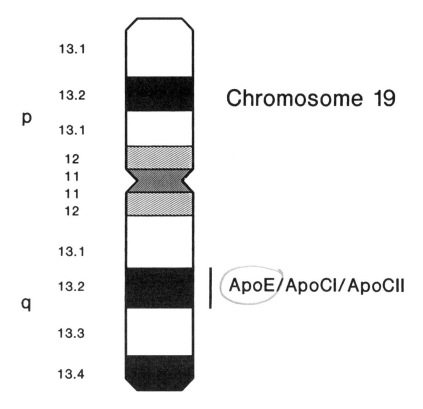

Figure 2–2.   Chromosome 19, with the location of the APOE gene indicated.

Hyslop et al. 1990). Thus the search continued for genes on other chromosomes. Success was reported in 1992, with the finding of linkage of early-onset FAD in several families to markers in the mid portion of the long arm of chromosome 14 (Schellenberg et al. 1992b) (Figure 2–3). This finding was rapidly confirmed by other investigators; chromosome 14 appears to be the most common genetic site underlying the early-onset form of FAD (Mullan et al. 1992; St. George-Hyslop et al. 1992; Van Broeckhoven et al. 1992). In fact, the original four FAD kindreds suggesting evidence of linkage to chromosome 21 markers are now known to be chromosome 14–linked kindreds (St. George-Hyslop et al. 1987, 1992).

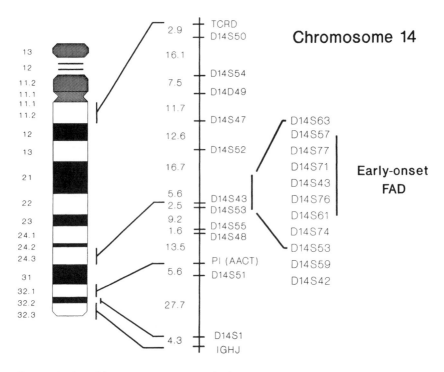

Figure 2–3.   Chromosome 14, with the region containing a gene responsible for early-onset FAD in many families indicated.

   The FAD gene is in band 14q24, close to marker D14S43 and somewhere in the region between D14S61 and D14S63, and within 2–3 cM of marker D14S77 (Figure 2–3). Candidate genes in this general region are being screened for possible implication in FAD. Two genes in this region, *alpha-1 antichymotrypsin* and *cathepsin G,* can be eliminated based on their position on chromosome 14 and frequent recombinations in the FAD families. Also, the c-FOS gene in this region has been sequenced and no mutations were identified in FAD subjects (Bonnycastle et al. 1993).
   In 1995 the chromosome 14 FAD gene was discovered by Sherrington et al. (1995) and named *presenilin 1* (PS-1). The gene has 10 exons and codes for a 467 amino acid protein that is predicted to have 7 to 10 hydrophobic transmembrane domains. The normal

function of the protein and its precise role in the pathogenesis of AD are presently unknown. More than 25 mutations in more than 30 families of different ethnic backgrounds have been reported in the PS-1 gene (Alzheimer's Disease Collaborative Group 1995).

Clinical phenotype comparisons of various forms of FAD are also under way. In earlier studies only occasional differences among FAD kindreds could be observed (e.g., age at onset, ethnic background, neurological examination findings, and neuropathological changes) but these could not be related to specific genetic subtypes of the disease (Bird et al. 1989). Now comparisons can be made among APP mutation families, chromosome 14–linked families, and individuals with various APOE allele genotypes. Several large FAD kindreds are now known to show chromosome 14 linkage (Foncin et al. 1985; Goudsmit et al. 1981; Martin et al. 1991; Nechiporuk et al. 1993; Nee et al. 1983).

Lampe and colleagues (1994) have described in detail the clinical and pathologic findings in one such chromosome 14–linked FAD kindred (Figure 2–4) and compared them with similar reports of families with APP mutation. Features commonly seen in individuals with 14q FAD include early onset (almost always before the

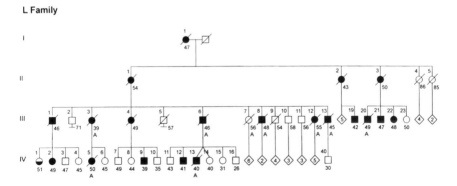

Figure 2–4. Pedigree of a large, four-generation family with early-onset FAD demonstrating linkage to chromosome 14q markers (Lampe et al. 1994). *A* indicates autopsy.

age of 50 years), early progressive aphasia, early appearing myoclonus and generalized seizures, paratonia, cortical atrophy, numerous amyloid plaques, extensive neurofibrillary tangle formation, and prominent amyloid angiopathy (Table 2–1). These clinical characteristics are often so striking and relentlessly progressive that they may be confused with Creutzfeldt-Jakob disease (Haltia et al. 1994). Comparisons of this 14q FAD family with three reported APP codon 717 mutation kindreds suggested several distinctions: prominent progressive aphasia, myoclonus, seizures, and paratonia were all apparently less prevalent in the families with APP 717 mutation, with language function predominantly spared over the initial disease course. Mean age at onset appears to be earlier in chromosome 14–linked FAD than in FAD with APP mutations (42 years versus 54 years, respectively; Mullan et al. 1993a) (Table 2–2). Disease duration may also generally be shorter in the chromosome 14 families (mean 5.8 years ± 2.5 in the L family of Lampe et al. 1994). Further delineation of the phenotypic similarities and differences among and between the various genetic sub-

---

Table 2–1.   Chromosome 14/PS-1 FAD

Clinical aspects (Lampe et al. 1994)

- Early onset (40s)
- Early dysphasia
- Early myoclonus
- Early seizures
- Prominent paratonia
- Short duration (6 years)

Table 2–2.   FAD clinical course

	Chromosome 14/PS-1	APP
Mean onset age[a]	42.5 ± 5.6 years	53.9 ± 6.6 years
Duration[b]	5.8 ± 2.5 years (mean)	6–11.8 years (range)

[a]Mullan et al. 1993.
[b]Lampe et al. 1994.

types of FAD may eventually correlate with important underlying biochemical differences.

It is also now possible to provide presymptomatic diagnosis of AD in the chromosome 14–linked families using direct DNA analysis of the PS-1 gene. Such testing raises numerous clinical and ethical dilemmas that remain to be resolved (Hersch et al. 1994; Bird and Bennett 1995). Thus far, PS-1 gene testing is not commercially available and is only done on a research basis.

Of additional note is that the chromosome 14 locus does not appear to be responsible for the disease in the majority of late-onset FAD families (Schellenberg et al. 1993).

Other Genes for FAD

There remain additional families with AD in which no evidence for linkage to chromosome 21, 14, or 19 is seen (Lannfelt et al. 1993). The best example of such families are the Volga German FAD kindreds (Bird et al. 1988, 1992). This cluster of families represents a genetic founder effect in which the presently affected individuals are all the distant descendants of a single early ancestor with AD who presumably migrated from central Germany to the Volga River region of Russia in the mid-eighteenth century. These families have clinically and neuropathologically typical AD with early, intermediate, and late age at onset.

In 1995 it was determined that the gene for FAD in Volga German (VG) kindreds showed linkage to a region on the long arm of chromosome 1 (Levy-Lahad et al. 1995a) (Figure 2–5). Because of this gene's close homology to the chromosome 14/PS-1 gene, the chromosome 1 FAD gene was quickly identified and has been termed *presenilin 2* (PS-2) (Levy-Lahad et al. 1995b). Several VG patients with dementia were determined to represent phenocopies, that is, individuals with sporadic AD who did not carry the PS-2 mutation. It is also important to note that the age at onset in the PS-2 VG families varies from 45 to 75 years, demonstrating that mutations in the PS-2 gene can result in both early- and late-

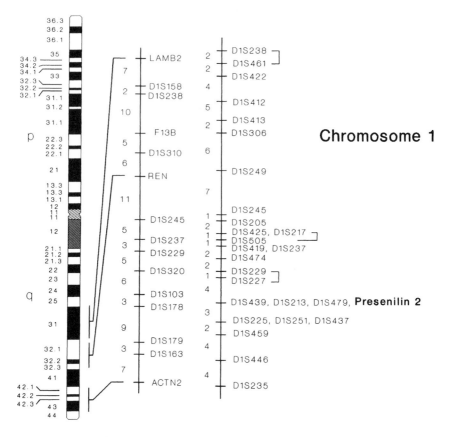

Figure 2–5. Chromosome 1 showing the region containing a gene for FAD (PS-2) in some Volga German kindreds.

onset AD (Bird et al. 1996). An Italian family with a different mutation in the PS-2 gene has also been described (Rogaev et al. 1995).

In summary, AD can now be considered a syndrome with multiple probable causes (Figure 2–6). These include several different genes and numerous possible but unproven environmental causes. It may be that the most common form of so-called sporadic AD is a multifactorial disorder resulting from a combination of predisposing genetic factors, aging of the nervous system, and exposure to one or more environmental agents.

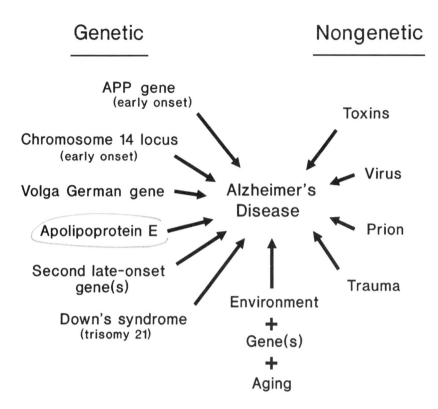

Figure 2–6. Numerous known and hypothetical influences related to the pathogenesis of AD. Several of the genetic factors are well documented. The chromosome 14 gene is presenilin 1, and the Volga German gene is presenilin 2. The nongenetic factors are speculative. The most common form of AD in the population may be the result of predisposing genes interacting with aging and yet-to-be-determined environmental agents.

References

Alzheimer's Disease Collaborative Group: The structure of the presenilin 1 (S1820) gene and identification of six novel mutations in early onset AD families. Nat Genet 11:219–222, 1995

Bird TD, Bennett RL: Why do DNA testing? practical and ethical implications of new neurogenetic tests. Ann Neurol 38:141–146, 1995

Bird TD, Lampe TH, Nemens EJ, et al: Familial Alzheimer's disease in

American descendants of the Volga Germans: probable genetic founder effect. Ann Neurol 23:25–31, 1988

Bird TD, Sumi SM, Nemens EJ, et al: Phenotypic heterogeneity in familial Alzheimer's disease: a study of 24 kindreds. Ann Neurol 25:12–25, 1989

Bird TD, Nemens EM, Nochlin D, et al: Familial Alzheimer's disease in Germans from Russia: a model of genetic heterogeneity in Alzheimer's disease, in Heterogeneity of Alzheimer's Disease. Edited by Boller F, Forette F, Khachaturian Z, et al. Berlin and Heidelberg, Springer-Verlag, 1992, pp 118–129

Bird TD, Levy-Lahad E, Poorkaj P, et al: Wide range of onset for chromosome 1 related familial Alzheimer disease. Ann Neurol 40:932–936, 1996

Bonnycastle LLC, Yu CE, Wijsman EM, et al: The c-fos gene and early-onset familial Alzheimer's disease. Neurosci Lett 160:33–36, 1993

Cook RH, Ward BE, Austin JH: Studies in aging of the brain, IV: familial Alzheimer disease: relation to transmissible dementia, aneuploidy, and microtubular defects. Neurology 29:1402–1412, 1979

✗ Corder EH, Saunders AM, Strittmatter WJ, et al: Gene dose of apolipoprotein E type 4 allele and the risk of Alzheimer's disease in late onset families. Science 261:921–923, 1993

Foncin JF, Salmon D, Supino-Viterbo V, et al: Presenile Alzheimer's disease in a large kindred. Rev Neurol 141:194–202, 1985

Goate A, Chartier-Harlin M, Mullan M, et al: Segregation of a missense mutation in the amyloid precursor protein gene with familial Alzheimer's disease. Nature 349:704–706, 1991

Goudsmit J, White BJ, Weitkamp LR, et al: Familial Alzheimer's disease in two kindreds of the same geographic and ethnic origin. J Neurol Sci 49:78–89, 1981

Haltia M, Viitanen M, Sulkava R, et al: Chromosome 14-encoded Alzheimer's disease: genetic and clinicopathological description. Ann Neurol 36:362–367, 1994

Hersch S, Jones R, Koroshetz W, et al: The neurogenetics genie: testing for the Huntington's disease mutation. Neurology 44:1369–1373, 1994

Karlinsky H, Vaula G, Haines JL, et al: Molecular and prospective phenotypic characterization of a pedigree with familial Alzheimer's disease and a missense mutation in codon 717 of the β-amyloid precursor protein gene. Neurology 42:1445–1453, 1992

Lampe TH, Bird TD, Nochlin D, et al: Phenotype of chromosome 14-linked familial Alzheimer's disease in a large kindred. Ann Neurol 36:368–378, 1994

Lannfelt L, Lilius L, Appelgren H, et al: No linkage to chromosome 14 in Swedish Alzheimer's disease families. Nat Genet 4:218–219, 1993

Lannfelt L, Axelman K, Lilius L, et al: Genetic counseling in a Swedish Alzheimer family with amyloid precursor protein mutation. Am J Hum Genet 56:332–335, 1995

Larson T, Sjogren T, Jacobson G, et al: Senile dementia: a clinical, sociomedical and genetic study. Acta Psychiatr Scand 39(suppl 167): S1–S259, 1963

Levy E, Carman MD, Fernandez-Madrid IJ, et al: Mutation of the Alzheimer's disease amyloid gene in hereditary cerebral hemorrhage, Dutch type. Science 248:1124–1126, 1990

Levy-Lahad E, Wasco W, Poorkaj P, et al: A candidate gene for the chromosome 1 familial Alzheimer's disease locus. Science 269:973–977, 1995a

Levy-Lahad E, Wijsman EM, Nemens E, et al: A familial Alzheimer's disease locus on chromosome 1. Science 269:970–973, 1995b

Martin JJ, Gheuens J, Bruyland M, et al: Early-onset Alzheimer's disease in 2 large Belgian families. Neurology 41:62–68, 1991

Mullan M, Houlden H, Windelspecht M, et al: A locus for familial early-onset Alzheimer's disease on the long arm of chromosome 14, proximal to the I1-antichymotrypsin gene. Nat Genet 2:340–342, 1992

Mullan M, Houlden H, Crawford F, et al: Age of onset in familial early onset Alzheimer's disease correlates with genetic aetiology. Am J Med Genet (Neuropsych Genet) 48:129–130, 1993a

Mullan M, Tsuji S, Miki T, et al: Clinical comparison of Alzheimer's disease in pedigrees with the codon 717 val ile mutation in the amyloid precursor protein gene. Neurobiol Aging 14:407–419, 1993b

Nechiporuk A, Fain P, Kort E, et al: Linkage of familial Alzheimer disease to chromosome 14 in two large early-onset pedigrees: effects of marker allele frequencies on lod scores. Am J Med Genet (Neuropsych Genet) 48:63–66, 1993

Nee LE, Polinsky RJ, Eldridge R, Weingartner H, et al: A family with histologically confirmed Alzheimer's disease. Arch Neurol 40:203–208, 1983

✳ Pericak-Vance MA, Bebout JL, Gaskell Jr PC, et al: Linkage studies in familial Alzheimer disease: evidence for chromosome 19 linkage. Am J Hum Genet 48:1034–1050, 1991

Rogaev EI, Sherrington R, Rogaeva E, et al: Familial Alzheimer's disease in kindreds with missense mutations in a gene on chromosome 1 related to the Alzheimer's disease type 3 gene. Nature 376:775–778, 1995

Roses AD: Apolipoprotein E affects the rate of Alzheimer disease expression: J-amyloid burden is a secondary consequence dependent on APOE genotype and duration of disease. J Neuropathol Exp Neurol 53:429–437, 1994

Schellenberg GD, Deeb SS, Boehnke M, et al: Association of an apolipoprotein CII allele with familial dementia of the Alzheimer type. J Neurogenet 4:97–108, 1987

Schellenberg GD, Bird TD, Wijsman EM, et al: Absence of linkage of chromosome 21q21 markers to familial Alzheimer's disease. Science 241: 1507–1510, 1988

Schellenberg GD, Anderson L, O'Dahl S, et al: APP_{717}, APP_{693}, and PRIP gene mutations are rare in Alzheimer disease. Am J Hum Genet 49: 511–517, 1991a

Schellenberg GD, Pericak-Vance MA, Wijsman EM, et al: Linkage analysis of familial Alzheimer disease, using chromosome 21 markers. Am J Hum Genet 48:563–583, 1991b

* Schellenberg GD, Boehnke M, Wijsman EM, et al: Genetic association and linkage analysis of the apolipoprotein CII locus and familial Alzheimer's disease. Ann Neurol 31:223–227, 1992a

Schellenberg GD, Bird TD, Wijsman EM, et al: Genetic linkage evidence for a familial Alzheimer's disease locus on chromosome 14. Science 258:668–671, 1992b

Schellenberg GD, Payami H, Wijsman EM, et al: Chromosome 14 and late-onset familial Alzheimer disease (FAD). Am J Hum Genet 53:619–628, 1993

Schottky J: Uber prasenile Verblodungen. Zeitschrift Gesamte Neurologie Psychiatrie 140:333–397, 1932

Sherrington R, Rogaev E, Liang Y, et al: Cloning of a gene bearing missense mutations in early onset familial Alzheimer's disease. Nature 375: 754–760, 1995

Sjogren T, Sjogren H, Lindgren AGH: Morbus Alzheimer and morbus pick. Acta Psychiatr Scand Suppl 82:1–139, 1952

St. George-Hyslop PH: Recent advances in the molecular genetics of Alzheimer's disease. Neuroscience 1:171–175, 1993

St. George-Hyslop PH, Tanzi RE, Polinsky RJ, et al: The genetic defect causing familial Alzheimer's disease maps on chromosome 21. Science 235:885–890, 1987

St. George-Hyslop PH, Haines JK, Farrer LA, et al: Genetic linkage studies suggest that Alzheimer's disease is not a single homogeneous disorder. Nature 347:194–197, 1990

St. George-Hyslop P, Haines J, Rogaev E, et al: Genetic evidence for a novel familial Alzheimer's disease locus on chromosome 14. Nat Genet 2: 330–334, 1992

Strittmatter WJ, Saunders AM, Schmechel D, et al: Apolipoprotein E: high-avidity binding to J-amyloid and increased frequency of type 4 allele in late-onset familial Alzheimer disease. Proc Natl Acad Sci U S A 90: 1977–1981, 1993

Van Broeckhoven C, Backhovens H, Cruts M, et al: Mapping of a gene predisposing to early-onset Alzheimer's disease to chromosome 14q24.3. Nat Genet 2:335–339, 1992

Van Duijn CM, Clayton D, Chandra V, et al: Familial aggregation of Alzheimer's disease and related disorders: a collaborative reanalysis of case-control studies. Int J Epidemiol 20(suppl 2):S13–S20, 1991

CHAPTER

3

Cellular Production of Amyloid β-Protein: A Direct Route to the Mechanism and Treatment of Alzheimer's Disease

Dennis J. Selkoe, M.D.

Progressive cerebral dysfunction in AD and adult Down's syndrome is accompanied by the formation of innumerable extracellular amyloid deposits in the form of senile plaques and microvascular amyloid. The amyloid fibrils are composed of the 40–42 residue amyloid β-protein (Aβ), a fragment of the integral membrane polypeptide, β-amyloid precursor protein (βAPP). Evidence from several laboratories has shown that amorphous, largely nonfilamentous deposits of Aβ (diffuse or preamyloid plaques) precede the development of fibrillary amyloid, dystrophic neurites, neurofibrillary tangles, and other cytopathological changes in Down's syndrome and, by inference, in AD. This finding suggests that β-amyloidosis, like certain other human amyloidoses, does not occur secondary to local cellular pathology (e.g., dystrophic neurites) but rather precedes it. The clearest evidence that the processing

43

of βAPP into Aβ can actually cause AD has come from the identification by several laboratories of missense mutations in the βAPP gene within and flanking the Aβ region in affected members of certain families having AD or hereditary cerebral hemorrhage with amyloidosis of the Dutch type. Additional strong support comes from the progressive Alzheimer-like neuritic plaque formation found in a line of transgenic mice overexpressing a familial AD (FAD)-linked mutant form of βAPP (Games et al. 1995).

The mechanism of proteolytic release of the Aβ fragment from βAPP is poorly understood. Because the normal secretion of the large extramembranous portion of βAPP (APP$_s$) from cells involves a proteolytic cleavage within Aβ, we searched for evidence of an alternate pathway of βAPP processing that leaves Aβ intact. In view of the presence of a consensus sequence (NPXY) in the cytoplasmic tail of βAPP that could mediate internalization of the protein from the cell surface and its targeting to endosomes or lysosomes, we looked specifically for evidence of endocytotic trafficking of βAPP. Incubation of an antibody to the extracellular region of βAPP with living human cells led to binding of the antibody to cell-surface βAPP and trafficking of the antigen antibody complex to endosomes or lysosomes (Haass et al. 1992a). The resultant βAPP-immunoreactive pattern closely resembled that seen after incubating the same cells with rhodamine-tagged albumin, a marker for fluid-phase endocytosis. Late endosomes or lysosomes purified from the cells by step-gradient centrifugation contained abundant full-length βAPP plus an array of low molecular weight, C-terminal fragments ranging from ~10 to 22 kDa, most of which are of a size and immunoreactivity that suggest that they contain the intact Aβ peptide (Haass et al. 1992a). Similar potentially amyloidogenic C-terminal fragments had been detected previously in whole lysates of βAPP-expressing cells (Caporaso et al. 1992; Cole et al. 1989; Golde et al. 1992). These various results provide evidence that some βAPP molecules are normally reinternalized from the cell surface and targeted to lysosomes. This second cellular pathway for βAPP processing (the first described was the α-secretase pathway [Esch et al. 1990; Sisodia et al. 1990]) is capable of producing potentially amyloidogenic fragments. Studies by Koo and Squazzo (1994) have shown directly that at least a portion of secreted Aβ is generated during early endocytic trafficking of βAPP. However, it is not yet clear to what extent the endocytic pathway, an alternative proteolytic cleavage other than that by α-secretase occurring within the secretory pathway (Seubert et al. 1993), or a combination of these two routes, is responsible for Aβ formation in different cell types.

During the courses of the aforementioned studies, we searched for evidence of the production and release of the Aβ peptide itself during normal cellular metabolism, based in part on the hypothesis that some Aβ deposits (e.g., those in capillary walls and the subpial cortex) might arise from a circulating (plasma or cerebrospinal fluid [CSF]) source of the peptide. To this end, a series of antibodies to Aβ were used to screen the conditioned media of several cell types for the presence of soluble Aβ. These experiments demonstrated that Aβ is continuously produced as a soluble 4-kDa peptide and is released into the media of normal cells (Haass et al. 1992b). In simultaneously conducted experiments, Aβ was detected in CSF in addition to various cultured cell media (Seubert et al. 1992; Shoji et al. 1992) and in plasma (Seubert et al. 1992). The form in CSF has been purified and sequenced, confirming that it is authentic Aβ (Seubert et al. 1992), whereas the plasma form has clearly been detected immunohistochemically but not yet fully characterized at the structural level. Aβ peptides with heterogeneous N- and C-termini are now known to be released by all βAPP-expressing cells studied to date under normal culture conditions (Busciglio et al. 1993; Haass et al. 1992b, 1993, 1994; Seubert et al. 1992; Shoji et al. 1992; Suzuki et al. 1994). Aβ in culture supernatants is soluble and generally present in high picomolar to low nanomolar concentrations (Seubert et al. 1992). Pulse-chase and biological toxin experiments have suggested that Aβ production follows full maturation of βAPP and involves an acidic compartment other than lysosomes, for example, early endosomes or the late Golgi (Haass et al. 1993). The two proteolytic cleavages generating Aβ (designated β-secretase and γ-secretase cleavages, respectively) may therefore occur in part in an acidic vesicle near the cell surface, after which Aβ is rapidly released into the medium, with little Aβ detected intracellularly (Haass et al. 1992b, 1993).

The relevance of such in vitro Aβ production to the pathogenesis of AD is demonstrated by the finding that a βAPP missense mutation causing a Swedish form of FAD, when expressed in cultured cells, leads to a marked increase in Aβ production (Citron et al. 1992). Moreover, primary fibroblasts cultured from the skin of living subjects with this Swedish form show hypersecretion of Aβ, and this can be seen at least a decade before onset of clinical symptoms (Citron et al. 1994). The amyloidogenic mechanism of three other FAD-linked βAPP mutations, the mutations of βAPP_{717val}, have now been shown to involve increased production of the longer (42-residue), more amyloidogenic form of Aβ (Haass et al. 1994a). Also, mutation at βAPP_{692Ala} that causes both AD and hemorrhagic amyloid angiopathy has been found to lead to increased Aβ secretion, particularly of N-terminally truncated forms (Haass et al. 1994a).

Because cell-surface βAPP molecules appear to provide one source of precursors for Aβ production, it is important to understand the precise pathway and kinetics of cell-surface βAPP trafficking. To this end, we have applied biochemical and morphological methods to βAPP-transfected Chinese hamster ovary cells. By binding a labeled monoclonal βAPP antibody to living cells, we demonstrated that some surface βAPP molecules were rapidly secreted into the medium with a $t_{1/2}$ under 10 minutes. At the same time, some surface βAPP was rapidly internalized. A cell line transfected with a deletion construct lacking the βAPP cytoplasmic tail showed enhanced secretion and a corresponding decrease in internalization, as expected. Using immunofluorescence and immunoelectron microscopy, βAPP was shown to be rapidly internalized via coated pits and vesicles, after which the molecules were transported to endosomes, prelysosomes, and lysosomes. Using a modified immunodetection protocol, we directly demonstrated the rapid recycling (within 5 to 10 minutes) of endocytosed βAPP to the cell surface and the ultimate targeting of a portion of βAPP to lysosomes. Because endocytosis of cell-surface βAPP has been shown to be one route for the constitutive production of Aβ (Koo and Squazzo 1994), the recycling pathway for cell-surface βAPP delineated in these studies is a probable route for production of the critical Aβ fragment. However, other routes are being demonstrated at this writing.

Because the β-secretase cleavage of βAPP to generate the Aβ N-terminus appears to occur before γ-secretase cleavage generating the C-terminus, it is important to characterize the substrate requirement of the β-secretase or secretases and ultimately identify the responsible protease or proteases. Thus we have mutagenized βAPP by placing stop codons within or at the end of the transmembrane domain or by substituting various amino acids for the wild-type Met and Asp at the P_1 and P_1' positions. These and related experiments have led to the conclusion that β-secretase-type cleavage requires a membrane-anchored βAPP substrate but can tolerate shifts in the distance of the hydrolyzed peptide bond from the membrane, in contrast to findings reported for α-secretase-type cleavage. The major β-secretase-type protease appears to have a minimum recognition region of Val669 to Ala673 ($βAPP_{770}$); most substitutions in this sequence strongly decrease or eliminate Aβ production when expressed in intact human cells. Only the Swedish FAD mutation (Lys670 Asn/Met671 Leu) strongly increases Aβ production. Moreover, in the Swedish mutant, but not in wild-type βAPP, the entire cytoplasmic tail with its reinternalization signals can be deleted without affecting the β-secretase cleavage, consistent with the concept that Aβ-generating cleavage of this mutant form occurs in a different cellular compartment than that of wild-type molecules. Although our experiments demonstrate a high degree of sequence specificity for the β-secretase cleavage in intact neural and nonneural cells, analogous mutagenesis experiments around the Aβ C-terminus suggest that the unknown protease or proteases cleaving here (i.e., γ-secretase[s]) do not show much peptide bond specificity. Our results about the characteristics of these cleavages have implications for current intensive approaches to develop assays for and identify and purify enzymes with β-secretase or γ-secretase activity.

The cellular trafficking of βAPP is of interest not only because it should provide information about where within the cell the critical Aβ-generating cleavages occur but also because it provides more general knowledge about the mechanisms for trafficking of membrane-spanning proteins that are both inserted as holoproteins at the cell surface and serve as the precursors of various secreted derivatives. We have previously reported that βAPP undergoes highly polarized sorting in Madin-Darby canine kidney (MDCK) epithelial cells, a well characterized model system for studying protein trafficking in polarized cells. βAPP is trafficked principally to the basolateral surface of MDCK cells, and the major soluble derivative (APP$_s$) and Aβ are preferentially secreted from the basolateral surface (Haass et al. 1994b). In more recent studies, we have extended this work by conducting an analysis of the sorting signals in the βAPP cytoplasmic tail in MDCK cells, using cDNA constructs containing a variety of deletions and substitutions.

Deletion of the last 32 amino acids (residues 664–695) of the βAPP cytoplasmic tail had no influence on either the constitutive ~90% level of basolateral sorting of surface βAPP or the strong basolateral secretion of APP$_s$, Aβ, and p3. However, deleting the last 42 amino acids (residues 654–695) or changing tyrosine 653 to alanine altered the distribution of cell-surface βAPP so that ~40%–50% of the molecules were inserted apically. In parallel, Aβ was not secreted from both surfaces. Surprisingly, this change in surface βAPP had no influence on the basolateral secretion of APP$_s$ and p3. This result suggests that most βAPP molecules that give rise to APP$_s$ in MDCK cells are cleaved intracellularly before reaching the surface. Consistent with this conclusion, we readily detected intracellular APP$_s$ in carbonate extracts of isolated membrane vesicles. Moreover, ammonium chloride treatment resulted in the equal secretion of APP$_s$ into both compartments, as occurs with other nonmembranous, basolaterally secreted proteins, but it did not influence the polarity of cell-surface βAPP. These results demonstrate that in epithelial cells two independent mechanisms mediate the polarized trafficking of βAPP holoprotein and its major secreted derivative (APP$_s$) and that Aβ peptides are derived in part from βAPP holoprotein targeted to the cell surface by a signal that includes tyrosine 653.

The studies summarized demonstrate the usefulness of cultured cells expressing normal or mutant βAPP molecules for deciphering both the proteolytic processing and the intercellular trafficking of βAPP. In addition to their utility in such studies, cells constitutively secreting Aβ might be useful for examining the critical issue of the aggregation of the soluble Aβ monomer into its potentially neurotoxic aggregated (polymeric) form under physiological conditions.

Attempts to model the cytotoxicity of Aβ in vitro using synthetic peptides have shown that soluble, monomeric Aβ is relatively inert, whereas aggregated, polymeric Aβ reproducibly exerts a variety of neurotoxic effects. The processes that initiate the conversion of soluble Aβ to a polymeric, toxic state are of great interest, but most studies of this conversion have employed high doses (10^{-3} to 10^{-5} M) of synthetic Aβ peptides under nonphysiological conditions. We have found that Chinese hamster ovary cells expressing endogenous or transfected amyloid β-protein precursor (βPP) spontaneously form small amounts ($<10^{-9}$ M) of Aβ oligomers from their constitutively secreted Aβ monomers under normal culture conditions. The identity of these low oligomers (primarily dimers and trimers) was confirmed by selective and specific immunoprecipitation with a panel of Aβ antibodies, by electrophoretic comigration with synthetic Aβ oligomers and by amino acid sequencing. The oligomeric Aβ species comprised ~10%–20% of the total immunoprecipitable Aβ in these cultures. A truncated Aβ species beginning at Arg 5 was found to be enriched in the oligomers, suggesting that N-terminal heterogeneity can influence Aβ oligomerization in this system. Addition of Congo red (10 μm) during metabolic labeling of the cells led to increased monomeric and decreased oligomeric Aβ. Similarly, Aβ multimers have recently been detected in another cell type but in lower amounts. The ability to detect and quantitate oligomers of secreted Aβ peptides in cell culture should now enable dynamic studies of the critical process of initial Aβ aggregation under physiological conditions and could potentially be used to screen and characterize compounds that inhibit Aβ polymerization.

The studies summarized here, as well as similar studies being conducted in numerous other laboratories, demonstrate that the regulation of Aβ production, secretion, and extracellular aggregation can be effectively studied under controlled conditions in a variety of cultured cells. Such work can provide information about βAPP processing and the economy of Aβ under physiological conditions that can complement analyses of the processes in vivo. Moreover, cells stably expressing wild-type or mutant βAPP provide an excellent screening system to identify potentially therapeutic compounds that decrease Aβ production or enhance its clearance. Positive compounds identified by in vitro screening can then be tested in in vivo models of AD, such as the recently described βAPP-overexpressing transgenic mouse (Games et al. 1995).

References

Busciglio J, Gabuzda DH, Matsudaira P, et al: Generation of β-amyloid in the secretory pathway in neuronal and nonneuronal cells. Proc Natl Acad Sci U S A 90:2092–2096, 1993

Caporaso GL, Gandy SE, Buxbaum JD, et al: Chloroquine inhibits intracellular degradation but not secretion of Alzheimer β/A4 amyloid precursor protein. Proc Natl Acad Sci U S A 89:2252–2256, 1992

Citron M, Oltersdorf T, Haass C, et al: Mutation of the β-amyloid precursor protein in familial Alzheimer's disease increases β-protein production. Nature 360:672–674, 1992

Citron M, Vigo-Pelfrey C, Teplow DB, et al: Excessive production of amyloid β-protein by peripheral cells of symptomatic and presymptomatic patients carrying the Swedish familial Alzheimer's disease mutation. Proc Natl Acad Sci U S A 91:11993–11997, 1994

Cole GM, Huynh TV, Saitoh T: Evidence for lysosomal processing of beta-amyloid precursor in cultured cells. Neurochem Res 14:933–939, 1989

Esch FS, Keim PS, Beattie EC, et al: Cleavage of amyloid β-peptide during constitutive processing of its precursor. Science 248:1122–1124, 1990

Games D, Adams D, Alessandrini R, et al: Alzheimer-type neuropathology in transgenic mice overexpressing V717F β-amyloid precursor protein. Nature 373:523–527, 1995

Golde TE, Estus S, Younkin LH, et al: Processing of the amyloid protein precursor to potentially amyloidogenic carboxyl-terminal derivatives. Science 255:728–730, 1992

Haass C, Koo EH, Mellon A, et al: Targeting of cell-surface β-amyloid precursor protein to lysosomes: alternative processing into amyloid-bearing fragments. Nature 357:500–503, 1992a

Haass C, Schlossmacher MG, Hung AY, et al: Amyloid β-peptide is produced by cultured cells during normal metabolism. Nature 359:322–325, 1992b

Haass C, Hung AY, Schlossmacher MG, et al: β-Amyloid peptide and a 3-kDa fragment are derived by distinct cellular mechanisms. J Biol Chem 268:3021–3024, 1993

Haass C, Hung AY, Selkoe DJ, et al: Mutations associated with a locus for familial Alzheimer's disease result in alternative processing of amyloid β-protein precursor. J Biol Chem 269:17741–17748, 1994a

Haass C, Koo EH, Teplow DB, et al: Polarized secretion of β-amyloid precursor protein and amyloid β-peptide in MDCK cells. Proc Natl Acad Sci U S A 91:1564–1568, 1994b

Koo EH, Squazzo S: Evidence that production and release of amyloid β-protein involves the endocytic pathway. J Biol Chem 269:17386–17389, 1994

Seubert P, Vigo-Pelfrey C, Esch F, et al: Isolation and quantitation of soluble Alzheimer's β-peptide from biological fluids. Nature 359:325–327, 1992

Seubert P, Oltersdorf T, Lee MG, et al: Secretion of β-amyloid precursor protein cleaved at the amino-terminus of the β-amyloid peptide. Nature 361:260–263, 1993

Shoji M, Golde TE, Ghiso J, et al: Production of the Alzheimer amyloid β protein by normal proteolytic processing. Science 258:126–129, 1992

Sisodia SS, Koo EH, Beyreuther K, et al: Evidence that β-amyloid protein in Alzheimer's disease is not derived by normal processing. Science 248:492–495, 1990

Suzuki N, Cheung TT, Cai X-D, et al: An increased percentage of long amyloid β protein secreted by familial amyloid β protein precursor (βAPP717) mutants. Science 264:1336–1340, 1994

4

Regulation of β-Amyloid Metabolism in Alzheimer's Disease

Samuel E. Gandy, M.D., Ph.D.

Alzheimer's disease (AD) is characterized by an intracranial amyloidosis that develops in an age-dependent manner and that appears to be dependent on the production of Aβ-amyloid by proteolysis of its integral membrane precursor, the Alzheimer Aβ-amyloid precursor protein (APP). Evidence causally linking APP to AD has been provided by the discovery of mutations within the APP coding sequence that segregate with disease phenotypes in autosomal dominant familial cerebral amyloidoses, including some types of familial AD (FAD). Though FAD is rare (<10% of all AD), the characteristic clinicopathologic features—amyloid plaques, neurofibrillary tangles, synaptic and neuronal loss, neurotransmitter deficits, and dementia—are apparently indistinguishable when FAD

This work was supported by USPHS Grant AG-11508. The author is the recipient of a Cornell Scholar Award in the Biomedical Sciences.

The author thanks Drs. Paul Greengard, Dennis Selkoe, and Sangram Sisodia for their critical reading of this chapter.

is compared with typical, common, nonfamilial, or sporadic AD (SAD).

The characterization and regulation of pathways for the cellular processing of APP have been characterized extensively and recent data demonstrate that soluble Aβ-amyloid is released from various cells and tissues in the course of normal cellular metabolism. To date, studies of APP catabolic intermediates and soluble Aβ-amyloid in SAD tissues and fluids have not provided specific SAD-associated changes in APP metabolism. However, studies of some clinically relevant mutant APP molecules from FAD families have yielded evidence that APP mutations can lead to enhanced generation or aggregability of Aβ-amyloid, consistent with a pathogenic role in AD.

In addition, genetic loci for FAD that are distinct from the immediate regulatory and coding regions of the APP gene have been discovered, indicating that defects in molecules other than APP can also specify cerebral amyloidogenesis and FAD. It remains to be elucidated which, if any, of these rare genetic causes of AD is most relevant to our understanding of typical, common SAD.

Alzheimer's Disease Is Associated With an Intracranial Amyloidosis

Amyloid is a generic description applied to a heterogeneous class of tissue protein precipitates that have the common feature of beta-pleated sheet secondary structure, a characteristic that confers affinity for the histochemical dye Congo red (Tomlinson and Corsellis 1984). Amyloids may be deposited in a general manner throughout the body (systemic amyloids) or confined to a particular organ (e.g., cerebral amyloid). AD is characterized by clinical evidence of cognitive failure in association with cerebral amyloidosis, cerebral intraneuronal neurofibrillary pathology, neuronal and synaptic loss, and neurotransmitter deficits (Tomlinson and Corsellis 1984). The cerebral amyloid of AD is deposited around meningeal and cerebral vessels, as well as in gray matter. In gray matter, the deposits coalesce into structures known as plaques. Parenchymal amyloid plaques are distributed in brain in a characteristic fashion, differentially affecting the various cerebral and cerebellar lobes and cortical laminae.

The main constituent of cerebrovascular amyloid was purified and sequenced by Glenner and Wong in 1984. This 40–42 amino acid polypeptide, designated β protein (Glenner and Wong 1984a,b) (or, according to Masters and colleagues [1985], A4; now standardized as Aβ by Husby et al. 1993), is derived from a 695–770 amino acid precursor, termed the Aβ-amyloid precursor protein (APP) (Figure 4–1), which was discovered by molecular cloning (Goldgaber et al. 1987; Kang et al. 1987; Kitaguchi et al. 1988; Ponte et al. 1988; Robakis et al. 1987; Tanzi et al. 1987, 1988).

APP Structure Gives Clues to Some of Its Functions

The deduced amino acid sequence of APP predicts a protein with a single transmembrane domain (Goldgaber et al. 1987; Kang et al. 1987; Kitaguchi et al. 1988; Ponte et al. 1988; Robakis et al. 1987; Tanzi et al. 1987, 1988). Isoform diversity is generated by alternative mRNA splicing, and isoforms of 751 and 770 amino acids include a protease inhibitor domain (Kunitz-type protease inhibitor domain, or KPI [Kitaguchi et al. 1988; Ponte et al. 1988; Tanzi et al. 1988]) in the extracellular region of the APP molecule. The ectodomains of the protease inhibitor-bearing isoforms of APP are identical to molecules that had been identified previously based on their tight association with proteases and thus were designated protease nexin II (PN-II) (Oltersdorf et al. 1989; Van Nostrand and Cunningham 1987; Van Nostrand et al. 1989). Identical molecules are also present in the platelet alpha-granules, where they were described under the name of factor XIa inhibitor (XIaI) (Bush et al. 1990; Smith et al. 1990). Upon degranulation of the platelet, factor XIaI/PN-II/APP exerts an antiproteolytic effect on activated factor XIa at late steps of the coagulation cascade. Recent evidence

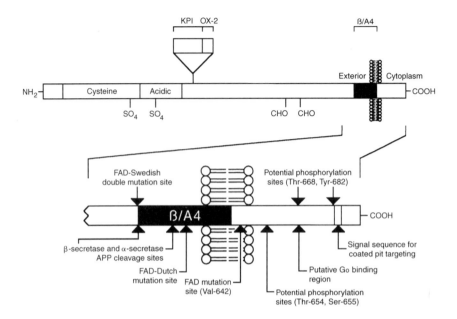

Figure 4–1. Structure of the Alzheimer Aβ-amyloid precursor protein (Courtesy of Dr. Gregg Caporaso; numbering according to APP$_{695}$, Kang et al. 1987. β/A4 domain = Aβ domain; see text or Husby et al. 1993).

suggests that KPI-lacking isoforms may also act as regulators of proteolysis (Miyazaki et al. 1993).

Other physiological roles for APP are as yet unknown, although evidence from several independent lines of inquiry suggests that APP may play a role in transmembrane signal transduction (Nishimoto et al. 1993) or calcium metabolism (Arispe et al. 1993; Mattson et al. 1993). In addition, potential functional motifs in APP have been recognized by the presence of consensus sequences or by experimental implication. Some of these motifs suggest a role in metal ion binding (Bush et al. 1992), heparin binding (Schubert et al. 1989), cell–cell interaction (Konig et al. 1992), or functioning as a receptor for a currently unrecognized ligand (Chen et al. 1990; Kang et al. 1987). In some investigations, Saitoh and colleagues have accumulated evidence that APP may play a role in regulating cell growth (Saitoh et al. 1989). Recently, novel APP-like proteins (APLPs) have been discovered (Slunt et al. 1994; Wasco et al. 1992,

1993), suggesting that APP may be a member of a larger family of related molecules. APLPs are highly homologous to APP and to each other, but they lack the Aβ-amyloid domain and therefore cannot serve as precursors to Aβ-amyloid.

APP Is Processed via Several Distinct Enzymatic and Subcellular Pathways

APP is initially synthesized and cotranslationally inserted into membranes in the endoplasmic reticulum (ER). Studies of APP metabolism in the presence of either brefeldin A or monensin have, to date, failed to implicate the ER as an important site for discrete proteolytic processing of APP (Caporaso et al. 1992a).

Following its exit from the ER, APP traverses the Golgi apparatus, where it is subjected to N- and O-glycosylation, tyrosyl sulfation, and sialylation (Oltersdorf et al. 1990; Weidemann et al. 1989). APP is also phosphorylated in both the extracellular and cytoplasmic domains, and preliminary evidence implies that some of these events may occur in an early compartment of the central vacuolar pathway (Knops et al. 1993). In addition, some APP molecules are chondroitin sulfated in their ectodomains (Shioi et al. 1992).

The proteolytic processing steps for APP have been a subject of intense interest, in part due to early evidence that excluded the possibility that AD was frequently associated with APP gene mutations or with disordered APP transcription (Koo et al. 1990). One attractive possibility, then, was that AD might be a disorder of APP processing. The likelihood of this possibility was strengthened by early evidence for an APP processing pathway that precluded Aβ-amyloid generation (Esch et al. 1990; Sisodia et al. 1990), implying that a defect in this pathway might underlie AD.

Several proteolytic cleavage products of APP processing have now been definitively identified by purification and sequencing. The first to be identified (Weidemann et al. 1989) was a fragment that results primarily from the cleavage occurring within the

Aβ-amyloid domain. A large amino-terminal (N-terminal) fragment of the APP extracellular domain (PN-II [Oltersdorf et al. 1989; Van Nostrand and Cunningham 1987; Van Nostrand et al. 1989], or s-APP or APPs, for soluble APP [Citron et al. 1992]), is released into the medium of cultured cells and into the cerebrospinal fluid (CSF) (Oltersdorf et al. 1990; Palmert et al. 1989; Weidemann et al. 1989), leaving associated with the cell a small nonamyloidogenic carboxyl-terminal (C-terminal) fragment. This pathway is currently desig-nated the α-secretory cleavage/release processing pathway for APP, so called because the (as-yet-undiscovered) enzyme that per-forms this nonamyloidogenic cleavage/release has been designated α-secretase (Esch et al. 1990; Seubert et al. 1993). Thus, one im-portant processing event in the biology of APP acts to preclude amyloidogenesis by proteolyzing APP within the Aβ-amyloid do-main.

The few details are available concerning the molecular nature of α-secretase, although it is very likely to be a member of a class of enzymes that regulates the "shedding" of ectodomains from a wide variety of transmembrane molecules, including growth factor pre-cursors, cell adhesion molecules, receptors, and ectoenzymes (Eh-lers and Riordan 1991). Surprisingly, these enzymes appear to act primarily at or near the cell surface and to specify cleavage of sub-strates at a certain distance from the plasma membrane, largely without regard for the primary sequence surrounding the cleavage site (Maruyama et al. 1991; Sahasrabudhe et al. 1992; Sisodia 1992). Based on studies of proteolytic processing of the TGF-α pre-cursor and the c-kit ligand precursors (which also appear to be cleaved by similar, cell-surface proteinase activities [Pandiella and Massagué 1991; Pandiella et al. 1992]), it appears that secretase-like activities may be heterogeneous at the molecular level (i.e., several individual proteinase species probably exist). This conclu-sion is based on the observation that, depending on the substrate assayed, slightly different protease inhibitor sensitivity profiles were obtained in studies of TGF-alpha secretase in side-by-side comparison with c-kit ligand family secretases. Intracellular signal transduction, especially via protein kinase C, is commonly an important regulatory mechanism for processing of molecules via secretase-like pathways (see following section). The possibility currently exists that the activities of secretases are regulated by the phosphorylation state of the enzymes themselves; if true, this would provide the first known examples of proteases whose activities are regulated by their states of phosphorylation.

Alternative Pathways of APP Metabolism Provide Clues to the Source of Aβ-Amyloid

Due to issues of peptide conformation, peptide aggregation, and antibody reagent insensitivity, the Aβ-amyloid molecule was not initially detected as a normal metabolite of APP in brain, CSF, or a cell culture system. In fact, until mid-1992, Aβ-amyloid was generally described as being an abnormal metabolite of APP. Instead, early clues into Aβ-amyloidogenesis were provided by the observation of electrophoretic microheterogeneity of C-terminal fragments of APP. Such microheterogeneity was detected in association with high-level overexpression of human APP using recombinant vaccinia viruses (Wolf et al. 1990), baculoviruses (Gandy et al. 1992a), or stable transfection (Golde et al. 1992), in association with supraphysiological levels of protein phosphorylation (Buxbaum et al. 1990), and in human cerebral vessels (Tamaoka et al. 1992) and cortex (Estus et al. 1992). Antigenic characterization of C-terminal fragments of APP in cerebral vessels (Tamaoka et al. 1992) and cortex (Estus et al. 1992), in transfected cells (Golde et al. 1992), and in the baculoviral overexpression system (Gandy et al. 1992a) provided the evidence to support the possibility of alternative cleavage of APP molecules, giving rise to C-terminal fragments containing the complete Aβ-amyloid sequence, which, in turn, might give rise to Aβ-amyloid. Protein sequencing of the various putative amyloidogenic C-terminal species (candidate intermediates in the pathway to Aβ-amyloid deposition) recently provided for their definitive identification (Cheung et al. 1994).

The alternative (i.e., non-intra-Aβ) cleavage suggested by this microheterogeneity prompted a search for additional intracellular routes for APP trafficking and cleavage. The existence of trafficking routes other than the α-secretory cleavage/release processing pathway was also suggested by the estimation that only about 20% of mature molecules are recovered as released molecules (in PC-12 cells) (Caporaso et al. 1992b). Since evidence failed to suggest the existence of an important degradative pathway for APP in the ER (Caporaso et al. 1992a), several groups undertook experiments to determine whether acidic (endosomal/lysosomal or trans-Golgi network) compartments of the cell were important in APP metabolism (Caporaso et al. 1992a; Cole et al. 1989; Golde et al. 1992; Haass et al. 1992a; Knops et al. 1992). The possibility of endosomal metabolism of APP was bolstered by the discovery of a clathrin-coated vesicle (CCV) targeting motif in the low-density lipoprotein (LDL) receptor (Chen et al. 1990). This motif, NPXY, was required for proper internalization of the LDL receptor and was also present in the sequence of the cytoplasmic tail of APP (Figure 4–1). The copurification of APP with CCVs was subsequently demonstrated directly (Nordstedt et al. 1993). The fact that APP contains an NPXY motif associates APP with a host of cell-surface receptors and suggests the possibility that APP may be a receptor for an as yet undiscovered or unrecognized ligand.

In other efforts to dissect the process of Aβ-amyloidogenesis, vesicle-neutralizing agents (such as chloroquine and ammonium chloride) were applied to cultured cells, and these compounds were associated with greatly enhanced recovery of full-length APP and an array of C-terminal fragments, including nonamyloidogenic and potentially amyloidogenic fragments (Caporaso et al. 1992a; Estus et al. 1992; Golde et al. 1992; Haass et al. 1992a; Knops et al. 1992). A similar array of fragments was recovered from purified lysosomes (Haass et al. 1992a). This led to the formulation that both the potentially amyloidogenic C-terminal fragments and Aβ-amyloid might be generated primarily in lysosomes. However, no Aβ-amyloid could be recovered from lysosomes (Haass et al. 1993), making this a less likely (but not impossible) scenario. The likelihood that

Aβ-amyloid is generated in lysosomes was further diminished by the observation that vesicular neutralization fails to consistently diminish Aβ-amyloid production in certain cell types (Busciglio et al. 1993; see also next section), although neutralization-induced stabilization of the standard array of potentially amyloidogenic C-terminal fragments is consistently apparent.

Aβ-Amyloid Is a Normal Constituent of Body Fluids and the Conditioned Medium of Cultured Cells

Until mid-1992, the prevailing notion of Aβ-amyloid was that of an abnormal, potentially toxic species, the production of which was perhaps relatively restricted to the brain in humans (and perhaps a few other species) and that occurred primarily in association with aging and AD. This concept became obsolete with the discovery by several groups that a soluble Aβ-amyloid species (presumably a forerunner of the aggregated fibrillar species that is deposited in senile plaque cores) is detectable in body fluids from various species and in the conditioned medium of cultured cells (Haass et al. 1992b; Seubert et al. 1992; Shoji et al. 1992) but is not detectable in the lysates of cultured cells.

This so-called soluble Aβ-amyloid is apparently generated in a cellular compartment distal to the ER since brefeldin abolishes its generation and does not result in its accumulation inside cells (Haass et al. 1993). Vesicular neutralization compounds are effective in inhibiting Aβ-amyloid release from some cell types (Shoji et al. 1992), but this is not true for all cell types studied (Busciglio et al. 1993). The precise cellular locus or loci involved in the amino (A)- and C-terminal cleavages responsible for Aβ-amyloid generation have not yet been unequivocally established. The consistent inability to recover Aβ-amyloid from cell lysates or from purified vesicles has led to a shift in focus away from the terminal degradative compartments of the cell (i.e., lysosomes) as possible sources for the generation of Aβ-amyloid. One important observation in this regard is that a CCV-targeting-incompetent APP molecule (i.e., NPXY-deleted APP) retains the ability to give rise to Aβ-amyloid (Haass et al. 1993). One plausible scenario for Aβ-amyloid production is that cleavage at the Aβ-amyloid A-terminus is catalyzed by β-secretase (see later section) in the precell surface limb of the constitutive secretory pathway, perhaps beginning in the trans-Golgi network (TGN). Cell-type-dependent variations in sensitivity of the TGN to neutralizing compounds may explain the observed dissociability of Aβ-amyloid generation from the apparent stabilization by these compounds of potentially amyloidogenic C-terminal fragments.

Still unexplained is the cellular mechanism by which the C-terminus of Aβ-amyloid is generated, since this region of the APP molecule resides within an intramembranous domain. A plausible and conventional scenario for this step might involve the trafficking of APP or a potentially amyloidogenic fragment into a multivesicular body where vesiculated APP or an APP fragment may be liberated from the bilayer (Gandy et al. 1992b). This is supported by ultrastructural evidence that multivesicular bodies are immunoreactive for APP epitopes (Caporaso et al. 1994). Once the cleavage has occurred, which generates the C-terminus of Aβ-amyloid, fusion with the plasma membrane of a multivesicular body containing wholly intraluminal Aβ-amyloid could effect release of Aβ-amyloid into the extracellular space.

Evidence Suggests the Existence of an Enzyme, β-Secretase, That Cleaves APP at the N-Terminus of the Aβ-Amyloid Domain

The possibility of heterogeneous cleavage along the constitutive secretory pathway (i.e., cleavage in the pre–cell-surface pathway or at the cell surface) was initially discounted (Golde et al. 1992). However, Seubert and colleagues (1992) extended this line of investigation and succeeded in preparing an antibody that was specific for the free methionyl residue that would reside at the predicted C-terminus of such an alternatively cleaved and released attenuated PN-II-like (or APP-like) molecule. This species was successfully detected as a trace component of the PN-II/APPs pool of cleaved and released APP ectodomains. The importance of this activity, designated β-secretase, was subsequently strengthened by the discovery that a pathogenic FAD mutation in APP results in dramatic increases in Aβ-amyloid generation, which is probably attributable to an increase in β-secretase-type cleavage of the mutant APP (probably because the mutant APP is a better substrate for β-secretase than is wild-type APP).

APP Mutations Underlie Some Familial Cerebral Amyloidoses

Certain mutations associated with familial cerebral amyloidoses have been identified within or near the Aβ-amyloid region of the coding sequence of the APP gene. These mutations segregate with the clinical phenotypes of either hereditary cerebral hemorrhage with amyloidosis, Dutch type (HCHWAD or FAD-Dutch; Figure 4–1) (Levy et al. 1990; Van Broeckhoven et al. 1990; van Duinen et al. 1987), or more typical FAD (Figure 4–1) (Chartier-Harlin et al. 1991; Goate et al. 1991; Mullan et al. 1992a; Murrell et al. 1991; Naruse et al. 1991) and provide support for the notion that aberrant APP metabolism is a key feature of AD.

In FAD-Dutch, an uncharged glutamine residue is substituted for a charged glutamate residue at position 693 of APP_{770}. This mutated residue is located in the extracellular region of APP, within the Aβ-amyloid domain, where it apparently exerts its proamyloidogenic effect by generating Aβ-amyloid molecules that bear enhanced aggregation properties (Wisniewski et al. 1991).

Mutations in APP that are apparently pathogenic for more typical FAD have also been discovered. In the first discovered FAD mutation (Goate et al. 1991), an isoleucine residue is substituted for a valine residue at position 717 of APP_{770}, within the transmembrane domain (or at position 642 of APP_{695}, as indicated in Figure 4–1), at a position just downstream from the C-terminus of the Aβ-amyloid domain. Although a conservative substitution, the mutation segregates with FAD in pedigrees of American, European, and Asian origins, arguing against the possibility that the mutations represent irrelevant polymorphisms. Other pedigrees have been discovered in which affected members have either phenylalanyl (Murrell et al. 1991) or glycyl (Chartier-Harlin et al. 1991) residues at this position. Neuropathological examination has verified the similarity of these individuals to typical SAD neuropathology (reviewed by Rossor 1992; see also Cairns et al. 1993; Ghetti et al. 1992; Kennedy et al. 1993; Lantos et al. 1992; Mann et al. 1992). The 717 mutant APPs (residue 717 in APP_{770} is equivalent to residue 642 in APP_{695} [Figure 4–1]) are the most common of the FAD-causing APP mutations, and the mechanism by which these mutant APPs exert their effects appears to lie in their production of C-terminally extended, hyperhydrophobic, and thus hyperaggregable, Aβ-amyloid molecules (Suzuki et al. 1994a).

Another FAD pedigree has been discovered and has also proven to be informative in elucidating the cell biological consequences of the pathogenic mutation. In a large Swedish kindred, tandem missense mutations occur at the N-terminus of the Aβ-amyloid domain (Mullan et al. 1992a). Transfection of cultured cells with APP molecules containing the Swedish missense mutations results in the production of six- to eightfold excess soluble Aβ-amyloid above that generated from wild-type APP (Cai et al. 1993; Citron et al. 1992). This is the first (and, to date, only) example of AD apparently caused by excessive Aβ-amyloid production. Based on the models of FAD-APP[717(or 642)], FAD-Dutch, and FAD-Swedish, an important issue for clarification in sporadic AD will be to establish whether hyperaggregation or hyperproduction of Aβ-amyloid (or neither) is an important predisposing factor to this much more commonly encountered clinical entity.

Signal Transduction via Protein Phosphorylation Regulates the Relative Utilization of APP Processing Pathways

As noted, the protease that cleaves APP within the Aβ-amyloid domain, as part of the nonamyloidogenic cleavage/release pathway (α-secretase), and the proteases that cleave APP at other sites within the molecule to generate Aβ-amyloid (β-secretase and perhaps others), have not yet been identified. Nevertheless, some progress has been made toward understanding the regulation of APP cleavage. For example, the relative utilization of the various alternative APP processing pathways appears to be at least partially cell-type determined, with transfected AtT20 cells secreting virtually all APP molecules (Overly et al. 1991), whereas glia release little or none (Haass et al. 1991). In neuronal-like cells, the state of differentiation also plays a role in determining the relative utilization of the pathways (Baskin et al. 1992; Hung et al. 1992), with the differentiated neuronal phenotype being associated with relatively diminished basal utilization of the nonamyloidogenic α-secretase cleavage/release pathway (Hung et al. 1992).

Certain signal transduction systems that involve protein phosphorylation are potent regulators of APP cleavage, acting in some cases, perhaps, by altering the relative activity of nonamyloidogenic cleavage by α-secretase. The role of protein kinase C (PKC) in this process has received the most attention. In many types of cultured cells, activation of PKC by phorbol esters dramatically stimulates APP proteolysis (Buxbaum et al. 1990) and cleavage/release (Caporaso et al. 1992b; Gillespie et al. 1992; Sinha and Lieberburg 1992) via the α-secretase pathway. PKC-stimulated α-secretory cleavage of APP may also be induced by the application of neurotransmitters and other first messenger compounds whose receptors are linked to PKC (Buxbaum et al. 1992; Lahiri et al. 1992; Nitsch et al. 1992). Okadaic acid, an inhibitor of protein phosphatases 1 and 2A (Cohen et al. 1990), also increases APP proteolysis and release via the α-secretase pathway (Buxbaum et

al. 1990; Caporaso et al. 1992b). Thus, either stimulation of PKC
or inhibition of protein phosphatases 1 and 2A is sufficient to produce a dramatic acceleration of nonamyloidogenic APP degradation. Furthermore, this PKC-activated processing can be demonstrated to occur at the expense of amyloidogenic APP degradation,
resulting in diminished generation of Aβ-amyloid (Buxbaum et al.
1993; Hung et al. 1993; S. Sinha, personal communication).

   These results suggest that defects in signal-dependent regulation of APP cleavage may contribute to the pathogenesis of AD, a
possibility supported by evidence that deficits in cholinergic neurotransmission (Davies and Maloney 1976) and in PKC activity
(Cole et al. 1988; Masliah et al. 1991; Van Huynh et al. 1989) accompany AD. By extension, then, the possibility exists that pharmacological modulation of APP metabolism via signal transduction
might be therapeutically beneficial in individuals with AD (Gandy
and Greengard 1992; Gandy et al. 1991, 1992b). Complicating
these notions, however, is the observation that PKC is also a potent
regulator of APP expression (Goldgaber et al. 1989), although these
pleiotropic effects of PKC may be dissociable at the level of the PKC
isoenzyme involved (Hata et al. 1993). In addition to the attention
to regulation of the nonamyloidogenic α-secretase pathway as a
source of candidate etiologic defects and therapeutic opportunities, it may also be fruitful to study the potentially amyloidogenic
β-secretase pathway in an analogous fashion. Further work will be
required to elucidate the importance of signal transduction systems
as important candidate defects or therapeutic targets in AD. The
enormous pharmacological experience with compounds that affect
signal transduction makes such an approach particularly attractive
for targeting therapy. The probable causal relationship between aberrant protein phosphorylation and neurofibrillary tangle formation (another component of Alzheimer structural pathology) adds
to the attractiveness of protein phosphorylation pathways as potential therapeutic targets in AD.

   The mechanism by which stimulation or inhibition of intracellular protein phosphorylation regulates the processing of APP (including evaluation of the effect of changing the phosphorylation
state of APP per se) remains to be fully elucidated. Protein kinase

C rapidly phosphorylates a seryl residue in the cytoplasmic domain of APP (Figure 4–1), using either a synthetic peptide (Gandy et al. 1988; Suzuki et al. 1992) or APP holoprotein (Suzuki et al. 1992) as substrate. Moreover, APP species are phosphorylated on this and other seryl and threonyl residues in intact cells and in brain (Hung and Selkoe 1994; Knops et al. 1993; M. Oishi et al., personal communication; Suzuki et al. 1994b). Characterization of the various APP residues phosphorylated in intact cells is under way to determine which sites of phosphorylation are utilized and the possible existence of novel APP phosphorylation sites and APP kinases (Hung and Selkoe 1994; Knops et al. 1993; M. Oishi et al., personal communication; Suzuki et al. 1994b). Once the sites for APP phosphorylation in intact cells are established, analysis of the processing of phosphorylation-site mutant APP molecules can be used to elucidate the role of direct phosphorylation of APP.

This approach has already been applied to certain cytoplasmic phosphorylation sites in APP (da Cruz e Silva et al. 1993; Hung and Selkoe 1994; Vitek et al., personal communication). These experiments have demonstrated that changes in the phosphorylation state of the APP cytoplasmic domain are not necessary for the phenomenon of phosphorylation-regulated α-secretory cleavage of APP to occur. These observations have led to the proposal that proteins of the processing–cleavage–release pathway may be phosphoprotein mediators of regulated or activated processing.

Activation of proteolysis by phosphorylation has been demonstrated for a number of integral membrane proteins, including the polyimmunoglobulin receptor (pIgR) (Casanova et al. 1990), the transforming growth factor-alpha (TGF-α) precursor (Pandiella and Massagué 1991), and the receptor for colony-stimulating factor-1 (CSF1R) (Downing et al. 1989). Direct phosphorylation of pIgR appears to be crucial to the activation of its trafficking and processing; phosphorylation of the TGF-α precursor has not been demonstrated; CSF1R is known to be a phosphoprotein, but the relationship between its phosphorylation and its proteolysis has not yet been established.

In general terms, the possible mechanisms for activated processing of integral molecules can be conceptualized as involving either activation or redistribution of either the substrate (i.e., APP) or the enzyme (i.e., secretase). Based on the APP cytoplasmic tail mutational analyses described previously (da Cruz e Silva et al. 1993; Hung and Selkoe 1994; Vitek et al., personal communication), the substrate activation model (Gandy et al. 1988, 1991, 1992b) is inadequate to completely explain activated processing of APP. Furthermore, in recent immunofluorescent studies of APP in cultured cells that were incubated in the absence or presence of PKC-activating phorbol esters (Caporaso et al. 1994), no obvious phorbol-dependent redistribution of APP immunoreactivity was apparent at steady state. A more detailed analysis of APP distribution following PKC activation is under way, as suggested by Luini and De Matteis's (1993) PKC-regulated constitutive pathway model.

Along a similar line of investigation, Bosenberg and colleagues (1993) have succeeded in demonstrating apparently faithful activated processing of TGF-α precursor in porated cells in the virtual absence of cytosol, and in the presence of N-ethylmaleimide or 2.5 M NaCl. The preservation of activated processing under such conditions suggests that extensive vesicular trafficking is probably not required for some aspects of activated processing and is consistent with a model of enzyme activation by direct phosphorylation. Studies are under way to determine whether activated APP processing has similar features and which regulatory steps are most important for regulated cleavage of APP.

Beyond Aβ-Amyloid: Other Molecular Factors in Amyloidogenesis and Factors Differentiating Aging-Related Cerebral Amyloidosis From Alzheimer's Disease

Since APP can be metabolized along several nonamyloidogenic or potentially amyloidogenic pathways, AD might be a clinicopathologic phenotype due to a metabolic imbalance of the relative utilization of nonamyloidogenic pathway(s) versus potentially amyloidogenic pathway(s). To examine a possible correlation between APP metabolic pathway utilization and AD, some investigators have sought to identify AD-related changes in APP metabolism. Diminished levels of the large N-terminal fragment of APP have been reported in CSF from patients with AD and from patients with the cerebrovascular Aβ-amyloidosis HCHWAD or FAD-Dutch (Van Nostrand et al. 1992a,b). According to these reports, decreased levels of the released APP N-terminal fragment were characteristic of the CSF from AD and FAD-Dutch patients but not that from age-matched controls, although there was some overlap between AD patients and patients with non–Alzheimer-type dementia. To date, however, AD-specific changes in the levels of potentially amyloidogenic C-terminal fragments have not been observed either in AD cortex (Estus et al. 1992; Nordstedt et al. 1991) or in FAD-Dutch vessels (J. Ghiso and B. Frangione, unpublished observations). Further, as noted in a preceding section, the metabolism of some mutant APP molecules and their C-terminal fragments in transfected cells appears to proceed in standard fashion (Cai et al. 1993; Felsenstein and Lewis-Higgins 1993) (including apparently "normal" secretory cleavage), unperturbed by the presence of either the $APP_{Val717Ile}$ FAD mutation or the Glu-to-Gln FAD-Dutch mutation.

CSF levels of soluble Aβ-amyloid in normal aging and AD have been investigated to determine whether a correlation exists between CSF-soluble Aβ-amyloid levels and the predisposition to AD. An initial study failed to detect an obvious relationship (Shoji et al. 1992), and that observation recently has been confirmed (Wisniewski et al. 1993). Thus, there appear to be other important factors—perhaps downstream events in the metabolism of APP fragments or soluble Aβ-amyloid—that play key roles in Aβ-fibrillogenesis. In support of this latter possibility is the evidence that an important effect of the FAD-Dutch mutation is to accelerate Aβ-amyloid fibril formation (Wisniewski et al. 1991). Other factors contributing to Aβ-amyloid deposition and fibril formation may include the processing of soluble Aβ-amyloid into an aggregated form (Burdick et al. 1992; Dyrks et al. 1992) or the association of Aβ-amyloid with other molecules, such as α-1-antichymotrypsin (Abraham et al. 1988), heparan sulfate proteoglycan (Snow et al.

1994), apolipoprotein E (Wisniewski and Frangione 1992; Stritt-matter et al. 1993), and P component (Wisniewski and Frangione 1992). In addition, deposited Aβ-amyloid plaques may serve as nucleation foci and act to recruit additional Aβ-amyloid deposition (Maggio et al. 1992).

Events beyond Aβ-amyloid deposition may also be crucial in determining the eventual toxicity of Aβ-amyloid plaques. While aggregation of Aβ-amyloid is important for in vitro models of neurotoxicity (Mattson and Rydel 1992; Pike et al. 1993), the relevance of these phenomena for the pathogenesis of AD is unclear, since Aβ-amyloid deposits may occur in normal aging, in the absence of any evident proximate neuronal injury (Berg et al. 1993; Crystal et al. 1988; Delaere et al. 1993; Masliah et al. 1990). This suggests that other events must distinguish simple cerebral amyloidosis from full-blown AD. One intriguing possible contributing factor is the association of complement components with Aβ-amyloid (Rogers et al. 1992). In cerebellum, where Aβ-amyloid deposits appear to cause no injury, plaques are apparently free of associated complement, whereas in the forebrain, complement associates with plaques, perhaps becoming activated and injuring the surrounding cells (Lue and Rogers 1992). Other, as yet undiscovered, plaque-associated molecules may also play important roles.

It is also possible that Alzheimer neuropathology may be an end product that can develop through a host of independent initiating molecular abnormalities, analogous to the manner in which either disorders of oxygen radical metabolism (Rosen et al. 1993) or of cytoskeletal protein expression (Brady 1993; Cote et al. 1993; Xu et al. 1993) can lead to a clinicopathologic picture of motor neuron disease. Similarly, in the case of AD, it is unknown whether, for example, in some situations, cytoskeletal phosphorylation abnormalities could be initiating events and Aβ-amyloid deposits could occur secondarily. In support of this possibility is the recent demonstration that toxin- or lesion-induced nerve-terminal degeneration can be associated with altered, potentially amyloidogenic APP metabolism (Iverfeldt et al. 1993). Further, Aβ-amyloid deposition may "decorate" the periphery of amyloid plaques primarily composed of prion protein (Ikeda et al. 1993).

The most promising leads for furthering our understanding of the molecular pathology of AD beyond APP metabolism lie in elucidating the role of apolipoprotein E allelic variation in determining predisposition to increased cerebral amyloidosis (Schmechel et al. 1993) and SAD (Saunders et al. 1993) and in the recent discovery of the gene, presenilin-1, which resides on chromosome 14, that causes the most common form of FAD (Sherrington et al. 1995). The mechanism of how this mutant gene causes AD is entirely unknown: It may regulate APP expression or degradation or neurofibrillary components or may eventually point in an entirely unexpected direction. In any event, discovery of the presenilin-1 gene will eventually prove to be an important step toward the unraveling of the molecular basis of typical, common SAD, and this information offers the most promise for ultimately providing us with a full understanding of AD and enabling its rational treatment.

References

Abraham CR, Selkoe DJ, Potter H: Immunochemical identification of the serine protease inhibitor α_1-antichymotrypsin in the brain amyloid deposits of Alzheimer's disease. Cell 52:487–501, 1988

Arispe N, Rojas E, Pollard HB: Alzheimer disease amyloid β protein forms calcium channels in bilayer membranes: blockade by tromethamine and aluminum. Proc Natl Acad Sci U S A 90:567–571, 1993

Baskin F, Rosenberg R, Davis RM: Morphological differentiation and proteoglycan synthesis regulate Alzheimer amyloid precursor protein processing in PC-12 and human astrocyte cultures. J Neurosci Res 32:274–279, 1992

Berg L, McKeel DW, Miller JP, et al: Neuropathological indexes of Alzheimer's disease in demented and nondemented persons aged 80 years and older. Arch Neurol 50:349–358, 1993

Bosenberg MW, Pandiella A, Massagué J: Activated release of membrane-anchored TGF-alpha in the absence of cytosol. J Cell Biol 122:95–101, 1993

Brady ST: Motor neurons and neurofilaments in sickness and in health. Cell 73:1–3, 1993

Burdick D, Soreghan B, Kwon M, et al: Assembly and aggregation properties of synthetic Alzheimer's A4/β amyloid peptide analogs. J Biol Chem 267:546–554, 1992

Busciglio J, Gabuzda DH, Matsudaira P, et al: Generation of β-amyloid in the secretory pathway in neuronal and nonneuronal cells. Proc Natl Acad Sci U S A 90:2092–2096, 1993

Bush AI, Martins RN, Rumble B, et al: The amyloid precursor protein of Alzheimer's disease is released by human platelets. J Biol Chem 265:15977–15983, 1990

Bush AI, White S, Thomas LD, et al: An abnormality of plasma amyloid protein precursor in Alzheimer's disease. Ann Neurol 32:57–65, 1992

Buxbaum JD, Gandy SE, Cicchetti P, et al: Processing of Alzheimer β/A4 amyloid precursor protein: modulation by agents that regulate protein phosphorylation. Proc Natl Acad Sci U S A 87:6003–6006, 1990

Buxbaum JD, Oishi M, Chen HI, et al: Cholinergic agonists and interleukin 1 regulate processing and secretion of the Alzheimer β/A4 amyloid protein precursor. Proc Natl Acad Sci U S A 89:10075–10078, 1992

Buxbaum JD, Koo EH, Greengard P: Protein phosphorylation inhibits production of Alzheimer amyloid β/A4 peptide. Proc Natl Acad Sci U S A 90:9195–9198, 1993

Cai X-D, Golde TE, Younkin SG: Release of excess amyloid β protein from a mutant amyloid β protein precursor. Science 259:514–516, 1993

Cairns NJ, Chadwick A, Lantos PL, et al: βA4 protein deposition in familial Alzheimer's disease with the mutation in codon 717 of the βA4 amyloid precursor protein gene and sporadic Alzheimer's disease. Neurosci Lett 149:137–140, 1993

Caporaso GL, Gandy SE, Buxbaum JD, et al: Chloroquine inhibits intracellular degradation but not secretion of Alzheimer β/A4 amyloid precursor protein. Proc Natl Acad Sci U S A 89:2252–2256, 1992a

Caporaso GL, Gandy SE, Buxbaum JD, et al: Protein phosphorylation regulates secretion of Alzheimer β/A4 amyloid precursor protein. Proc Natl Acad Sci U S A 89:3055–3059, 1992b

Caporaso G, Takei K, Gandy S, et al: Morphologic and biochemical analysis of the intracellular trafficking of the Alzheimer β/A4 amyloid precursor protein. J Neurosci 14:3122–3138, 1994

Casanova JE, Breitfeld PP, Ross SA, et al: Phosphorylation of the polymeric immunoglobulin receptor required for its efficient transcytosis. Science 248:742–745, 1990

Chartier-Harlin M-C, Crawford F, Houlden H, et al: Early-onset Alzheimer's disease caused by mutations at codon 717 of the β-amyloid precursor protein gene. Nature 353:844–846, 1991

Chen W-J, Goldstein JL, Brown MS: NPXY, a sequence often found in cytoplasmic tails, is required for coated pit-mediated internalization of the low density lipoprotein receptor. J Biol Chem 265:3116–3123, 1990

Cheung TT, Ghiso J, Shoji M, et al: Characterization by radiosequencing of the carboxyl-terminal derivatives produced from normal and mutant amyloid β protein precursors. Amyloid 1:30–38, 1994

Citron M, Oltersdorf T, Haass C, et al: Mutation of the β-amyloid precursor protein in familial Alzheimer's disease increases β-protein production. Nature 360:672–674, 1992

Cohen P, Holmes CFB, Tsukitani Y: Okadaic acid: a new probe for the study of cellular regulation. Trends Biochem Sci 15:98–102, 1990

Cole G, Dobkins KR, Hansen LA, et al: Decreased levels of protein kinase C in Alzheimer brain. Brain Res 452:165–174, 1988

Cole GM, Huynh TV, Saitoh T: Reduced protein kinase C immunoreactivity and altered protein phosphorylation in Alzheimer's disease fibroblasts. Neurochem Res 14:933–939, 1989

Cote F, Collard J-F, Julien J-P: Progressive neuronopathy in transgenic mice expressing the human neurofilament heavy gene: a mouse model of amyotrophic lateral sclerosis. Cell 73:35–46, 1993

Crystal H, Dickson D, Fuld P, et al: Clinico-pathologic studies in dementia: nondemented subjects with pathologically confirmed Alzheimer's disease. Neurology 38:1682–1687, 1988

da Cruz e Silva O, Iverfeldt K, Oltersdorf T, et al: Regulated cleavage of Alzheimer β-amyloid precursor protein in the absence of the cytoplasmic tail. Neuroscience 57:873–877, 1993

Davies P, Maloney AJF: Selective loss of central cholinergic neurons in Alzheimer's disease. Lancet 2:1403, 1976

Delaere P, He Y, Fayet G, et al: βA4 deposits are constant in the brain of the oldest old: an immunocytochemical study of 20 French centenarians. Neurobiol Aging 14:191–194, 1993

Downing JR, Roussel MF, Sherr CJ: Ligand and protein kinase C downmodulate the colony-stimulating factor 1 receptor by independent mechanisms. Mol Cell Biol 9:2890–2896, 1989

Dyrks T, Dyrks E, Hartmann T, et al: Amyloidogenicity of βA4 and βA4-bearing fragments by metal catalyzed oxidation. J Biol Chem 267:18210–18217, 1992

Ehlers MRW, Riordan JF: Membrane proteins with soluble counterparts: role of proteolysis in the release of transmembrane proteins. Biochemistry 30:10065–10074, 1991

Esch FS, Keim PS, Beattie EC, et al: Cleavage of amyloid β peptide during constitutive processing of its precursor. Science 248:1122–1124, 1990

Estus S, Golde T, Kunishita T, et al: Potentially amyloidogenic, carboxyl-terminal derivatives of the amyloid protein precursor. Science 255: 726–728, 1992

Felsenstein K, Lewis-Higgins L: Processing of the β-amyloid precursor protein carrying the familial, Dutch-type, and a novel recombinant C-terminal mutation. Neurosci Lett 152:185–189, 1993

Gandy S, Czernik AJ, Greengard P: Phosphorylation of Alzheimer disease amyloid precursor peptide by protein kinase C and Ca^{2+}/calmodulin-dependent protein kinase II. Proc Natl Acad Sci U S A 85:6218–6221, 1988

Gandy SE, Buxbaum JD, Greengard P: Signal transduction and the pathobiology of Alzheimer's disease, in Alzheimer's Disease: Basic Mechanisms, Diagnosis and Therapeutic Strategies. Edited by Iqbal K, Crapper McLachlan DR, Winblad B, Wisniewski HM. New York, Wiley, 1991, pp 155–172

Gandy S, Greengard P: Amyloidogenesis in Alzheimer's disease: some possible therapeutic opportunities. Trends Pharmacol Sci 13:108–113, 1992

Gandy SE, Bhasin R, Ramabhadran TV, et al: Alzheimer β/A4-amyloid precursor protein: evidence for putative amyloidogenic fragment. J Neurochem 58:383–386, 1992a

Gandy SE, Buxbaum JD, Greengard P: A cell biological approach to the therapy of Alzheimer-type cerebral βA4-amyloidosis, in Alzheimer's Disease: New Treatment Strategies. Edited by Khachaturian ZS, Blass JP. New York, Marcel Dekker 1992b, pp 175–192

Ghetti B, Murrell J, Benson M D, et al: Spectrum of amyloid β-protein immunoreactivity in hereditary Alzheimer disease with a guanine to thymine missense change at position 1924 of the APP gene. Neurosci Lett 571:133–139, 1992

Gillespie SL, Golde TE, Younkin SG: Secretory processing of the Alzheimer amyloid β/A4 protein precursor is increased by protein phosphorylation. Biochem Biophys Res Commun 187:1285–1290, 1992

Glenner GG, Wong CW: Alzheimer's disease: initial report of the purification and characterization of a novel cerebrovascular amyloid protein. Biochem Biophys Res Commun 120:885–890, 1984a

Glenner GG, Wong CW: Alzheimer's disease and Down's syndrome: sharing of a unique cerebrovascular amyloid fibril protein. Biochem Biophys Res Commun 122:1131–1135, 1984b

Goate A, Chartier-Harlin M-C, Mullan M, et al: Segregation of a missense mutation in the amyloid precursor protein gene with familial Alzheimer's disease. Nature 349:704–706, 1991

Golde TE, Estus S, Younkin LH, et al: Processing of the amyloid protein precursor to potentially amyloidogenic derivatives. Science 255:728–730, 1992

Goldgaber D, Lerman MI, McBride OW, et al: Characterization and chromosomal localization of a cDNA encoding brain amyloid of Alzheimer's disease. Science 235:877–880, 1987

Goldgaber D, Harris HW, Hla T, et al: Interleukin 1 regulates synthesis of amyloid β-protein precursor mRNA in human endothelial cells. Proc Natl Acad Sci U S A 86:7606–7610, 1989

Haass C, Hung AY, Selkoe DJ: Processing of β-amyloid precursor protein in microglia and astrocytes favors an internal localization over constitutive secretion. J Neurosci 11:3783–3793, 1991

Haass C, Koo EH, Mellon A, et al: Targeting of cell-surface β-amyloid precursor protein to lysosomes: alternative processing into amyloid-bearing fragments. Nature 357:500–503, 1992a

Haass C, Schlossmacher MG, Hung AY, et al: Amyloid β-peptide is produced by cultured cells during normal metabolism. Nature 359:322–325, 1992b

Haass C, Hung AY, Schlossmacher MG, et al: β-amyloid peptide and a 3-kDa fragment are derived by distinct cellular mechanisms. J Biol Chem 268:3021–3024, 1993

Hata A, Akita Y, Suzuki K, et al: Functional divergence of protein kinase C family members. J Biol Chem 268:9122–9129, 1993

Hung AY, Selkoe DJ: Selective ectodomain phosphorylation and regulated cleavage of β-amyloid precursor protein. EMBO J 13:534–542, 1994

Hung AY, Koo EH, Haass C, et al: Increased expression of β-amyloid precursor protein during neuronal differentiation is not accompanied by secretory cleavage. Proc Natl Acad Sci U S A 89:9439–9443, 1992

Hung AY, Haass C, Nitsch RM, et al: Activation of protein kinase C inhibits cellular production of the amyloid β-protein. J Biol Chem 268:22959–22962, 1993

Husby G, Araki S, Benditt EP, et al: Nomenclature of amyloid and amyloidosis. Bull World Health Organ 71:105–108, 1993

Ikeda S, Yanagisawa N, Glenner G, et al: Gerstmann-Straussler-Scheinker disease showing β-protein amyloid deposits in the peripheral regions of PrP-immunoreactive amyloid plaques. Neurodegeneration 1:281–288, 1993

Iverfeldt K, Walaas SI, Greengard P: Altered processing of Alzheimer amyloid precursor protein in response to neuronal degeneration. Proc Natl Acad Sci U S A 90:4146–4150, 1993

Kang J, Lemaire H-G, Unterbeck A, et al: The precursor of Alzheimer's disease amyloid A4 protein resembles a cell-surface receptor. Nature 325:733–736, 1987

Kennedy AM, Newman S, McCaddon A, et al: Familial Alzheimer's disease: a pedigree with a mis-sense mutation in the amyloid precursor protein gene (amyloid precursor protein 717 valine to glycine). Brain 116: 309–324, 1993

Kitaguchi N, Takahashi Y, Tokushima Y, et al: Novel precursor of Alzheimer's disease amyloid protein shows protease inhibitory activity. Nature 331:530–532, 1988

Knops J, Lieberburg I, Sinha S: Evidence for a nonsecretory, acidic degradation pathway for amyloid precursor protein in 293 cells. J Biol Chem 267:16022–16024, 1992

Knops J, Gandy S, Greengard P, et al: Serine phosphorylation of the secreted extracellular domain of APP. Biochem Biophys Res Commun 197:380–385, 1993

Konig G, Monning U, Czeck C, et al: Identification and expression of a novel alternative splice form of the βA4 amyloid precursor protein. (APP) mRNA in leucocytes and brain microglial cells. J Biol Chem 267:10804–10809, 1992

Koo E, Sisodia S, Cork L, et al: Differential expression of amyloid precursor protein mRNAs in cases of Alzheimer's disease and in aged nonhuman primates. Neuron 2:97–104, 1990

Lahiri DK, Nall C, Farlow M: The cholinergic agonist carbachol reduces intracellular β-amyloid precursor protein in PC 12 and C6 cells. Biochem Int 28:853–860, 1992

Lantos PL, Luthert PJ, Hanger D, et al: Familial Alzheimer's disease with the amyloid precursor protein position 717 mutation and sporadic Alzheimer's disease have the same cytoskeletal pathology. Neurosci Lett 137:221–224, 1992

Levy E, Carmen MD, Fernandez-Madrid IJ, et al: Mutation of the Alzheimer's disease amyloid gene in hereditary cerebral hemorrhage, Dutch type. Science 248:1124–1126, 1990

Lue L-F, Rogers J: Full complement activation fails in diffuse plaques of the Alzheimer's disease cerebellum. Dementia 3:308–313, 1992

Luini A, De Matteis MA: Receptor-mediated regulation of constitutive secretion. Trends Cell Biol 3:290–292, 1993

Maggio JE, Stimson ER, Ghilard JR, et al: Reversible in vitro growth of Alzheimer disease β-amyloid plaques by deposition of labeled amyloid peptide. Proc Natl Acad Sci U S A 89:5462–5466, 1992

Mann DMA, Jones D, Snowden JS, et al: Pathological changes in the brain of a patient with familial Alzheimer's disease having a missense mutation at codon 717 in the amyloid precursor protein gene. Neurosci Lett 137:225–228, 1992

Maruyama K, Kametani F, Usami M, et al: "Secretase," Alzheimer amyloid protein precursor secreting enzyme is not sequence specific. Biochem Biophys Res Commun 179:1670–1676, 1991

Masliah E, Terry RD, Mallory M, et al: Diffuse plaques do not accentuate synapse loss in Alzheimer's disease. Am J Pathol 137:1293–1297, 1990

Masliah E, Cole GM, Hansen LA, et al: Protein kinase C alteration is an early biochemical marker in Alzheimer's disease. J Neurosci 11:2759–2767, 1991

Masters CL, Simms G, Weinman NA, et al: Amyloid plaque core protein in Alzheimer disease and Down syndrome. Proc Natl Acad Sci U S A 82:4245–4249, 1985

Mattson MP, Rydel R: β-amyloid precursor protein and Alzheimer's disease: the peptide plot thickens. Neurobiol Aging 13:617–621, 1992

Mattson MP, Cheng B, Culwell AR, et al: Evidence for excitoprotective and intraneuronal calcium-regulating roles for secreted forms of the β-amyloid precursor protein. Neuron 10:243–254, 1993

Miyazaki K, Hasegawa M, Funahashi K, et al: A metalloproteinase inhibitor domain in Alzheimer amyloid protein precursor. Nature 362:839–841, 1993

Mullan M, Crawford F, Axelman K, et al: A pathogenic mutation for probable Alzheimer's disease in the APP gene at the N-terminus of β-amyloid. Nat Genet 1:345–347, 1992a

Murrell J, Farlow M, Ghetti B, et al: A mutation in the amyloid precursor protein associated with hereditary Alzheimer disease. Science 254:97–99, 1991

Naruse S, Igarashi S, Kobayashi H, et al: Mis-sense mutation Val-Ile in exon 17 of amyloid precursor protein gene in Japanese familial Alzheimer's disease. Lancet 337:978–979, 1991

Nishimoto I, Okamoto T, Matsuura Y, et al: Alzheimer amyloid protein precursor complexes with brain GTP-binding protein G_o. Nature 362: 75–79, 1993

Nitsch RM, Slack BE, Wurtman RJ, et al: Release of Alzheimer amyloid precursor derivatives stimulated by activation of muscarinic acetylcholine receptors. Science 258:304–307, 1992

Nordstedt C, Gandy SE, Alafuzoff I, et al: Alzheimer β/A4 amyloid precursor protein in human brain: aging-associated increases in holoprotein and in a proteolytic fragment. Proc Natl Acad Sci U S A 88: 8910–8914, 1991

Nordstedt C, Caporaso GL, Thyberg J, et al: Identification of the Alzheimer β/A4 amyloid precursor protein in clathrin-coated vesicles purified from PC12 cells. J Biol Chem 268:608–612, 1993

Oltersdorf T, Fritz LC, Schenk DB, et al: The secreted form of the Alzheimer's amyloid precursor protein with the Kunitz domain is protease nexin-II. Nature 341:144–147, 1989

Oltersdorf T, Ward PJ, Henriksson T, et al: The Alzheimer amyloid precursor protein: identification of a stable intermediate in the biosynthetic/degradative pathway. J Biol Chem 265:4492–4497, 1990

Overly CC, Fritz LC, Lieberburg I, et al: The β-amyloid precursor protein is not processed by the regulated secretory pathway. Biochem Biophys Res Commun 181:513–519, 1991

Palmert MR, Berman Podlisny M, Witker DS, et al: The β-amyloid protein precursor of Alzheimer disease has soluble derivatives found in human brain and cerebrospinal fluid. Proc Natl Acad Sci U S A 86:6338–6342, 1989

Pandiella A, Massagué J: Cleavage of the membrane precursor for transforming growth factor α is a regulated process. Proc Natl Acad Sci U S A 88:1726–1730, 1991

Pandiella A, Bosenberg MW, Huang EJ, et al: Cleavage of membrane-anchored growth factors involves distinct protease activities regulated through common mechanisms. J Biol Chem 267:24028–24033, 1992

Pike CJ, Burdick D, Walencewicz AJ, et al: Neurodegeneration induced by β-amyloid peptides in vitro: the role of peptide assembly state. J Neurosci 13:1676–1687, 1993

Ponte P, Gonzalez-DeWhitt P, Schilling J, et al: A new A4 amyloid mRNA contains a domain homologous to serine proteinase inhibitors. Nature 331:525–527, 1988

Robakis NK, Ramakrishna N, Wolfe G, et al: Molecular cloning and characterization of a cDNA encoding the cerebrovascular and neuritic plaque amyloid peptides. Proc Natl Acad Sci U S A 84:4190–4194, 1987

Rogers J, Cooper NR, Webster S, et al: Complement activation by β-amyloid in Alzheimer disease. Proc Natl Acad Sci U S A 89:10016–10020, 1992

Rosen DR, Siddique T, Patterson D, et al: Mutations in Cu/Zn superoxide dismutase gene are associated with familial amyotrophic lateral sclerosis. Nature 362:59–62, 1993

Rossor M: Familial Alzheimer's disease, in Baillere's Clinical Neurology: Unusual Dementias. Edited by Rossor M. Philadelphia, Baillere Tindall, 1992, pp 517–534

Sahasrabudhe SR, Spruyt MA, Muenkel HA, et al: Release of aminoterminal fragments from amyloid precursor protein reporter and mutated derivatives in cultured cells. J Biol Chem 267:25602–25608, 1992

Saitoh T, Sundsmo M, Roch J-M, et al: Secreted form of amyloid β protein precursor is involved in the growth regulation of fibroblasts. Cell 58:615–622, 1989

Saunders AM, Strittmatter WJ, Schmechel D, et al: Association of apolipoprotein E allele ε4 with late-onset familial and sporadic Alzheimer's disease. Neurology 43:1467–1472, 1993

Schmechel DE, Saunders AM, Strittmatter WJ, et al: Increased amyloid β-peptide deposition in cerebral cortex as a consequence of apolipoprotein E genotype in late-onset Alzheimer disease. Proc Natl Acad Sci U S A 90:9649–9653, 1993

Schubert D, LaCorbiere M, Saitoh T, et al: Characterization of an amyloid β precursor protein that binds heparin and contains tyrosine sulfate. Proc Natl Acad Sci U S A 86:2066–2069, 1989

Seubert P, Vigo-Pelfrey C, Esch F, et al: Isolation and quantification of soluble Alzheimer's β-peptide from biological fluids. Nature 359:325–327, 1992

Seubert P, Oltersdorf T, Lee MG, et al: Secretion of β-amyloid precursor protein cleaved at the amino terminus of the β-amyloid peptide. Nature 361:260–263, 1993

Sherrington R, Rogaev EI, Liang Y, et al: Cloning of a gene bearing missense mutations in early-onset familial Alzheimer's disease. Nature 375:754–760, 1995

Shioi J, Anderson JP, Ripellino JA, et al: Chondroitin sulfate proteoglycan
    form of the Alzheimer's β-amyloid precursor. J Biol Chem 267:13819–
    13822, 1992
Shoji M, Golde TE, Ghiso J, et al: Production of the Alzheimer amyloid β
    protein by normal proteolytic processing. Science 258:126–129, 1992
Sinha S, Lieberburg I: Normal metabolism of the amyloid precursor pro-
    tein (APP). Neurodegeneration 1:169–175, 1992
Sisodia SS: β-amyloid precursor protein cleavage by a membrane-bound
    protease. Proc Natl Acad Sci U S A 89:6075–6079, 1992
Sisodia SS, Koo EH, Beyreuther K, et al: Evidence that β-amyloid protein
    in Alzheimer's disease is not derived by normal processing. Science
    248:492–495, 1990
Slunt HH, Thinakaran G, Von Koch C, et al: Expression of a ubiquitous
    cross-reactive homologue of the mouse β-amyloid precursor protein
    (APP) J Biol Chem 269:2637–2644, 1994
Smith RP, Higuchi DA, Broze GJ Jr: Platelet coagulation factor XI_a-
    inhibitor, a form of Alzheimer amyloid precursor protein. Science
    248:1126–1128, 1990
Snow AD, Sekiguchi R, Nochlin D, et al: An important role of heparan
    sulfate proteoglycan (Perlecan) in a model system for the deposition
    and persistence of fibrillar Aβ-amyloid in rat brain. Neuron 12:219–
    234, 1994
Strittmatter WJ, Saunders AM, Schmechel D, et al: Apolipoprotein E: high-
    avidity binding to β-amyloid and increased frequency of type 4 allele
    in late-onset familial Alzheimer disease. Proc Natl Acad Sci U S A 90:
    1977–1981, 1993
Suzuki T, Nairn AC, Gandy SE, et al: Phosphorylation of Alzheimer amy-
    loid precursor protein by protein kinase C. Neuroscience 48:755–761,
    1992
Suzuki N, Cheung TT, Cai X-D, et al: An increased percentage of long
    amyloid beta protein secreted by familial amyloid beta protein pre-
    cursor (βAPP717) mutants. Science 264:1336–1340, 1994a
Suzuki T, Oishi M, Marshak DR, et al: Cell cycle-dependent regulation of
    the phosphorylation and metabolism of the Alzheimer amyloid pre-
    cursor protein. EMBO J 13:1114–1122, 1994b
Tamaoka A, Kalaria RN, Lieberburg I, et al: Identification of a stable frag-
    ment of the Alzheimer amyloid precursor containing the β-protein in
    brain microvessels. Proc Natl Acad Sci U S A 89:1345–1349, 1992
Tanzi RE, Gusella JF, Watkins PC, et al: Amyloid β protein gene: cDNA,

mRNA distribution, and genetic linkage near the Alzheimer locus. Science 235:880–884, 1987

Tanzi RE, McClatchey AI, Lamperti ED, et al: Protease inhibitor domain encoded by an amyloid protein precursor mRNA associated with Alzheimer's disease. Nature 331:528–530, 1988

Tomlinson BE, Corsellis JAN: Ageing and the dementias, in Greenfield's Neuropathology, 4th Edition. Edited by Adams JH, Corsellis JAN, Duchen LW. New York, Wiley, 1984, pp 951–1025

Van Broeckhoven C, Haan J, Bakker E, et al: Amyloid β protein precursor gene and hereditary cerebral hemorrhage with amyloidosis (Dutch). Science 248:1120–1122, 1990

Van Broeckhoven C, Backhovens H, Cruts M, et al: Mapping of a gene predisposing to early-onset Alzheimer's disease to chromosome 14q24.3. Nat Genet 2:335–339, 1992

van Duinen SG, Castaño EM, Prelli F, et al: Hereditary cerebral hemorrhage with amyloidosis in patients of Dutch origin is related to Alzheimer disease. Proc Natl Acad Sci U S A 84:5991–5994, 1987

Van Huynh T, Cole G, Katzman R, et al: Reduced protein kinase C immunoreactivity and altered protein phosphorylation in Alzheimer's disease fibroblasts. Arch Neurol 46:1195–1199, 1989

Van Nostrand WE, Cunningham DD: Purification of protease nexin II from human fibroblasts. J Biol Chem 262:8508–8514, 1987

Van Nostrand WE, Wagner SL, Suzuki M, et al: Protease nexin-II, a potent antichymotrypsin, shows identity to amyloid β-protein precursor. Nature 341:546–549, 1989

Van Nostrand WE, Wagner SL, Haan J, et al: Alzheimer's disease and hereditary cerebral hemorrhage with amyloidosis-Dutch type share a decrease in cerebrospinal fluid levels of amyloid β-protein precursor. Ann Neurol 32:215–218, 1992a

Van Nostrand W, Wagner S, Shankle WR, et al: Decreased levels of soluble amyloid β-protein precursor in cerebrospinal fluid of live Alzheimer disease patients. Proc Natl Acad Sci U S A 89:2551–2555, 1992b

Wasco W, Bupp K, Magendantz M, et al: Identification of a mouse brain cDNA that encodes a protein related to the Alzheimer disease-associated amyloid β protein precursor. Proc Natl Acad Sci U S A 89: 10758–10762, 1992

Wasco W, Gurubhagavatula S, Paradis MD, et al: Isolation and characterization of APLP2 encoding a homologue of the Alzheimer's associated amyloid β protein precursor. Nat Genet 5:95–100, 1993

Weidemann A, König G, Bunke D, et al: Identification, biogenesis, and localization of precursors of Alzheimer's disease A4 amyloid protein. Cell 57:115–126, 1989

Wisniewski T, Ghiso J, Frangione B: Peptides homologous to the amyloid protein of Alzheimer's disease containing a glutamine for glutamic acid substitution have accelerated amyloid fibril formation. Biochem Biophys Res Commun 179:1247–1254, 1991

Wisniewski T, Frangione B: Apolipoprotein E: a pathological chaperone in patients with cerebral and systemic amyloid. Neurosci Lett 135:235–238, 1992

Wisniewski T, Wegiel J, Wisniewski HM, et al: Alzheimer's amyloid β subunit is present in preamyloid deposits and in CSF. Neurology 43:A422, 1993

Wolf D, Quon D, Wang Y, et al: Identification and characterization of C-terminal fragments of the β-amyloid precursor produced in cell culture. EMBO J 9:2079–2084, 1990

Xu Z, Cork LC, Griffin JW, et al: Increased expression of neurofilament subunit NF-L produces morphological alterations that resemble the pathology of human motor neuron disease. Cell 73:23–33, 1993

5

Prion Diseases: The Spectrum of Etiologic and Pathogenic Mechanisms

Stephen J. DeArmond, M.D., Ph.D.

The human prion diseases include Creutzfeldt-Jakob disease (CJD), Gerstmann-Sträussler-Scheinker syndrome (GSS), fatal familial insomnia (FFI), and kuru. The most important prion diseases occur in animals because of their economic impact and the worry that they might transmit to humans; these include scrapie of sheep, which has been known for perhaps a thousand years, and bovine spongiform encephalopathy (BSE), which was inadvertently transmitted to cattle in the early 1980s in Great Britain through scrapie-contaminated feed and bone meal (Wilesmith 1993).

This work was supported by grants from the National Institutes of Health (NS14069, AG08967, AG02132, NS22786, and AG10770) and the American Health Assistance Foundation, as well as by a gift from the Sherman Fairchild Foundation.

The Discovery of Prions

Originally sporadic, familial, and iatrogenic CJD and GSS were grouped together because they shared in common spongiform degeneration of gray matter and transmissibility and, therefore, were once designated the transmissible spongiform encephalopathies (TSEs). Fifteen years ago, Stanley Prusiner's proposal that an infectious agent capable of transmitting the TSEs might consist of a protein and nothing else (Prusiner 1982) was met with a good deal of skepticism. At the time, the notion was heretical because the prevailing dogma held that infectious agents required genetic material composed of nucleic acid (DNA or RNA) to propagate in a host. Later, many remained similarly dubious when it was suggested that prions could underlie dominantly inherited disorders such as familial CJD and GSS in addition to those disorders acquired by infection (Hsiao et al. 1989a, 1990, 1994). Such dual behavior of a host-encoded protein was then unknown to science. Nor was the resistance to the prion hypothesis abated when the experimental data suggested that prions multiply in an incredible way: They convert normal cellular PrP molecules, designated PrP^C, into pathogenic ones, designated PrP^{Sc} or PrP^{CJD}, simply by inducing the benign ones to change their conformation.

However, during the past 15 years, a wealth of experimental and clinical data has made a convincing case that the prion protein and prions underlie the etiology and pathogenesis of all forms of prion diseases. The most significant discovery was made by Prusiner when he and his colleagues found that the infectious agent that transmits scrapie consists almost exclusively of a single protease resistant 27–30-kDa protein, designated PrP 27–30 (McKinley et al. 1983; Prusiner 1982). Subsequently it was found that PrP27–30 is produced in vitro from a 33–35-kDa precursor, designated PrP^{Sc}, by limited proteolysis (Oesch et al. 1985; Prusiner et al. 1984). Highly purified preparations of the scrapie agent do not contain viral nucleic acid; rather, they contain small fragments of nucleic acid 40 to 80 nucleotides in length that new studies, to be described in this chapter, suggest are contaminants entrapped during the purification procedure (Meyer et al. 1991). For these reasons, the infectious particle that transmits scrapie was called a prion (pronounced "pree-on") to distinguish it from conventional infectious agents.

Formation of PrP^{Sc} From PrP^{C}

From studies of cell lines that remain stably infected with scrapie after multiple passages in culture, it has been found that PrP^{Sc} is derived from the constitutively expressed normal PrP isoform, PrP^{C}, as the result of a posttranslational process that involves a profound conformational change (Pan et al. 1993). The majority of PrP^{C} becomes attached to the outer surface of these cells by a glycolipid anchor (GPI anchor) after it passes through the Golgi. Like other GPI-anchored proteins, mouse (Mo) PrP^{C} returns into the cell through cholesterol-rich caveolae (Ying et al. 1992). In mouse neuroblastoma cells that express chicken PrP^{C} for use as a traceable PrP^{C} marker, it appears that some PrP^{C} is also internalized through clathrin-coated pits. In either case, a small proportion is endocytosed and degraded while the majority is recycled to the cell surface along with other proteins and lipids of the endosome (Shyng et al. 1994). In pulse-chase experiments, PrP^{C} in uninfected cells is rapidly labeled by a radioactive amino acid tracer and appears to be degraded in about 6 hours (Borchelt et al. 1990; Caughey et al. 1989). In scrapie-infected cells, labeling of PrP^{Sc} is delayed by about 1 hour after the pulse and increases to a maximum during the time period when the PrP^{C} pool loses the tracer (Borchelt et al. 1990). Over the next 24 hours, there is little or no loss of tracer from the PrP^{Sc} pool. These results argue that PrP^{Sc} is derived from PrP^{C}, but, unlike PrP^{C}, PrP^{Sc} is not degraded and accumulates in the cell. Immunoelectron microscopy studies indicate that PrP^{Sc} accumulates in structures believed to be secondary lysosomes containing "myelin" figures (i.e., layers of phospholipid-rich membranes) (McKinley et al. 1991).

In vivo, the same process appears to occur most probably in central nervous system (CNS) neurons since they express the highest levels of PrP mRNA (DeArmond et al. 1992; Kretzschmar et al. 1986a). Following intracerebral inoculation of an animal with prions, PrP^{Sc} begins to accumulate exponentially in the brain, usually at the site of inoculation (Jendroska et al. 1991). Of interest, PrP^{Sc} concentration is proportional to the scrapie infectivity titer, consistent with the hypothesis that it is a component of the prion. Furthermore, the characteristic neuropathological features of prion diseases, which are spongiform degeneration of neurons, nerve cell loss, and reactive astrocytic gliosis, colocalize with the sites of PrP^{Sc} accumulation, consistent with the hypothesis that PrP^{Sc} accumulation causes neuronal dysfunction and neuropathology (DeArmond and Prusiner 1993).

Similarities and Differences Between PrP^{Sc} and PrP^{C}

Multiple attempts over several years to find a chemical difference that could distinguish PrP^{Sc} from PrP^{C} have failed. PrP^{Sc} and PrP^{C} have identical molecular weights of 33 to 35 kDa. They have the same amino acid sequence and similar N-linked carbohydrate side chains and GPI anchors (Stahl et al. 1992, 1993). In spite of these similarities, PrP^{Sc}, and similarly PrP^{CJD}, which accumulates in human prion diseases, can be distinguished from PrP^{C} in several ways. PrP^{Sc} is associated with scrapie infectivity whereas PrP^{C} is not. PrP^{C} is completely digested by limited exposure to proteinase K, whereas PrP^{Sc} and PrP^{CJD} are partially digested to a 27- to 30-kDa protein designated PrP 27–30, which is equally infectious as PrP^{Sc}. PrP 27–30 derived from PrP^{Sc} or PrP^{CJD} aggregates into rodlike structures when exposed to detergents that are morphologically indistinguishable from many purified amyloids both ultrastructurally and tinctorially.

The only known posttranslational modification of PrP^{C} that occurs during its transformation into PrP^{Sc} is the acquisition of β-sheet conformation. The first indication that PrP^{Sc} is rich in β-sheet came from the demonstration that PrP 27–30 forms amyloid since all known amyloids possess a high β-sheet content (Prusiner et al. 1983). PrP^{Sc} is 43% β-sheet and 30% α-helix, whereas PrP^{C} is 3%

β-sheet and 42% α-helix (Pan et al. 1993; Safar et al. 1993). PrP 27–30 has an even higher β-sheet content (54%) and lower α-helix content (21%) than PrP^{Sc}, which presumably accounts for its propensity to form into amyloid rods (Caughey et al. 1991; Gasset et al. 1993). Similarly, limited proteolysis of PrP^{Sc} and PrP^{CJD}, both of which possess high β-sheet content, presumably accounts at least in part for cerebral amyloidogenesis in prion diseases.

Accumulation of PrP^{Sc} Causes Neuronal Dysfunction

In addition to forming into an infectious particle, accumulation of PrP^{Sc} in the brain causes neuronal dysfunction and the clinically relevant neuropathology (DeArmond and Prusiner 1993). The first evidence to support this view was a finding that amyloid plaques in scrapie, CJD, and GSS are composed of protease-resistant PrP (DeArmond et al. 1985; Prusiner and DeArmond 1987; Roberts et al. 1988; Snow et al. 1989). The amyloidogenic propensity of PrP^{Sc} and ΔPrP is no doubt related to their high β-sheet content since all amyloids are composed of proteins in a β-sheet configuration. Most cases of CJD (90%–95%) do not contain amyloid; the amyloid load in CJD and scrapie, when it occurs, as well as in GSS, is insufficient to account for the severity of clinical signs and death. Rather, there are multiple reasons to believe that the pathogenesis of neuronal dysfunction in prion diseases is related to accumulation of abnormal PrP. Spongiform degeneration of gray matter and reactive astrocytic gliosis colocalize precisely with sites of PrP^{Sc} accumulation in scrapie (DeArmond et al. 1987; Hecker et al. 1992) and follow within a few weeks of its accumulation (Jendroska et al. 1991). However, one of the strongest arguments is the discovery that neuronal dysfunction, spongiform degeneration, and cerebral amyloidosis are linked to mutations of the *PRNP* gene.

In total numbers, CJD is rarely acquired by infection. CJD is the most common human prion disease; 80%–90% of CJD cases appear to occur spontaneously and sporadically and are not caused by a prion infection or a mutation of the PrP gene (see following sections).

Prion Diseases Acquired by Infection

The human disorders in particular have puzzled physicians and scientists because they are the most complicated of all neurodegenerative disorders presenting as sporadic and dominantly inherited disorders like Alzheimer's disease (AD) while also being infectious. Although all these disorders are transmissible, only a small number of human cases actually appear to be acquired by infection. Kuru was spread among the Fore people of New Guinea by endocannibalism and, in Western civilization, a small number of CJD cases have been acquired by invasive medical procedures (iatrogenic CJD) (Brown et al. 1992). Thirty medical-dental caregivers have died of CJD (Berger and David 1993); however, none of these have been linked with certainty to patient care (Ridley and Baker 1993). Furthermore, the incidence of CJD among health care providers is the same as for the general population.

More recently, 10 young (less than 40 years of age) unrelated individuals in England died of a new variant of CJD (Will et al. 1996). The evidence that these cases were acquired by infection include 1) the young age of the victims (the mean age at onset for sporadic CJD is 60–65 years); 2) the atypical clinical presentation, beginning with peripheral nerve signs and symptoms; and 3) the atypical neuropathological features. The neuropathological changes are unique and have not been described for other cases of iatrogenic, sporadic, or familial CJD. The hallmark of this new variant is the presence of numerous kuru-type (spiked-ball) amyloid plaques in the cerebral cortex. More than 10 can be found in some medium-powered microscope fields. In addition, each of these plaques or small clusters of plaques is frequently surrounded by neuropil vacuoles. None of the 10 subjects were related or had mutations of the PrP gene. The young age, the atypical features, and the occurrence exclusively in England have argued for an infectious etiology. Incubation times for kuru in New Guinea and for iatrogenic CJD caused by CJD-contaminated human growth hormone preparations have been 5 or more years as a rule. The onset of the new CJD variant in 1994–1995 argues for a time of exposure to environmental prions that corresponds to the height of the bovine spongiform encephalopathy (BSE) of dairy and beef cattle in Great Britain. While there is as of yet no definitive proof that the unusual CJD epidemic in England was caused by BSE, it is the only current explanation.

Genetically Determined Prion Diseases

Of human prion diseases, 10%–15% are dominantly inherited. In the past, there were only two named diseases included among the familial transmissible spongiform encephalopathies: familial CJD and GSS. FFI was added more recently because of its unique clinical features and distribution of pathology. Familial CJD and GSS are distinguished primarily by their neuropathological characteristics. In familial CJD, the main features are spongiform degeneration of cortical and subcortical gray regions (status spongiosis), with few or no PrP amyloid plaques. In GSS, there are numerous prion protein–containing amyloid and preamyloid plaques in the cerebellum, cerebral cortex, and basal ganglia, with variable amounts of spongiform degeneration of gray matter. Molecular genetics has linked all familial CJD and GSS cases to mutations of the prion protein gene (Figure 5–1), designated the *PRNP* gene and located on the short arm of chromosome 20 (Sparkes et al. 1986). Eleven mutations have been discovered. Mutated prion protein is designated ΔPrP. Sufficient genetic linkage has been found with 5 of the 11, to demonstrate a causal relationship between the mutation and CNS neurodegeneration (Dlouhy et al. 1992; Gabizon et al. 1993; Hsiao et al. 1989a; Petersen et al. 1992; Poulter et al. 1992). Some investigators prefer to use the term *prion disease* followed by the mutation in parentheses because it precisely identifies the molecular lesion and does not depend on matching clinical and neuropathological features in the pedigree with one of the named diseases. In practice, however, most investigators continue

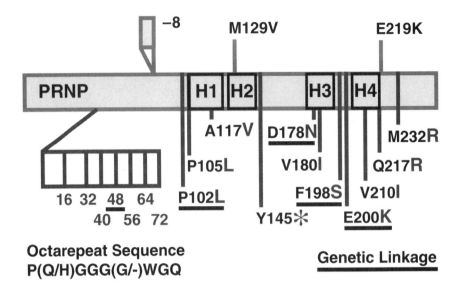

Figure 5–1. Mutations that segregate with dominantly inherited prion diseases (below) and wild-type polymorphisms (above) of the human prion protein gene (*PRNP*). The locations of the four putative α-helical domains are shown as boxes in the open reading frame (ORF) labeled H1 through H4 (Huang et al. 1994). The wild-type *PRNP* gene ORF contains five octarepeats from codons 51–91 (Kretzschmar et al. 1992). Deletion of a single octarepeat at codon 81 or 82 is not associated with prion disease (Laplanche et al. 1990; Palmer et al. 1993; Puckett et al. 1991; Vnencak-Jones and Phillips 1992). The normal distribution of the common polymorphism coded at codon 129 in the United States, United Kingdom, and France is M/V = 51%, M/M = 38%, and V/V = 11% (Brown et al. 1992; Collinge et al. 1991a). The methionine (Met) allotype at codon 129 appears to be more prevalent among normal Japanese (M:V = 0.958:0.043) relative to the U.S. and European populations (M:V = 0.625:0.375) (Miyazono et al. 1992). Homozygosity for Met or valine (Val) at codon 129 appears to increase susceptibility to sporadic CJD (Collinge et al. 1991a) and to iatrogenic CJD (Brown et al. 1992; Collinge et al. 1991b). References to individual disorders can be found in the text. (The figure was generated by Stanley Prusiner.)

* indicates stop codon

to name the disorder in each pedigree in which a new mutation has been discovered as either familial CJD or GSS depending on the dominant neuropathological features.

The *PRNP* mutation in the original family described by Gerstmann, Sträussler, and Scheinker (Gerstmann et al. 1936) is at codon 102 and leads to a nonconservative amino acid substitution of a proline (P) for a leucine (L) (Kretzschmar et al. 1991). This form of GSS is therefore designated GSS(P102L) regardless of the pedigree (Hsiao et al. 1989a,b). This and three other mutations in different pedigrees with GSS-like disorders occur in the region of the first two putative α-helical regions of the PrP molecule (Figure 5–1). Two of these are at codons 105 and 117, and the third occurs at codon 145 (Doh-ura et al. 1989; Goldfarb et al. 1990a; Goldgaber et al. 1989; Kitamoto et al. 1993b). The 145 mutation results in formation of a stop codon and leads to the synthesis of truncated PrP (Kitamoto et al. 1993a) (normal human PrP is 254 amino acids) (Kretzschmar et al. 1986b). Two other mutations at codons 198 and 217 in the third and fourth α-helical domains produce unusual GSS-like syndromes with abundant PrP amyloid plaques but also neurofibrillary degeneration of neurons and senile plaque formation (Dlouhy et al. 1992; Hsiao et al. 1992). The amyloid cores of the senile plaques in these families are composed of prion protein and not the Aβ peptide of AD or aging, suggesting a link between the pathogenesis of these familial prion disorders and AD (Ghetti et al. 1989). Although they have been designated GSS with neurofibrillary tangles, in reality the unusual blending of the neuropathological features of AD and prion disease go beyond the strict criteria for GSS as originally described (Seitelberger 1981).

The familial occurrence of CJD-like clinicopathologic syndromes has been linked to insertions of variable numbers of octapeptide repeats in the amino-terminal (N-terminal) domain of PrP (Goldfarb et al. 1991a; Owen et al. 1989, 1990) and to mutations at codons 178, 180, 200, 210, and 232 in the region of the third and fourth α-helical domains (Gabizon et al. 1991; Goldfarb et al. 1990b, 1991c, 1992a; Hsiao et al. 1991; Kitamoto et al. 1993b; Ripoll et al. 1993). The codon 200 mutation, CJD(E200K), among Libyan Jews represents the largest focus of CJD in the world, with an incidence about 100 times greater than the worldwide incidence (Gabizon et al. 1993; Neugut et al. 1979). The E200K mutation has arisen independently multiple times (Hsiao et al. 1991); it is found in unrelated families in Slovakia (Goldfarb et al. 1990c), Chile (Goldfarb et al. 1991b), and the United States (Bertoni et al. 1992).

The mutation at codon 178 resulting in an Asn-for-Asp substitution is particularly interesting because it is linked to both a typical CJD syndrome and to FFI (Goldfarb et al. 1992a; Medori et al. 1992a,b). Subsequently it was discovered that the *PRNP* allele carrying the 178 mutation in FFI also codes for a methionine (Met) polymorphism at codon 129, while the mutated allele in familial CJD (D178N) codes for valine (Val) at codon 129 (Goldfarb et al. 1992b). These findings demonstrate how a single amino acid difference in a mutated PrP molecule determines which population of neurons are vulnerable and the resulting clinical features. In FFI (D178N, M129), the neuropathology is confined largely to the mediodorsal and anterior ventral nuclei of the thalamus, whereas in familial CJD (D178N, V129) the neuropathology is widespread in the cerebral cortex and subcortical nuclei. FFI has been transmitted to rodents (Tateishi et al. 1995).

Sporadic CJD

Whereas familial prion diseases are very rare, with an incidence of about 1 per 10 million, neither a genetic nor infectious etiology can be identified to account for the vast majority of human prion disease cases. These cases are generally referred to as sporadic CJD and occur equally in men and women and with an incidence of one per million throughout the world. The clinical features that suggest the diagnosis include rapidly progressive dementia with extrapyramidal and/or cerebellar signs, myoclonic jerks, and a characteristic electroencephalogram (EEG). A presumptive diagnosis can be made when these clinical features are present and the neurohistopathology shows spongiform degeneration of the cerebral cortex and basal ganglia. The definitive diagnosis can be made today if one of the following four additional criteria are met: 1) the presence of kuru-type, PrP amyloid plaques in the molecular layer of the cerebellar cortex (however, these are only found in 5%–10% of CJD cases whereas they occur in 75% of kuru cases); 2) the presence of protease-resistant PrP, designated PrP^{CJD} (or PrP^{Sc} by some) by Western analysis (Bockman et al. 1987); 3) dot blot (Serban et al. 1990), histoblot of frozen tissue sections (Figure 5–2) (Taraboulos et al. 1992), or hydrolytic autoclaving immunohistochemistry of formalin fixed tissues (Muramoto et al. 1992); or 4) transmission to animals. Rarely, kuru-type amyloid plaques, often associated with amyloid angiopathy, occur in the cerebellum in cases of AD. These can be distinguished from the kuru plaques of prion disease by their immunoreactivity to Aβ peptide antibodies and failure to react with PrP-specific antibodies.

In the past, the definitive diagnosis of a sporadic, iatrogenic, or familial form of prion disease required showing transmissibility to animals. However, incubation times in primates range from 17 to

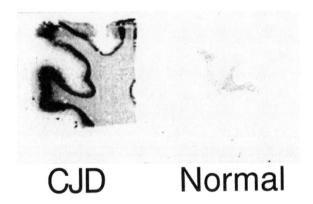

CJD   Normal

Figure 5–2. Identification of protease-resistant PrP^{CJD} on histoblots of the cerebral cortex in Creutzfeldt-Jakob disease (CJD). The histoblots are made by pressing unfixed frozen sections of cerebral cortex and underlying white matter onto nitrocellulose paper. The blotted sections are treated with proteinase K to eliminate PrP^{C}, followed by exposure to guanidinium to denature PrP^{CJD} and enhance binding of PrP-specific antibodies (Taraboulos et al. 1992). No immunostaining is found in normal brain. An intense signal is localized to the cerebral cortex in CJD cases.

64 months, and there are false-negative transmissions. In the National Institutes of Health (NIH) series, laboratory transmission rates were highest for iatrogenic CJD (100%), less for sporadic CJD (90%), and least for familial forms (68%) (Brown et al. 1994). Transmission rates varied considerably among familial prion diseases: CJD(E200K) was 85%, CJD(D178N, V129) was 70%, and GSS (P102L) was 38%. Stanley Prusiner's laboratory has developed a new transgenic (Tg) mouse that expresses a chimeric mouse (Mo) and human (Hu) PrP, designated Tg(MHu2M) (Telling et al. 1994). This appears to be a more efficient, more rapid, and less expensive bioassay. Incubation times are between 6 and 7 months with the current Tg(MHu2M) mice, with a 100% success rate. New Tg mouse lines expressing chimeric Mo/Hu PrP are being constructed in an attempt to greatly shorten incubation times and to eliminate any potential of the host species barrier to HuCJD and HuGSS prions (see later section).

The Etiology of Sporadic CJD

The molecular and cellular events that cause sporadic CJD are not known. One possible etiology is an acquired somatic mutation of the human prion protein gene, since multiple mutations of the *PRNP* gene are pathogenic and lead to the spontaneous formation of infectious particles. It is theoretically possible that a mutation in a single cell could trigger the self-perpetuating process of PrP^{Sc} formation. A second possible etiology is an age-related mismetabolism of PrP^{C} leading to its spontaneous conversion to PrP^{CJD}. The latter has been suggested by studies with Tg mice expressing high levels of normal wild-type (wt) PrP^{C} in which prions form spontaneously (Westaway et al. 1994).

Expanding the Range of Prion Protein Diseases

The pathological changes in prion protein disorders may not be confined to the CNS. PrP has been identified along with the Aβ peptide in the common age-related myopathy, inclusion body myositis (Askanas et al. 1993). Overexpression of PrP^C in Tg mice causes a similar age-related necrotizing myopathy (Westaway et al. 1994), and a myopathy was commonly found in scrapie of sheep, leading to the suggestion at one time that scrapie is a primary myopathy (Hulland 1958).

Transgenic Mice and the Molecular Pathogenesis of Genetic, Infectious, and Sporadic Prion Diseases

Acceptance of the prion hypothesis has been slow because each of the individual experiments and studies supporting it could be subjected to different interpretations. Ironically, the few remaining skeptics of the protein-only hypothesis generally cite the results of a single or very small number of experiments to refute it and deny or ignore the mountain of varied and consistent data that support the prion hypothesis. Today, the prion hypothesis is supported by a massive amount of data from multiple disciplines that, when viewed in aggregate, leave no other conclusion. Some of the most convincing evidence for the central role of PrP has come from Tg mouse studies. These have verified that human genetic forms of prion disease are due to mutations of the PrP gene (Hsiao et al. 1990); that prions form spontaneously in Tg mice expressing ΔPrP (Hsiao et al. 1994); that the host species barrier and different cliniconeuropathologic subtypes of scrapie are determined by the amino acid structure of PrP (Prusiner et al. 1990; Scott et al. 1989, 1993; Telling et al. 1994); and that all of the parameters that distinguish different scrapie prion isolates, including scrapie incubation time, the distribution of spongiform degeneration, and whether the PrP amyloid plaques' form can be manipulated by changing the amino acid sequence of PrP. Tg mice expressing a variety of PrP constructs have not only validated the prion hypothesis but have also given us new insights into the pathogenic mechanisms of all forms of prion diseases.

Tg(MoPrP-P101L) Mice Provide a Model for Human GSS(P102L)

Tg mouse lines expressing a mutant mouse PrP that mimics the codon 102 mutation linked to GSS in humans, designated Tg (MoPrP-P101L)H mice, were constructed (Hsiao et al. 1990). Codon 101 in mice is analogous to codon 102 in humans. Two Tg mouse lines expressing high (H) levels of the transgene product developed a spontaneous neurodegenerative disorder, with spongiform degeneration of gray matter and formation of PrP immunopositive amyloid plaques in multiple brain regions similar to those found in human GSS (Figure 5–3). Thus, the characteristic neuropathologic features of GSS were duplicated in these mice. A third line of Tg(MoPrP-P101L) mice expressing low levels of mutant PrP did not develop spontaneous CNS degeneration and were designated Tg196 (Hsiao et al. 1994).

Transmission of brain extracts from Tg(MoPrP-P101L)H mice to Syrian hamsters and Tg196 mice (Figure 5–3) expressing low levels of the transgene product has been achieved (Hsiao et al. 1994). Twelve of 164 Syrian hamsters (about 7%) and 73 of 152 Tg196 mice (about 40%) developed a scrapielike neurodegenerative disease after inoculation. These rates of transmission, although relatively low, are significant and different than the zero rate of transmission with normal brain homogenates from healthy CD-1 mice or non-Tg littermates. In contrast, only 2 of 97 Tg196 became ill following inoculation with normal homogenates and at greater than 500 days. Brain homogenates from clinically ill Tg (MoGSS-P101L)H mice did not transmit to CD-1 mice. Transmissions to Tg196 mice are of particular interest because these Tg mice also express the MoPrP-P101L transgene but at much lower copy numbers than the Tg mice, which developed diseases spontaneously, and do not develop a neurodegenerative disease spontaneously. One explanation for the relatively high rate of transmission to Tg196 from clinically ill Tg(MoPrP-P101L)H mice is that Tg196 expresses the same mutated PrP transgene product. The less-than-100% transmission rate of MoGSS from Tg(MoPrP-

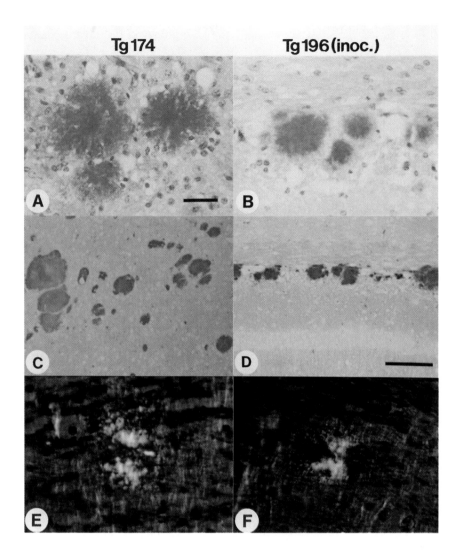

Figure 5–3. Spontaneous neurodegeneration with cerebral amyloidosis of the GSS type in Tg (MoPrP-P101L)H high expressor mice (Tg174) (A, C, E) and induced neurodegeneration with cerebral amyloidosis in low expressor Tg(MoPrP-P101L)L mice (Tg196 [inoculation]) (B, D, F) inoculated with prions from Tg174 mice. Similarities shared by the plaques were strong histochemical staining by the periodic acid-Schiff method (A and B), immunoreactivity with PrP-specific antibodies (C and D), and green-gold birefringence when stained with Congo red and viewed with polarized light (E and F). The main differences were that Tg174 plaques were primarily in the caudate nucleus and were as large as 90 μm, whereas those in inoculated Tg196 mice were primarily in the subcallosal region overlying the hippocampus and were smaller. (Bar in A = 50 μm for A, B, E, and F; bar in D = 100 μm for C and D.) From Hsiao et al. 1994.

P101L)H mice to other rodents is not unexpected since the rate of transmission of human GSS(P102L) to nonhuman primates is one of the lowest (38%) of all human prion diseases (Brown et al. 1994).

The Scrapie Phenotype

Several important characteristics of scrapie and scrapie prions were discovered during large-scale laboratory transmission of scrapie in sheep and goats and later within inbred mouse strains. Pattison and Millson (1961) were the first to recognize that there are distinct clinical patterns of scrapie in sheep and goats and that scrapie isolates from the CNS faithfully transmit these syndromes to other animals. The failure of transmission of a particular scrapie isolate to a different animal strain or species was designated the *host species barrier to scrapie*. More than 15 scrapie isolates (strains) have been identified in experimental scrapie in rodents (Bruce and Fraser 1991); they are distinguished by the host species barrier, by scrapie incubation time (the time from inoculation to onset of clinical signs), the distribution and intensity of spongiform degeneration in the nervous system, and whether amyloid plaques formed (Bruce et al. 1976; Fraser and Bruce 1973; Fraser and Dickinson 1973). All of these characteristics are faithfully reproduced during multiple sequential transmissions of a given prion isolate in animals with the same genotype but vary markedly or even fail when transferred to a different animal species (host species barrier). In a series of classical genetic studies with inbred mouse strains, Dickinson and Meikle (1971) showed that whether an animal strain has a long or short scrapie incubation time with a particular scrapie isolate is determined by a single host gene they designated the scrapie incubation time gene or *sinc* gene. Our own molecular studies of scrapie incubation time in Tg mice indicate that the *sinc* gene and the PrP gene in mice, designated *Prnp,* are the same (Carlson et al. 1986, 1994; Westaway et al. 1987).

Prion Propagation and the Host Barrier to Scrapie Infection Is Dependent on PrP Amino Acid Sequence

Two prion isolates to which there are well-defined host barriers are the RML isolate, Mo(RML) prion isolate, which is adapted to mice, and the Sc237 isolate, SHa(Sc237) prions, which is adapted to Syrian hamsters (Prusiner et al. 1990; Scott et al. 1989). When Syrian hamsters were inoculated in the thalamus with SHa(Sc237) prions, clinical signs of scrapie became detectable in ~75 days, whereas no Syrian hamsters became clinically ill in more than 500 days with Mo(RML) prions. Conversely, signs of scrapie were detectable in mice ~140 days after intrathalamic inoculation with Mo(RML) prions, but they did not develop signs of disease after more than 500 days when inoculated with SHa(Sc237) prions. That this barrier is due to amino acid differences between PrP^{Sc} in the prion and PrP^{C} of the host has been demonstrated in Tg mice expressing a variety of PrP transgenes.

The specificity of the interaction between PrP^{Sc} of the infecting prion and PrP^{C} of the host was first demonstrated in Tg(SHaPrP) mice that express both $SHaPrP^{C}$ and $MoPrP^{C}$ (Prusiner et al. 1990; Scott et al. 1989). When these animals were inoculated with SHa (Sc237) prions, only $SHaPrP^{Sc}$ was formed based on the characteristics of the neuropathology, the presence of $SHaPrP^{Sc}$ in the neuropil and in amyloid plaques, and the behavior of the newly formed prions that had characteristics of Sc237 prions (e.g., they infected Syrian hamsters but not mice). In contrast, with Mo(RML), there was a different distribution of gray matter vacuolation, vacuolation of the white matter, and the absence of amyloid plaques that is characteristic of RML scrapie. Thus, Sc237 prions selectively interacted with $SHaPrP^{C}$ in these Tg(SHaPrP) mice, and RML prions selectively interacted with $MoPrP^{C}$.

These observations have greatly increased our understanding of the $PrP^{C}-PrP^{Sc}$ interactions that lead to formation of nascent PrP^{Sc} (Figure 5–4). The necessity for amino acid homology between PrP^{C} of the host and PrP^{Sc} within the prion is well established. Considerable data argue that a heterodimer consisting of

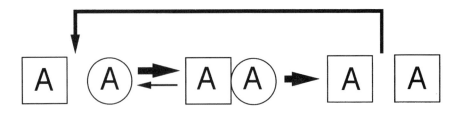

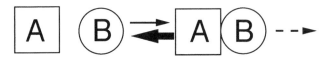

Figure 5–4. Schematic diagram illustrating the dimer hypothesis of prion propagation and the host species barrier to scrapie infection. Squares represent PrP^{Sc} and circles PrP^{C}. When there is sufficient amino acid homology between PrP^{Sc} (A) and PrP^{C} (A), dimer formation is favored and is followed by transformation of PrP^{C} (A) into a duplicate copy of PrP^{Sc} (A). In the absence of sufficient amino acid homology, PrP^{Sc} (A) tends not to bind to PrP^{C} (B), with the result that PrP^{C} (B) is not transformed into nascent PrP^{Sc} (A).

PrP^{C} and PrP^{Sc} is an intermediate in the formation of nascent prions. These results argue that the first step in the propagation of prions is an interaction of PrP^{Sc} of the infecting prion, with PrP^{C} expressed by the host. Thus, Tg mouse studies of the host species barrier argue strongly in favor of the protein-only hypothesis, just as the results from Tg (MoPrP-P101L) did.

Selective Vulnerability of Neurons as a Function of Prion Isolate and Sites of PrP^{Sc} Accumulation

Because PrP^{Sc} accumulation appears to cause spongiform degeneration and because the distribution of spongiform degeneration is one of the characteristics of the scrapie phenotype used to define each prion isolate, it follows that the distribution of PrP^{Sc} must also be characteristic of each prion isolate. This relationship was established with the development of the highly sensitive histoblot technique (Taraboulos et al. 1992). A frozen tissue section mounted on nitrocellulose paper can be treated harshly with proteinase K to completely digest PrP^C while preserving PrP^{Sc} or PrP^{CJD}. The remaining PrP^{Sc} can be denatured with guanidinium, which markedly increases its affinity for PrP antibodies. Earlier studies using PrP immunohistochemical techniques on aldehyde-fixed tissues were interpreted similarly, but the procedure used failed to eliminate PrP^C with certainty, and the intensity of PrP^{Sc} immunostaining was relatively weak (Bruce et al. 1989).

The histoblot technique has clearly revealed that the neuroanatomic location of PrP^{Sc} accumulation is unique for each scrapie prion isolate and not a function of scrapie incubation time when compared in animals with the same genotype (DeArmond and Prusiner 1993; DeArmond et al. 1993; Hecker et al. 1992). In comparing the kinetics of PrP^{Sc} accumulation in the brain of Syrian hamsters inoculated with either Sc237 or 139H prions, we found that its distribution at the time clinical signs became apparent was markedly different (Figure 5–5). Specifically, PrP^{Sc} was localized to fewer brain regions with Sc237 than with 139H; however, because scrapie incubation time was significantly longer with 139H, 170 days versus 70 days for Sc237, we could not rule out the possibility that the longer incubation time with 139H permitted the disease to spread nonspecifically to more brain regions rather than showing selective targeting. The influence of scrapie incubation time was eliminated in studies with Tg(SHaPrP)7 mice that express high levels of SHaPrP mRNA and have scrapie incubation times of ~50 days with both the Sc237 and 139H isolates (Hecker et al. 1992). After Sc237 prions were inoculated unilaterally into the thalamus, PrP^{Sc} accumulation was largely confined to selected nuclei in the thalamus, septum, and brain stem, whereas it was widely distributed throughout the CNS with 139H. With the Me7H isolate (Figure 5–5), PrP^{Sc} accumulation was even more restricted, being confined to the paraventricular nucleus of the thalamus, habenula, hypothalamus, zona incerta, nucleus accumbens septi, and peri-

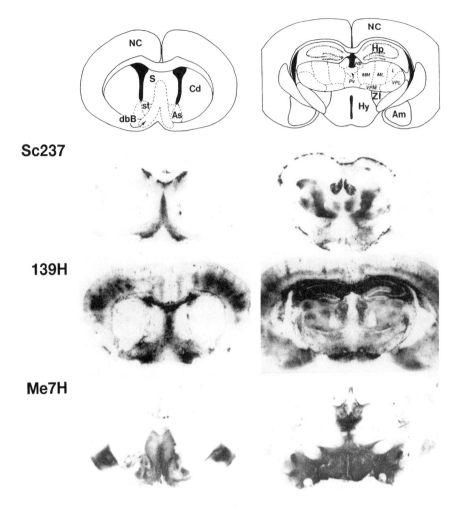

Figure 5–5. The distribution of PrP^{Sc} in the brains of Tg(SHaPrP) mice is significantly different for the Sc237, 139H, and Me7H prion isolates; however, some brain regions, such as the diagonal band of Broca (dbB), the hypothalamus (Hy), and various brain stem nuclei (not shown), accumulate PrP^{Sc} regardless of the prion isolate. Am, amygdala; As, accumbens septi; Cd, caudate nucleus; dbB, diagonal band of Broca and medial septal nuclei; Hp, hippocampus; Hy, hypothalamus; NC, neocortex; S, septum; st, bed nucleus of the stria terminalis; ZI, zona incerta. Thalamic nuclei in italics: Hb, habenula; L, lateral; ML, medial pars lateralis; MM, medial pars medialis; pv, paraventricular; VPL and VPM, ventral posterior lateral and medial, respectively. Adapted from DeArmond et al. 1993.

aqueductal gray of the midbrain. These findings were all the more remarkable because scrapie incubation times with Me7H in Tg (SHaPrP)7 mice were about 185 days, and therefore the highly restricted distribution of PrP^{Sc} could not be attributed to insufficient time for prions to spread within the CNS.

Therefore, prion isolate–determined selective vulnerability of neurons is characterized by differential targeting of neuron populations for conversion of PrP^C to PrP^{Sc} and for accumulation of PrP^{Sc}. The molecular mechanism of differential neuron targeting is unknown. Given the possibility that PrP^{Sc} is the sole functional component of prions, one would assume that some aspect of its three-dimensional structure is different for each prion isolate and that these differences are recognized by neurons.

The selective vulnerability of the thalamus in FFI(D178N, M129) and of the cerebral cortex in CJD(D178N, V129) is the best example from nature of how a single amino acid difference in ΔPrP can influence neuronal targeting of disease. In laboratory scrapie, prion strain–determined targeting of neurons occurs even when the amino acid sequence of PrP^{Sc} in the prion and PrP^C of the host are the same. One possible structural difference that could account for targeting is the composition of the two-carbohydrate tree side chains on the PrP molecule. In this regard, we have recently found that each neuron population synthesizes different PrP isoforms, each with the same amino acid sequence but with different degrees of sialation of their carbohydrate trees (S. J. DeArmond et al., in preparation). Interestingly, a single carbohydrate residue difference determines whether *E. Coli* infects the urinary tract (Lindstedt et al. 1991).

Artificial Prions Formed
From Chimeric SHa/MoPrP^C

The homotypic interaction of PrP^{Sc} with PrP^C was also demonstrated in Tg mice expressing chimeric PrP^C containing amino acid sequences from both SHa and MoPrP (Scott et al. 1993). Two chimeric constructs were made on the MoPrP background, one containing two amino acid substitutions from SHa at codons 108 and 111 designated MHM2 PrP and the other containing three additional substitutions at codons 138, 154, and 169 designated MH2M. Three Tg mouse lines expressing the former construct, Tg(MHM2) mice, were resistant to SHa(Sc237) derived from Syrian hamsters similar to non-Tg mice; however, all Tg mice expressing the transgene with 5 SHa amino acid substitutions, Tg(MH2M) mice, became clinically ill with SHa(Sc237) prions, supporting the view that the host species barrier is related to the amino acid sequence of both PrP^C and PrP^{Sc}. When the resulting prions, designated MH2M (Sc237), were passaged back into Syrian hamsters, the hamsters developed scrapie characterized by distribution of PrP^{Sc} similar to, although not identical with, that caused by SHa(Sc237). Mouse-derived RML prions, Mo(RML), also produced scrapie in the Tg (MH2M) mice. Although Mo(RML) prions do not infect Syrian hamsters, inoculation of brain homogenates infected with Mo(RML) prions from Tg(MH2M) mice into Syrian hamsters produced scrapie, indicating that MH2M(RML) prions had been formed. Furthermore, the pattern of PrP^{Sc} accumulation in Syrian hamster brain was unique, suggesting that the artificial prion created by the chimeric transgene was a new scrapie prion isolate. Particularly unique aspects of the PrP^{Sc} pattern were its dense accumulation along the hippocampal fissure and subpially at the periphery of the brain. Both the MH2M(RML) and MH2M(Sc237) prions also transmitted to CD-1 mice.

The successful transmission of Sc237 prions composed of SHaPrP^{Sc} into these animals argues that the amino acid homology in the region of the first two putative α-helical domains of the PrP molecule are sufficient for dimerization. SHaPrP differs from MoPrP by 16 amino acids in total (Westaway et al. 1987). Conversely, total amino acid homology in the first two α-helical domains is not necessary for dimerization since RML prions composed of MoPrP^{Sc} also interacted with the chimeric MH2MPrP^C. Finding that RML prions composed of MH2MPrP^{Sc} were able to cross the host barrier in Syrian hamsters and produce a new form of scrapie supports the hypothesis that the properties of prion isolates (strains) are determined by the amino acid sequence of the host prion protein.

Amino Acid Sequence Homology Is Insufficient for Crossing the Prion Species Barrier Between Humans and Mice

It became evident that there is another factor or set of factors that determine whether a prion isolate will initiate the transformation of PrP^C to nascent PrP^{Sc} when it was found that transmission of HuCJD prions to Tg(HuPrP) mice, which express whole $HuPrP^C$, occurred in only ~10% of the inoculated mice, similar to our findings with non-Tg mice (Telling et al. 1994). Thus when two Tg (HuPrP) mouse lines were inoculated intrathalamically with brain extracts from 18 patients who had died of sporadic CJD, iatrogenic CJD, familial CJD, or GSS over a 2.5-year period, only 14 of 169 Tg(HuPrP) mice became clinically ill (8.3%), which is similar to the 6 of 58 control non-Tg mice that had become clinically ill (10.3%). Incubation times were extremely long, ranging from 590 to 840 days for both Tg(HuPrP) and non-Tg mice.

Because of the successful transmission of scrapie with both SHa(Sc237) and Mo(RML) prions in Tg mice expressing chimeric $SHa/MoPrP^C$, a chimeric Hu/Mo transgene analogous to MH2M was constructed and designated MHu2M. The PrP^C coded by MHu2M differs from $MoPrP^C$ by nine amino acids between residues 96 and 167, the region of the first two putative α-helical domains of PrP. Tg(MHu2M) mice were inoculated with brain homogenates from two unrelated sporadic CJD patients and one iatrogenic CJD patient treated with human growth hormone. All 24 Tg(MHu2M) mice inoculated with the human prions developed clinical signs, with incubation periods ranging from 202 to 249 days. Histoblots revealed strong immunostaining for PrP^{Sc}, which correlated with the distribution of spongiform degeneration and reactive astrocytic gliosis.

The higher frequency of transmission of HuCJD prions to Tg (MHu2M) mice expressing chimeric Hu/MoPrP^C compared to Tg (HuPrP) mice expressing HuPrP^C or non-Tg mice that express only MoPrP^C has several implications. First, it argues that 100% amino acid sequence homology between PrP^{Sc} (or PrP^{CJD}) of the prion and PrP^C of the host is not sufficient to sustain the self-propagating process of PrP^C conversion into nascent PrP^{Sc}. In terms of the dimer hypothesis, it argues that PrP^{Sc}/PrP^C heterodimer formation by itself probably does not lead to spontaneous conversion of PrP^C to PrP^{Sc}. Secondly, efficient transmission of HuCJD prions to Tg mice expressing chimeric Hu/MoPrP^C is consistent with the importance of the first two putative α-helical domains for PrP^{Sc}(PrP^{CJD})/PrP^C dimerization. And thirdly, the efficient conversion of MHu2MPrP^C to MHu2MPrP^{Sc} initiated by HuCJD prions argues for the importance of the mouse PrP sequence. The last point argues that the conversion of PrP^C into PrP^{Sc} requires the active participation of a cellular factor that recognizes some residues of PrP^C specific for MoPrP (Figure 5–6). This mouse-specific factor is likely to be a protein, which we have provisionally designated protein X (Telling et al. 1994). Presumably, protein X is a chaperon-like molecule that forms a ternary complex with PrP^C and PrP^{Sc} and then catalyzes the conversion of PrP^C into PrP^{Sc}. We assume that there is a sizeable energy barrier that separates the α-helical conformational state of PrP^C from the β-sheet state of PrP^{Sc} (Cohen et al. 1994). Whether specific prion strain information is also transferred to nascent prions during the transformation of PrP^C into PrP^{Sc} remains to be established. The most likely explanation for the successful transmission of SHa(Sc237) prions to Tg(SHaPrP) mice expressing whole SHaPrP^C and the failure of transmission of HuCJD prions to Tg(HuPrP) mice expressing whole HuPrP^C is the relative degree of homology of SHaPrP and HuPrP with MoPrP: SHaPrP differs from MoPrP at 16 amino acids whereas HuPrP differs at 28 (Westaway et al. 1987).

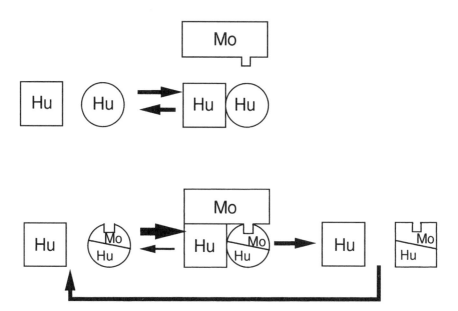

Figure 5–6. The "X-factor" hypothesis: A protein or a protein complex (rectangle with small projection) is required for the conversion of PrP^C (circles) into PrP^{Sc} (squares). The experience with propagation of human (Hu) CJD prions in Tg(MHu2M) mice is that efficient conversion of host PrP^C requires that the X factor recognize PrP^C of the PrP^C–PrP^{Sc} dimer (projection on rectangle fits in indentation in the Mo portion of the chimeric Mo/HuPrP^C).

Overexpression of wtPrP^C Results in Spontaneous Formation of Prions

Tg mice expressing a variety of normal wtPrP^C develop an age-related necrotizing myopathy (Westaway et al. 1994). In addition, we are testing whether prions form spontaneously in the brain of Tg mice overexpressing wtPrP^C. We have reported that brain homogenates from five Tg(SHaPrP) mice, which express the highest levels of SHaPrP^C, have transmitted a scrapielike neurological disorder to Syrian hamsters (Westaway et al. 1994). The many negative transmissions from control non-Tg mice argue against cross-contamination of the Tg(SHaPrP) inoculum. More recently, we have examined 11 new transmissions of Tg(SHaPrP) inocula into Syrian hamsters. Incubation times have varied from 113 to 369 days, with a mean of 188 days. Neurohistological examination shows mild to moderate spongiform degeneration of multiple brain regions; however, the most intense vacuolation occurred in the subiculum, in the cerebellar granule cell layer, and in deep cerebellar nuclei. There was an accompanying intense reactive astrocytic gliosis and Bergman radial gliosis. The distribution of the vacuolation was significantly different than that associated with any of the hamster-adapted prions (Sc237, 139H, or Me7H) used in our laboratories. Thus, the preliminary data argue that Tg(SHaPrP)7 mice that overexpress wtSHaPrP^C spontaneously form prions. Whether overexpression of PrP increases the probability of a pathologic somatic mutation or the spontaneous conversion of PrP^C into PrP^{Sc} occurs in these Tg(SHaPrP)7 mice is unknown. Overexpression or mismetabolism of PrP^C may be the etiology of some cases of sporadic CJD.

Prnp$^{0/0}$ Mice Neither Develop Scrapie nor Propagate Prions

Finally, strong evidence for the preeminence of PrP in the etiology and pathogenesis of prion diseases and their necessity for prion particle formation comes from mice in which the PrP gene has been ablated. These animals have normal life spans without any structural or behavioral abnormalities (Büeler et al. 1992). After inoculation with prions, they neither develop clinical or neuropathological features nor propagate prions. However, when a Syrian hamster (SHa) PrP transgene was introduced into *Prnp*$^{0/0}$ mice by crossing them with Tg(SHaPrP) mice, the Tg(SHaPrP)/*Prnp*$^{0/0}$ mice became susceptible to SHa prions but not to Mo prions (Büeler et al. 1993; Prusiner et al. 1993). These findings indicate that the absence of PrP^C expression is not the cause of neuronal dysfunction in scrapie; they also support the view that accumulation of PrP^{Sc} is responsible for CNS degeneration. Furthermore, these data indicate that prion propagation requires PrP^C. Finally, the transmission of scrapie with SHa prions containing $SHaPrP^{Sc}$ but not with prions containing $MoPrP^{Sc}$ to mice that express $SHaPrP^C$ but not $MoPrP^C$ supports the view that propagation of prions requires amino acid homology between the PrP^{Sc} of the prion and PrP^C of the host.

Conclusion: Different Etiologies and Pathogenic Mechanisms of Prion Diseases

The rapid advances in understanding the etiology and pathogenesis of CJD and GSS compared to other neurodegenerative diseases such as AD and Parkinson's disease have occurred in part because there are animal and tissue culture models of these diseases and in part because virtually all aspects of genetic, infectious, and possibly even sporadic prion diseases can be duplicated in Tg mice. Advances have also been rapid because all aspects of these diseases are causally related to one protein, PrP, in contrast to AD, in which at least four genes appear to play a role.

The key molecular factors in the pathogenesis of prion diseases reside in the properties of the prion protein and its interaction with a chaperon-like mechanism (molecule). They can be summarized as follows:

1. The PrP molecule can exist in one of two stable configurations: one with a high α-helical content and little or no β-sheet, exemplified by PrP^C, and one with a high β-sheet content and less α-helix, exemplified by PrP^{Sc} and ΔPrP.
2. A sizeable energy barrier separates the α-helical from the β-sheet state.

Three etiologic mechanisms that convert the structure of PrP to β-sheet and cause nerve cell dysfunction and formation of prions have been identified.

First, point mutations leading to nonconservative amino acid substitutions in the immediate vicinity of or within one of the four putative α-helical domains appear to destabilize PrP α-helices and foster spontaneous β-sheet formation. The highly amyloidogenic nature of several of the ΔPrPs testifies to their high β-sheet content. Additional enzymatic truncation of ΔPrP in vivo probably helps foster amyloid plaque formation much as limited proteolysis of PrP^{Sc} results in PrP27–30 with increased β-sheet content and amyloid rod formation in vitro. Whether the mechanisms of nerve cell dysfunction and neuropathology caused by ΔPrP accumulation are the same as for PrP^{Sc} accumulation is not known. It is also unknown whether ΔPrP forms a dimer with PrP^{C} and converts it to PrP^{Sc} in patients heterozygous for the mutation.

Secondly, overexpression of wild-type PrP^{C} in Tg mice not only causes an age-related necrotizing myopathy but also leads to spontaneous focal spongiform degeneration in the hippocampus and spontaneous formation of prions (Westaway et al. 1994). Although the infective prion particles in the overexpression syndrome have not been characterized structurally, it is reasonable to assume that the PrP comprising them has an increased β-sheet content. It appears that when PrP^{C} is overexpressed, a significant proportion is synthesized with a β-sheet structure, a significant proportion spontaneously crosses the energy barrier to β-sheet configuration, or the mechanisms that degrade PrP become overwhelmed and inadvertently divert a significant proportion of PrP^{C} into a pathway that converts its structure. The PrP overexpression syndrome suggests that mismetabolism of PrP^{C} can yield a pathogenic PrP molecule.

The third mechanism for acquisition of β-sheet structure is the one most synonymous with prion diseases, that is, by exposure of receptive cells to exogenous PrP^{Sc} in the form of prion particles. The evidence indicates that exogenous PrP^{Sc} forms a heterodimer with PrP^{C} expressed by the vulnerable host cell. The evidence also indicates that the PrP^C of the heterodimer is recognized by a chaperon-like molecule in the host cell that, like an enzyme, lowers the energy barrier separating the largely α-helical structure of PrP^C from the largely β-sheet structure of PrP^{Sc}; it also converts PrP^C into nascent PrP^{Sc} with a structure similar or identical to that of the original exogenous PrP^{Sc}.

Today, multiple questions remain to be answered, not about the validity of the prion hypothesis but about the details of the pathogenesis of each form of prion disease.

References

Askanas V, Bilak M, Engel WK, et al: Prion protein is abnormally accumulated in inclusion-body myositis. Neuroreport 5:25–28, 1993

Berger JR, David NJ: Creutzfeldt-Jakob disease in a physician: a review of the disorder in health care workers. Neurology 43:205–206, 1993

Bertoni JM, Brown P, Goldfarb L, et al: Familial Creutzfeldt-Jakob disease with the PRNP codon 200[lys] mutation and supranuclear palsy but without myoclonus or periodic EEG complexes (abstract). Neurology 42(4) (suppl 3):S350, 1992

Bockman JM, Prusiner SB, Tateishi J, Kingsbury DT: Immunoblotting of Creutzfeldt-Jakob disease prion proteins: host species-specific epitopes. Ann Neurol 21:589–595, 1987

Borchelt DR, Scott M, Taraboulos A, et al: Scrapie and cellular prion proteins differ in their kinetics of synthesis and topology in cultured cells. J Cell Biol 110:743–752, 1990

Brown P, Preece MA, Will RG: "Friendly fire" in medicine: hormones, homografts, and Creutzfeldt-Jakob disease. Lancet 340:24–27, 1992

Brown P, Gibbs CJ Jr, Rodgers-Johnson P, et al: Human spongiform encephalopathy: the National Institutes of Health series of 300 cases of experimentally transmitted disease. Ann Neurol 35:513–529, 1994

Bruce ME, Fraser H: Scrapie strain variation and its implications. Curr Top Microbiol Immunol 172:125–138, 1991

Bruce ME, Dickinson AG, Fraser H: Cerebral amyloidosis in scrapie in the mouse: effect of agent strain and mouse genotype. Neuropathol Appl Neurobiol 2:471–478, 1976

Bruce ME, McBride PA, Farquhar CF: Precise targeting of the pathology of the sialoglycoprotein, PrP, and vacuolar degeneration in mouse scrapie. Neurosci Lett 102:1–6, 1989

Büeler H, Fischer M, Lang Y, et al: Normal development and behaviour of mice lacking the neuronal cell-surface PrP protein. Nature 356:577–582, 1992

Büeler H, Aguzzi A, Sailer A, et al: Mice devoid of PrP are resistant to scrapie. Cell 73:1339–1347, 1993

Carlson GA, Kingsbury DT, Goodman PA, et al: Linkage of prion protein and scrapie incubation time genes. Cell 46:503–511, 1986

Carlson GA, Ebeling C, Yang S-L, et al: Prion isolate specified allotypic interactions between the cellular and scrapie prion proteins in congenic and transgenic mice. Proc Natl Acad Sci U S A 91:5690–5694, 1994

Caughey B, Race RE, Ernst D, et al: Prion protein biosynthesis in scrapie-infected and uninfected neuroblastoma cells. J Virol 63:175–181, 1989

Caughey BW, Dong A, Bhat KS, et al: Secondary structure analysis of the scrapie-associated protein PrP 27–30 in water by infrared spectroscopy. Biochemistry 30:7672–7680, 1991

Cohen FE, Pan K-M, Huang Z, et al: Structural clues to prion replication. Science 264:530–531, 1994

Collinge J, Palmer MS, Dryden AJ: Genetic predisposition to iatrogenic Creutzfeldt-Jakob disease. Lancet 337:1441–1442, 1991

Collinge J, Palmer M: Molecular genetics of inherited, sporadic and iatrogenic prion disease, in Prion Diseases in Humans and Animals. Edited by Prusiner S, Collinge J, Powell J, et al. London, Ellis Horwood, 1992, pp 95–119

DeArmond SJ, Prusiner SB: The neurochemistry of prion diseases. J Neurochem 61:1589–1601, 1993

DeArmond SJ, McKinley MP, Barry RA, et al: Identification of prion amyloid filaments in scrapie-infected brain. Cell 41:221–235, 1985

DeArmond SJ, Mobley WC, DeMott DL, et al: Changes in the localization of brain prion proteins during scrapie infection. Neurology 37:1271–1280, 1987

DeArmond SJ, Jendroska K, Yang S-L, et al: Scrapie prion protein accumulation correlates with neuropathology and incubation times in hamsters and transgenic mice, in Prion Diseases of Humans and Animals. Edited by Prusiner SB, Collinge J, Powell J, et al. London, Ellis Horwood, 1992, pp 483–496

DeArmond SJ, Yang S-L, Lee A, et al: Three scrapie prion isolates exhibit different accumulation patterns of the prion protein scrapie isoform. Proc Natl Acad Sci U S A 90:6449–6453, 1993

Dickinson AG, Meikle VMH: Host-genotype and agent effects in scrapie incubation: change in allelic interaction with different strains of agent. Mol Gen Genet 112:73–79, 1971

Dlouhy SR, Hsiao K, Farlow MR, et al: Linkage of the Indiana kindred of Gerstmann-Sträussler-Scheinker disease to the prion protein gene. Nat Genet 1:64–67, 1992

Doh-ura K, Tateishi J, Sasaki H, et al: Pro→Leu change at position 102 of prion protein is the most common but not the sole mutation related to Gerstmann-Sträussler syndrome. Biochem Biophys Res Commun 163:974–979, 1989

Fraser H, Bruce ME: Argyrophilic plaques in mice inoculated with scrapie from particular sources. Lancet 1:617–618, 1973

Fraser H, Dickinson AG: Scrapie in mice. Agent-strain differences in the distribution and intensity of grey matter vacuolation. J Comp Pathol 83:29–40, 1973

Gabizon R, Meiner Z, Cass C, et al: Prion protein gene mutation in Libyan Jews with Creutzfeldt-Jakob disease (abstract). Neurology 41:160, 1991

Gabizon R, Rosenmann H, Meiner Z, et al: Mutation and polymorphism of the prion protein gene in Libyan Jews with Creutzfeldt-Jakob disease. Am J Hum Genet 33:828–835, 1993

Gasset M, Baldwin MA, Fletterick RJ, Prusiner SB: Perturbation of the secondary structure of the scrapie prion protein under conditions associated with changes in infectivity. Proc Natl Acad Sci U S A 90:1–5, 1993

Gerstmann J, Sträussler E, Scheinker I: Über eine eigenartige hereditär-familiäre Erkrankung des Zentralnervensystems zugleich ein Beitrag zur frage des vorzeitigen lokalen Alterns. Zeitschrift für Neurologie und Psychiatrie 154:736–762, 1936

Ghetti B, Tagliavini F, Masters CL, et al: Gerstmann-Sträussler-Scheinker disease, II: neurofibrillary tangles and plaques with PrP-amyloid coexist in an affected family. Neurology 39:1453–1461, 1989

Goldfarb LG, Brown P, Goldgaber D, et al: Creutzfeldt-Jakob disease and kuru patients lack a mutation consistently found in the Gerstmann-Sträussler-Scheinker syndrome. Exp Neurol 108:247–250, 1990a

Goldfarb L, Korczyn A, Brown P, et al: Mutation in codon 200 of scrapie amyloid precursor gene linked to Creutzfeldt-Jakob disease in Sephardic Jews of Libyan and non-Libyan origin. Lancet 336:637–638, 1990b

Goldfarb LG, Mitrova E, Brown P, et al: Mutation in codon 200 of scrapie amyloid protein gene in two clusters of Creutzfeldt-Jakob disease in Slovakia. Lancet 336:514–515, 1990c

Goldfarb LG, Brown P, McCombie WR, et al: Transmissible familial Creutzfeldt-Jakob disease associated with five, seven, and eight extra octapeptide coding repeats in the *PRNP* gene. Proc Natl Acad Sci U S A 88:10926–10930, 1991a

Goldfarb LG, Brown P, Mitrova E, et al: Creutzfeldt-Jacob disease associated with the PRNP codon 200[Lys] mutation: an analysis of 45 families. Eur J Epidemiol 7:477–486, 1991b

Goldfarb LG, Haltia M, Brown P, et al: New mutation in scrapie amyloid precursor gene (at codon 178) in Finnish Creutzfeldt-Jakob kindred (letter). Lancet 337:425, 1991c

Goldfarb LG, Brown P, Haltia M, et al: Creutzfeldt-Jakob disease cosegregates with the codon 178[Asn] PRNP mutation in families of European origin. Ann Neurol 31:274–281, 1992a

Goldfarb LG, Petersen RB, Tabaton M, et al: Fatal familial insomnia and familial Creutzfeldt-Jakob disease: disease phenotype determined by a DNA polymorphism. Science 258:806–808, 1992b

Goldgaber D, Goldfarb LG, Brown P, et al: Mutations in familial Creutzfeldt-Jakob disease and Gerstmann-Sträussler-Scheinker's syndrome. Exp Neurol 106:204–206, 1989

Hecker R, Taraboulos A, Scott M, et al: Replication of distinct prion isolates is region specific in brains of transgenic mice and hamsters. Genes Dev 6:1213–1228, 1992

Hsiao K, Baker HF, Crow TJ, et al: Linkage of a prion protein missense variant to Gerstmann-Sträussler syndrome. Nature 338:342–345, 1989a

Hsiao KK, Doh-ura K, Kitamoto T, et al: A prion protein amino acid substitution in ataxic Gerstmann-Sträussler syndrome (abstract). Ann Neurol 26:137, 1989b

Hsiao KK, Scott M, Foster D, et al: Spontaneous neurodegeneration in transgenic mice with mutant prion protein. Science 250:1587–1590, 1990

Hsiao K, Meiner Z, Kahana E, et al: Mutation of the prion protein in Libyan Jews with Creutzfeldt-Jakob disease. N Engl J Med 324:1091–1097, 1991

Hsiao K, Dlouhy S, Farlow MR, et al: Mutant prion proteins in Gerstmann-Sträussler-Scheinker disease with neurofibrillary tangles. Nat Genet 1:68–71, 1992

Hsiao KK, Groth D, Scott M, et al: Serial transmission in rodents of neurodegeneration from transgenic mice expressing mutant prion protein. Proc Natl Acad Sci U S A 91:9126–9130, 1994

Huang Z, Gabriel J-M, Baldwin MA, et al: Proposed three-dimensional structure for the cellular prion protein. Proc Natl Acad Sci U S A 91: 7139–7143, 1994

Hulland TJ: The skeletal muscle of sheep affected with scrapie. J Comp Path 68:264–274, 1958

Jendroska K, Heinzel FP, Torchia M, et al: Proteinase-resistant prion protein accumulation in Syrian hamster brain correlates with regional pathology and scrapie infectivity. Neurology 41:1482–1490, 1991

Kitamoto T, Iizuka R, Tateishi J: An amber mutation of prion protein in Gerstmann-Sträussler syndrome with mutant PrP plaques. Biochem Biophys Res Commun 192:525–531, 1993a

Kitamoto T, Ohta M, Doh-ura K, et al: Novel missense variants of prion protein in Creutzfeldt-Jakob disease or Gerstmann-Sträussler syndrome. Biochem Biophys Res Commun 191:709–714, 1993b

Kretzschmar HA, Prusiner SB, Stowring LE, DeArmond SJ: Scrapie prion proteins are synthesized in neurons. Am J Pathol 122:1–5, 1986a

Kretzschmar HA, Stowring LE, Westaway D, et al: Molecular cloning of a human prion protein cDNA. DNA 5:315–324, 1986b

Kretzschmar HA, Honold G, Seitelberger F, et al: Prion protein mutation in family first reported by Gerstmann, Straussler, and Scheinker (letter). Lancet 337:1160, 1991

Kretzschmar HA, Neumann M, Riethmüller G, Prusiner SB: Molecular cloning of a mink prion protein gene. J Gen Virol 73:2757–2761, 1992

Laplanche J-L, Chatelain J, Launay J-M, et al: Deletion in prion protein gene in a Moroccan family. Nucleic Acids Res 18:6745, 1990

Lindstedt R, Larson G, Falk P, et al: The receptor repertoire defines the host range for attaching Escherichia coli strains that recognize globo-A. Infect Immun 59:1086–1092, 1991

McKinley MP, Bolton DC, Prusiner SB: A protease-resistant protein is a structural component of the scrapie prion. Cell 35:57–62, 1983

McKinley MP, Taraboulos A, Kenaga L, et al: Ultrastructural localization of scrapie prion proteins in cytoplasmic vesicles of infected cultured cells. Lab Invest 65:622–630, 1991

Medori R, Montagna P, Tritschler HJ, et al: Fatal familial insomnia: a second kindred with mutation of prion protein gene at codon 178. Neurology 42:669–670, 1992a

Medori R, Tritschler H-J, LeBlanc A, et al: Fatal familial insomnia, a prion disease with a mutation at codon 178 of the prion protein gene. N Engl J Med 326:444–449, 1992b

Meyer N, Rosenbaum V, Schmidt B, et al: Search for a putative scrapie genome in purified prion fractions reveals a paucity of nucleic acids. J Gen Virol 72:37–49, 1991

Miyazono M, Kitamoto T, Doh-ura K, et al: Creutzfeldt-Jakob disease with codon 129 polymorphism (Valine): a comparative study of patients with codon 102 point mutation or without mutations. Acta Neuropathol 84:349–354, 1992

Muramoto T, Kitamoto T, Tateishi J, Goto I: The sequential development of abnormal prion protein accumulation in mice with Creutzfeldt-Jakob disease. Am J Pathol 140:1411–1420, 1992

Neugut RH, Neugut AI, Kahana E, et al: Creutzfeldt-Jakob disease: familial clustering among Libyan-born Israelis. Neurology 29:225–231, 1979

Oesch B, Westaway D, Wälchli M, et al: A cellular gene encodes scrapie PrP 27–30 protein. Cell 40:735–746, 1985

Owen F, Poulter M, Lofthouse R, et al: Insertion in prion protein gene in familial Creutzfeldt-Jakob disease. Lancet 1:51–52, 1989

Owen F, Poulter M, Shah T, et al: An in-frame insertion in the prion protein gene in familial Creutzfeldt-Jakob disease. Molecular Brain Research 7:273–276, 1990

Palmer MS, Mahal SP, Campbell TA, et al: Deletions in the prion protein gene are not associated with CJD. Hum Mol Genet 2:541–544, 1993

Pan K-M, Baldwin M, Nguyen J, et al: Conversion of a-helices into b-sheets features in the formation of the scrapie prion proteins. Proc Natl Acad Sci U S A 90:10962–10966, 1993

Pattison IH, Millson GC: Experimental transmission of scrapie to goats and sheep by the oral route. J Comp Pathol 71:171–176, 1961

Petersen RB, Tabaton M, Berg L, et al: Analysis of the prion protein gene in thalamic dementia. Neurology 42:1859–1863, 1992

Poulter M, Baker HF, Frith CD, et al: Inherited prion disease with 144 base pair gene insertion, I: genealogical and molecular studies. Brain 115: 675–685, 1992

Prusiner SB: Novel proteinaceous infectious particles cause scrapie. Science 216:136–144, 1982

Prusiner SB, DeArmond SJ: Biology of disease: prions causing nervous system degeneration. Lab Invest 56:349–363, 1987

Prusiner SB, McKinley MP, Bowman KA, et al: Scrapie prions aggregate to form amyloid-like birefringent rods. Cell 35:349–358, 1983

Prusiner SB, Groth DF, Bolton DC, et al: Purification and structural studies of a major scrapie prion protein. Cell 38:127–134, 1984

Prusiner SB, Scott M, Foster D, et al: Transgenetic studies implicate interactions between homologous PrP isoforms in scrapie prion replication. Cell 63:673–686, 1990

Prusiner SB, Groth D, Serban A, et al: Ablation of the prion protein (PrP) gene in mice prevents scrapie and facilitates production of anti-PrP antibodies. Proc Natl Acad Sci U S A 90:10608–10612, 1993

Puckett C, Concannon P, Casey C, Hood L: Genomic structure of the human prion protein gene. Am J Hum Genet 49:320–329, 1991

Ridley RM, Baker HF: Occupational risk of Creutzfeldt-Jakob disease. Lancet 341:641–642, 1993

Ripoll L, Laplanche J-L, Salzmann M, et al: A new point mutation in the prion protein gene at codon 210 in Creutzfeldt-Jakob disease. Neurology 43:1934–1938, 1993

Roberts GW, Lofthouse R, Allsop D, et al: CNS amyloid proteins in neurodegenerative diseases. Neurology 38:1534–1540, 1988

Safar J, Roller PP, Gajdusek DC, Gibbs CJ Jr: Conformational transitions, dissociation, and unfolding of scrapie amyloid (prion) protein. J Biol Chem 268:20276–20284, 1993

Scott M, Foster D, Mirenda C, et al: Transgenic mice expressing hamster prion protein produce species-specific scrapie infectivity and amyloid plaques. Cell 59:847–857, 1989

Scott M, Groth D, Foster D, et al: Propagation of prions with artificial properties in transgenic mice expressing chimeric PrP genes. Cell 73:979–988, 1993

Seitelberger F: Spinocerebellar ataxia with dementia and plaque-like deposits (Sträussler's disease), in Handbook of Clinical Neurology, Vol 42. Edited by Vinken PJ, Bruyn GW. Amsterdam, North-Holland, 1981, pp 182–183

Serban D, Taraboulos A, DeArmond SJ, Prusiner SB: Rapid detection of Creutzfeldt-Jakob disease and scrapie prion proteins. Neurology 40:110–117, 1990

Shyng S-L, Heuser JE, Harris DA: A glycolipid-anchored prion protein is endocytosed via clathrin-coated pits. J Cell Biol 125:1239–1250, 1994

Snow AD, Kisilevsky R, Willmer J, et al: Sulfated glycosaminoglycans in amyloid plaques of prion diseases. Acta Neuropathol (Berl) 77:337–342, 1989

Sparkes RS, Simon M, Cohn VH, et al: Assignment of the human and mouse prion protein genes to homologous chromosomes. Proc Natl Acad Sci U S A 83:7358–7362, 1986

Stahl N, Baldwin MA, Hecker R, et al: Glycosylinositol phospholipid anchors of the scrapie and cellular prion proteins contain sialic acid. Biochemistry 31:5043–5053, 1992

Stahl N, Baldwin MA, Teplow DB, et al: Structural analysis of the scrapie prion protein using mass spectrometry and amino acid sequencing. Biochemistry 32:1991–2002, 1993

Taraboulos A, Jendroska K, Serban D, et al: Regional mapping of prion proteins in brains. Proc Natl Acad Sci U S A 89:7620–7624, 1992

Tateishi J, Brown P, Kitamoto T, et al: First experimental transmission of fatal familial insomnia. Nature 376:434–435, 1995

Telling GC, Scott M, Hsiao KK, et al: Transmission of Creutzfeldt-Jakob disease from humans to transgenic mice expressing chimeric human-mouse prion protein. Proc Natl Acad Sci U S A 91:9936–9940, 1994

Vnencak-Jones CL, Phillips JA: Identification of heterogeneous PrP gene deletions in controls by detection of allele-specific heteroduplexes (DASH). Am J Hum Genet 50:871–872, 1992

Westaway D, Goodman PA, Mirenda CA, et al: Distinct prion proteins in short and long scrapie incubation period mice. Cell 51:651–662, 1987

Westaway D, DeArmond SJ, Cayetano-Canlas J, et al: Degeneration of skeletal muscle, peripheral nerves, and the central nervous system in transgenic mice overexpressing wild-type prion proteins. Cell 76:117–129, 1994

Wilesmith JW: Epidemiology of bovine spongiform encephalopathy and related diseases. Arch Virol 7(suppl):S245–S254, 1993

Will RG, Ironside JW, Zeidler M, et al: A new variant of Creutzfeldt-Jakob disease in the UK [see comments]. Lancet 347:921–925, 1996

Ying Y-S, Anderson RGW, Rothberg KG: Each caveola contains multiple glycosyl-phosphatidylinositol-anchored membrane proteins. Cold Spring Harb Symp Quant Biol 57:593–604, 1992

6

Studies of Aβ Amyloidogenesis in Model Systems of Alzheimer's Disease

Gopal Thinakaran, Ph.D., Lee J. Martin, Ph.D., David R. Borchelt, Ph.D., Samuel E. Gandy, M.D., Ph.D., Sangram S. Sisodia, Ph.D., and Donald L. Price, M.D.

Introduction

Alzheimer's disease (AD), characterized by amyloid deposits and evidence of dysfunction/death of specific populations of nerve cells,

The authors thank Drs. Bruce T. Lamb, John D. Gearhart, Lary C. Walker, Linda C. Cork, Mary Lou Voytko, Molly V. Wagster, Edward H. Koo, Karen K. Hsiao, Jocelyn Bachevalier, and Mortimer Mishkin for helpful discussions of some of our work cited in this review.

These investigations are supported by grants from the U.S. Public Health Service (NIH AG 05146, NS 20471, AG 10491, NS 07179) as well as the Adler Foundation, the Alzheimer's Association, the American Health Assistance Foundation, is the most common cause of dementia in the elderly (Evans et al. 1989; Khachaturian 1985; McKhann et al. 1984). The clinical phenotype reflects the distribution and nature of pathological processes that involve specific regions of the brain. Affected nerve cells exhibit cytoskeletal abnormalities, and deposits of the β-amyloid protein (Aβ) occur in neocortex and hippocampus. To clarify the roles of etiological factors and pathogenetic mechanisms of AD, investigators have turned to the development of model systems. This review focuses on studies of Aβ amyloidogenesis and on the current status of work on animal models that recapitulate certain features of the pathology of AD, particularly amyloidogenesis.

A major histopathological hallmark of AD is the presence of amyloid deposits in the brain; the principal component of amyloid is Aβ, a 39–43 amino acid peptide derived from amyloid precursor proteins (APP). In cultured cells, APP mature through the constitutive secretory pathway, and some cell surface–bound APP are cleaved within the Aβ domain, an event that precludes Aβ amyloidogenesis. Additional pathways of APP processing include an endosomal–lysosomal pathway that generates a complex set of APP-related membrane-bound fragments, some of which contain the entire Aβ sequence, and a pathway that generates Aβ peptides. Molecular genetic investigations have identified a variety of mutations in the APP gene that segregate with early-onset familial AD (FAD). Several of these mutations appear to influence APP processing and result in the production of higher levels or longer Aβ-related peptides that are inherently more fibrillogenic. Although a variety of lines of evidence implicates APP/Aβ in AD, the mechanism or mechanisms by which Aβ influences the biology and vulnerability of neural cells is not fully clear.

Investigations of animal models have focused on aged nonhuman

and the Metropolitan Life Foundation. Drs. Price, Martin, and Borchelt are the recipients of a Leadership and Excellence in Alzheimer's Disease (LEAD) award (NIH AG 07914). Dr. Price is the recipient of a Javits Neuroscience Investigator Award (NIH NS 10580). Dr. Sisodia is the recipient of a Zenith Award from the Alzheimer's Association.

primates and APP transgenic mice. Aged nonhuman primates develop memory deficits and brain abnormalities, including amyloid deposits, senile plaques, and neurites, often occurring in proximity to Aβ deposits. Transgenic strategies (i.e., conventional cDNA and yeast artificial chromosome–embryonic stem [YAC–ES] cell methods) have been used to create mice that express the human APP gene with and without AD-linked APP mutations. One line of mice that exhibits amyloid deposits in the brain has been developed.

APP and Aβ

The brains of subjects with AD show deposits of extracellular Aβ, a 39–43 amino acid peptide comprised of 11–15 amino acids of the transmembrane domain and 28 amino acids of the extracellular domain of larger APP (Glenner and Wong 1984; Kang et al. 1987; Kitaguchi et al. 1988; Ponte et al. 1988; Tanzi et al. 1988). The APP gene, encompassing ~400 kilobases of DNA (Lamb et al. 1993), gives rise to alternatively spliced APP mRNA that encode Aβ-containing proteins of 695, 714, 751, and 770 amino acids (Kang et al. 1987; Kitaguchi et al. 1988; Ponte et al. 1988; Tanzi et al. 1988). Maturing through the constitutive secretory pathway, APP are modified by the addition of both *N*- and *O*-linked carbohydrates, phosphate, and sulfate moieties (Hung and Selkoe 1994; Oltersdorf et al. 1989; Weidemann et al. 1989). Varying levels of newly synthesized APP molecules appear at the cell surface (Haass et al. 1992a; Sisodia 1992; Weidemann et al. 1989); some of these molecules are cleaved endoproteolytically by APP α-secretase within the Aβ sequence (Anderson et al. 1991; Esch et al. 1990; Sisodia et al. 1990; Wang et al. 1991) to release the ectodomain of APP, including residues 1–16 of Aβ, into the medium. APP cleavage within the Aβ domain precludes the formation of Aβ. The presence of secreted APP isoforms that contain Aβ epitopes in cerebrospinal fluid suggests that similar processing events occur in vivo (Palmert et al. 1989a,b, 1990; Weidemann et al. 1989).

A fraction of cell-surface APP is also internalized and degraded via endosomal-lysosomal pathways (Cole et al. 1989; Golde et al. 1992; Haass et al. 1992a), resulting in the production of fragments that contain the entire Aβ region and APP carboxyl-terminus (C-terminus) (Golde et al. 1992; Haass et al. 1992a). However, several lines of evidence now suggest that the lysosomal degradation of APP is unlikely to contribute to the production of Aβ (Busciglio et al. 1993; Haass et al. 1992b, 1993). Studies (Citron et al. 1992; Haass et al. 1992b, 1993; Shoji et al. 1992) suggest that the re-internalization of APP from the cell surface may favor the generation of Aβ, and investigations demonstrating that Aβ can be generated from surface-labeled APP support this model (Koo and Squazzo 1994). Aβ peptides (Aβ1–40 and Aβ1–42 [43]) and truncated forms of Aβ are secreted constitutively by primary and tissue culture cells (Busciglio et al. 1993; Haass et al. 1992b; Scheuner et al. 1996; Seubert et al. 1992; Shoji et al. 1992) and are present in cerebrospinal fluid and plasma (Scheuner et al. 1996; Seubert et al. 1993; Shoji et al. 1992). Immunocytochemical and biochemical studies of the cortices of individuals with AD performed with antibodies uniquely specific for Aβ1–40 or Aβ1–42 revealed that Aβ deposition most likely begins with Aβ1–42(43) and not with Aβ1–40 (Gravina et al. 1995; Iwatsubo et al. 1994; Lemere et al. 1996).

Autosomal dominant linkage to missense mutations of APP has been demonstrated in a relatively small subset of patients with early-onset FAD (Goate et al. 1991; Mullan et al. 1992). In ~19 early-onset pedigrees, missense mutations generated amino acid substitutions at residue 717 (of APP-770) within the transmembrane domain of APP (Chartier-Harlin et al. 1991; Goate et al. 1991; Naruse et al. 1991). In one family with a mutation at codon 692 of APP resulting in a Gly-Ala substitution, biopsies from affected individuals disclosed diffuse deposits of Aβ, congophilic angiopathy, and scattered senile plaques but no neurofibrillary tangles (Hendricks et al. 1992). Finally, in two large, related families from Sweden (Mullan et al. 1992), a double mutation at codons 670 and 671 resulting in the substitution of Lys-Met to Asn-Leu was linked to early-onset AD.

Amyloidogenesis

Cellular transfection approaches have provided considerable insight regarding the mechanisms whereby mutations in APP affect the processing of APP and contribute to Aβ amyloidogenesis. Tissue culture cells expressing APP harboring the Swedish substitutions secrete higher levels of Aβ-containing peptides as compared to cells expressing wild-type constructs (Cai et al. 1993; Citron et al. 1992). Furthermore, because cells that express APP harboring the Swedish mutation secrete higher levels of Aβ, the level of secreted Aβ1–42 peptides increases accordingly (Suzuki et al. 1994). Additional studies of cells that express APP harboring the Ala-Gly substitution at amino acid 692 (Hendricks et al. 1992) reveal that α-secretase processing of this mutant polypeptide is inefficient and that secreted Aβ species exhibit considerable microheterogeneity, including the appearance of more hydrophobic species (Haass et al. 1994). Cells that express APP harboring 717 substitutions do not appear to secrete higher levels of Aβ but, rather, secrete a higher fraction of longer Aβ peptides (i.e., extending to Aβ residue 42) relative to cells that express wild-type APP (Suzuki et al. 1994).

The finding that APP-harboring FAD-linked mutations are processed to generate higher levels of longer Aβ peptides is of considerable interest, because physicochemical studies have indicated that amyloid formation is a nucleation-dependent phenomenon and that the C-terminus may be a critical determinant of the rate of amyloid formation (Jarrett and Lansbury 1993; Jarrett et al. 1993). These studies argue that Aβ1–42 and/or Aβ1–43, rather than Aβ1–40, may be the pathogenic proteins in AD. It is possible that the formation of Aβ1–40 can be seeded by trace amounts of Aβ1–42 fibrils (Jarrett and Lansbury 1993; Jarrett et al. 1993). In any event, the observation that APP mutations in early-onset FAD invariably flank the Aβ sequence suggests that altered processing of APP is central to the formation of amyloid in these individuals. The amino acid sequence of Aβ confers on it the possibility of spontaneous assembly into one of several biophysical forms (i.e., soluble, aggregated, fibrillar, and/or β-pleated Aβ conformations)

(Kirschner et al. 1987). Despite the obvious complexity of these alternative Aβ structures, high-resolution elucidation of various Aβ physical forms is lacking. One major contributor to the biophysical state of Aβ is peptide length, with Aβ1–42 exhibiting substantially more rapid and complete aggregation than Aβ1–40 (Burdick et al. 1992). In addition, Aβ1–42 fibrils can apparently act as nuclei, recruiting or seeding both Aβ1–40 and Aβ1–42 into a structured assembly (Jarrett et al. 1993). These phenomena appear to play a crucial role in AD because the longer Aβ1–42 is deposited preferentially early in the course of the disease (Iwatsubo et al. 1994). Moreover, in the cortices of individuals with Down's syndrome, Aβ deposition begins with Aβ 1–42 (43) and not Aβ 1–40 (Lemere et al. 1996).

The biophysical state of Aβ has been implicated as an explanation for the wide variability observed in its activity as a neurotoxin for cells in culture. Indeed, the aggregation state of Aβ has been reported by several independent groups to be a crucial factor in Aβ neurotoxic activity in cell culture (Busciglio et al. 1995; Pike et al. 1993; Simmons et al. 1994), and this neurotoxic activity can be mimicked by other aggregated or fibrillar amyloidogenic proteins that have primary sequences unrelated to Aβ (May et al. 1993). To date, the relevance of in vitro models of amyloid neurotoxicity, including Aβ amyloid, remains unclear for human AD. Efforts to extend this line of investigation to rodent and primate brains in vivo have met with highly inconsistent results (Price et al. 1992). Given the large number of substances associated with brain amyloid plaques in addition to Aβ (e.g., clusterin/apoβ [McGeer et al. 1992], heparan sulfate proteoglycans [Snow et al. 1988], and complement [Rogers et al. 1988]), it is entirely possible that more relevant mediators of important amyloid plaque bioactivity may be attributable to minor plaque component(s) and/or the brain's local responses to amyloid plaques (i.e., chronic active inflammation).

Presenilins and AD

Recently, mutations have been identified in two genes that cosegregate with affected members of FAD pedigrees: the presenilin-1

(PS-1) gene on chromosome 14 (Sherrington et al. 1995; St George-Hyslop et al. 1992) and the presenilin-2 (PS-2) gene on chromosome 1 (Levy-Lahad et al. 1995a,b; Rogaev et al. 1995). Although mutations in APP cosegregate with ~19 pedigrees with FAD, mutations in PS-1 are causative in nearly 50% of pedigrees with early onset-FAD (Schellenberg 1995). Approximately 35 missense mutations (Haass 1996; Van Broeckhoven 1995) and a point mutation upstream of a splice acceptor site that results in an in-frame deletion of exon 9 (PS-1–E9) (Perez-Tur et al. 1995) have been identified in the PS-1 gene in families with early-onset FAD. In addition, two missense mutations in the PS-2 gene have been identified in pedigrees with FAD of variable onset (Levy-Lahad et al. 1995b; Rogaev et al. 1995). Neither the normal functions of presenilin (PS) nor the mechanism or mechanisms by which FAD-linked mutations cause AD have been defined. The absence of nonsense or frameshift mutations that lead to truncated PS-1 and PS-2 supports the notion that AD is caused not by a loss but, rather, by the gain of deleterious function of mutant polypeptides.

PS-1 and PS-2 share extensive amino acid sequence identity and are predicted to contain seven (Sherrington et al. 1995) to nine (Slunt et al. 1995) transmembrane domains; the vast majority of mutations occur within, or immediately adjacent to, potential transmembrane helices. PS-1 is normally subject to endoproteolytic processing in vivo. The principal PS-1–related species that accumulate in brain and peripheral tissue and in cultured mammalian cells are amino-terminal (N-terminal) ~27 to 28 kD and C-terminal ~16 to 17 kD polypeptides (Thinakaran et al. 1996). In transgenic mice, PS-1 derivatives accumulate to saturable levels and to ~1:1 stoichiometry independent of the steady-state levels of transgene-derived human PS-1 mRNA (Thinakaran et al. 1996). Epitope mapping studies reveal that endoproteolytic cleavage likely occurs between PS-1 amino acids 260–320, a subdomain in which ~58% of FAD-linked missense mutations occur. This region also includes sequences known to be deleted in a PS-1 variant that lacks amino acids 290–319 (PS-1ΔE9) (Perez-Tur et al. 1995). Notably, PS-1ΔE9 is not subject to endoproteolytic cleavage in transfected mammalian cells and in lymphoblasts from an individual expressing this variant (Thinakaran et al. 1996). However, several missense mutations do not grossly affect the endoproteolytic processing of PS-1 (Borchelt et al. 1996).

The mechanism or mechanisms by which FAD-linked mutations in PS lead to AD is not fully understood. Lemere et al. (1996) have demonstrated massive Aβ42(43) deposits in the cerebral cortex and cerebellum of individuals with a PS-1–linked E280A mutation. Furthermore, sandwich ELISA assays revealed that conditioned medium from fibroblasts or plasma of affected members of pedigrees with PS-1/PS-2–linked mutations show a highly significant increase in the ratio of Aβ1–42(43)/Aβ1–40 relative to unaffected family members (Scheuner et al. 1996). These latter results are consistent with elevated ratios of Aβ1–42(43)/Aβ1–40 observed in the conditioned media of independent mouse neuroblastoma cell lines expressing FAD-linked A246E, M146L, or ΔE9 PS-1 variants relative to cells that express wild-type PS-1 (Borchelt et al. 1996). These findings strongly support the emerging view that PS-1 variants cause AD by increasing the extracellular concentration of Aβ1–42(43), the most amyloidogenic peptide species.

Animal Models of Amyloidogenesis

Aged Nonhuman Primates

Aged rhesus monkeys *(Macaca mulatta),* with a potential life span of more than 30 years (Tigges et al. 1988), have proved to be a useful model for investigations of age-associated Aβ amyloidogenesis. These animals show impaired performance on memory tasks (Bachevalier et al. 1991; Bartus et al. 1978, 1982; Presty et al. 1987; Rapp and Amaral 1989; Walker et al. 1988b) and exhibit some of the cellular and biochemical alterations that occur in the brains of aged humans and, to a greater extent, individuals with AD (Brizzee et al. 1980; Martin et al. 1991, 1994; Price and Sisodia 1994; Walker et al. 1988b; Wisniewski and Terry 1973a). Behavioral deficits that occur in aged nonhuman primates closely resemble those in aged humans (Bartus et al. 1978, 1979, 1980; Presty et al. 1987; Rapp and Amaral 1992; Walker et al. 1988b). The behavioral tasks were chosen on the basis of previous research showing that the successful performance of each task requires the integrity of relatively specific regions of brain (Bachevalier et al. 1991; Presty et al. 1987; Walker et al. 1988b). Cognitive and memory deficits in rhesus monkeys appear late in the second decade and become more evident in the mid-to-late twenties (Bachevalier et al. 1991; Walker et al. 1988b). Impairments in performance of certain spatial abilities occur in some animals in their late teens; however, in other test categories, behavior is not altered until the third decade of life. Visuospatial performance declines in some animals 16–19 years of age, whereas performance on a visual recognition memory task is altered only in a group of animals older than 25 years of age. Learning of object discriminations and simple motor skills is performed satisfactorily in all groups (Bachevalier et al. 1991). Monkeys that perform poorly on one task frequently are quite successful on another task. Variations in performance among aged animals and among tasks are similar to those observed in aged humans. The distributions and severities of lesions vary among different animals of the same age, and it is likely that performances on specific behavioral tasks are related, in some way yet to be determined, to patterns of these brain abnormalities in individual animals.

Aged monkeys provide an excellent model to examine alterations in the biology of APP that lead to Aβ amyloidogenesis. These animals develop senile plaques, comprised of neurites and deposits of Aβ, virtually identical to those that occur in aged humans and in individuals with AD (Abraham et al. 1989; Martin et al. 1991, 1994; Selkoe et al. 1987; Struble et al. 1985; Walker et al. 1987; Wisniewski and Terry 1973a,b). Early in the third decade of life, rhesus monkeys develop enlarged neurites (i.e., distal axons, nerve terminals, and dendrites) as well as preamyloid deposits in the parenchyma of cortex (Cork et al. 1990; Selkoe et al. 1987; Struble et al. 1982, 1985; Walker et al. 1988a; Wisniewski and Terry 1973b). These neurites are derived from cholinergic, monoaminergic, serotoninergic, GABAergic, and peptidergic populations of neurons (Kitt et al. 1984, 1985, 1989; Struble et al. 1984; Walker et al. 1985, 1987, 1988a), and, in individual plaques, neurites may be derived from more than one transmitter-specific system (Walker et al. 1988a). Neurites accumulate a variety of constituents, including membranous elements, mitochondria (some degenerating), lysosomes, APP, phosphorylated neurofilaments, acetylcholinesterase, transmitter markers, and synaptophysin (Martin et al. 1991, 1994). In individual plaques, APP- and synaptophysin-immunoreactive structures are often surrounded by a halo of distorted neuropil that, in adjacent sections, contains Aβ immunoreactivity. The presence of APP-like immunoreactivity in neuronal perikarya, axons, and some neurites within Aβ-containing plaques suggests that neurons can serve as one source for some of the Aβ deposited in the brains of these aged animals. Thus, parenchymal Aβ may, in part, be derived from APP in neurites, dendrites, and degenerating cell bodies. The proximity of Aβ to abnormal neuronal processes, reactive cells (including astrocytes and microglia), and elements suggests that several populations of cells, including neurons and nonneuronal cells, may participate in the formation of Aβ (Frackowiak et al. 1992; Martin et al. 1991; Masters et al. 1985a; Miyakawa et al. 1992; Wisniewski et al. 1992). As is the case in aged humans and in individuals with AD (Abraham et al. 1988), the serine protease inhibitor α_1-antichymotrypsin, derived, at least in part, from astrocytes (Koo et al. 1991), colocalizes with deposits of Aβ in the brains of aged rhesus monkeys (Abraham et al. 1989; Cork et al. 1990).

Transgenic Mice

Transgenic approaches can test directly whether the expression of exogenous wild-type or mutant APP or the expression of Aβ-containing fragments is involved in the pathogenesis of AD-type abnormalities (Price and Sisodia 1994; Sisodia and Price 1992). Over the past few years, several groups have attempted to produce mice with Aβ deposits using cDNA and YAC-based transgenic technologies. Some of these efforts are reviewed here.

LaFerla and colleagues (1995) generated a line of mice that carry a transgene encoding murine Aβ1–42 under the control of the 68-kD polypeptide neurofilament promoter (NF-L). Expression of the transgene was confirmed by Northern analysis and positive in situ hybridization in hippocampus and cerebral cortex. Neuropathological examination of these animals, which suffered seizures and died at higher rates than controls, showed extensive cell death, apoptosis, and intense gliosis in cerebral cortex and hippocampus. No senile plaques were identified by silver staining, but apparent extracellular Aβ immunostaining was detected in the neuropil. The finding that several missense mutations in APP are genetically linked to pedigrees with early-onset AD has led investigators to assess the phenotype of transgenic mice that overexpress mutant APP. Hsaio and colleagues (1995) created transgenic FVB mice that express myc epitope-tagged human APP-695 (HuAPP-695myc) or HuAPP-695myc harboring the APP-717 mutation placed under the transcriptional control of the hamster prion gene promoter. No developmental or pathological abnormalities were evident in wild-type animals despite abundant HuAPP-695myc expression in all neurons of the central nervous system; the level of total APP was elevated ~2.5-fold in wild-type lines. These animals developed behavioral disorders, including inactivity, agitation, neophobia, and seizures. Glucose utilization was diminished in cortical limbic areas, and animals died prematurely. The age at onset of illness decreased with increasing levels of brain APP. No extracellular amyloid has been detected, but there was significant gliosis. Because a similar neurological disorder develops naturally in older nontransgenic FVB mice, it has been argued that this disease may be an age- and strain-related dysfunction of the central nervous system exacerbated by the presence of the transgene. Mice that express mutant APP at levels similar to or slightly higher than wild-type expressors show markedly reduced life spans.

Transgenic mice that express high levels of human $717_{V \to F}$ mutant APP develop extracellular thioflavin S-positive Aβ deposits as well as neurites (Games et al. 1995). The construct used to generate these mice utilized the platelet-derived growth factor–β promoter driving a human APP minigene encoding the $APP_{717V \to F}$ mutation associated with FAD. The construct contained APP introns 6–8, allowing alternative splicing of exons 7 and 8. Southern blots disclosed ~40 copies of the transgene inserted at a single site and transmitted in a stable fashion. Levels of human APP mRNA and protein were significantly greater than endogenous APP transcript, and the three major splicing variants of APP were demonstrable. Significantly, levels of the transgene product were 10-fold higher than endogenous mouse APP. Moreover, a 4-kD $A\beta$-immunoreactive peptide was identified in the brains of these animals. By 8 months of age, $A\beta$ deposits were seen in the hippocampus, corpus callosum, and cerebral cortex; these deposits increased in number over time and ranged from diffuse irregular types to compacted plaques with cores. Amyloid deposits were stained by the thioflavin, Congo red, and Bielschowsky methods. Many plaques showed glial fibrillary acid protein–positive astrocytes as well as microglial cells. Although there were distorted neurites, often present in proximity to plaques, tau-positive neurites and neurofibrillary tangles were not present. To date, behavioral abnormalities have not been described, and no quantitative estimates of loss of neurons have been published. This work clearly shows that it is possible to create animals with some of the abnormalities that occur in human AD.

Finally, the overexpression of APP, as occurs in individuals with Down's syndrome, is thought to lead to the premature deposition of $A\beta$ in the brain (Cork et al. 1990; Giaccone et al. 1989; Glenner and Wong 1984; Masters et al. 1985a,b; Rumble et al. 1989). To mimic the trisomic APP dosage imbalance observed in individuals with Down's syndrome, a YAC containing ~650 kb of human genomic DNA, including the APP gene, was transfected into ES cells (Lamb et al. 1993). ES cells that contain stably integrated YAC DNA were microinjected into mouse blastocysts, and chimeric mice were generated. After breeding, it was established that human APP sequences were transmitted to the mouse germ line. Furthermore, human APP mRNA is actively transcribed in mouse tissue, and the splicing pattern of human APP transcripts in transgenic mouse tissue mirrored the endogenous pattern of alternatively spliced mRNA. Using antibodies specific for human APP, Western blot analysis of transgenic mouse brain extracts revealed that human APP contributed ~40% of total APP levels. No AD-type pathology was demonstrable in animals as old as two years (C. A. Kitt, B. T.

Lamb, D. L. Price, and J. D. Gearhart, unpublished observations, 1993). Ongoing additional breeding approaches are intended to increase human APP gene copy number and, hence, APP levels. The YAC-ES strategy is now being used to introduce modified human APP YAC that encode FAD mutations into the mouse germ line and to determine whether the presence of these mutations predisposes to Aβ deposition and, possibly, other brain abnormalities that occur in individuals with AD.

Over the next several years, it is virtually certain that additional lines of transgenic mice with APP mutations will be produced. Moreover, it will be interesting to analyze transgenic mice that overexpress apolipoprotein E4 (on an apolipoprotein E null background). Finally, it will be important to generate transgenic mice that express FAD-linked PS-1 or PS-2 variants recapitulating the clinical and pathological phenotypes of AD.

Conclusions

Over the past several years, significant progress has been made in understanding critical features of AD. This review focuses on APP, Aβ, and amyloidogenesis, as well as recent studies in animal models. Aβ is an ~4-kD peptide derived from APP, Aβ-containing type-I integral membrane glycoproteins of between 695 and 770 amino acids. The conservation of APP between species, the abundance of APP in the brain, the localization of APP in neurons (dendritic cell bodies and axons), and evidence that changes in APP biology (as occurs in AD) influence brain function have been interpreted to indicate that APP plays important roles in the biology of neural cells, but the functions of APP in the nervous system are not yet well defined. Mechanisms involved in the production of Aβ are not fully identified. It now appears that Aβ1–42(43) is the predominant Aβ species in amyloid deposits. Significantly, Aβ1–42(43) nucleates rapidly into amyloid fibrils and may serve as a seed for the aggregation and subsequent deposition of Aβ. Support for the idea that Aβ1–42(43) is critical for amyloid formation emerged recently from studies in which end-specific antibodies (i.e., reagents that recognize Aβ1–40 or Aβ1–42 uniquely) were utilized in immunocytochemical studies of the brains of individuals with AD. These studies demonstrated convincingly that the bulk of senile plaques consist of Aβ1–42.

Review of investigations in aged nonhuman primates and APP transgenic mice demonstrates the potential usefulness of animal models. At present, the nonhuman primate is very useful for examining selected brain abnormalities, including amyloid deposits, virtually identical to those occurring in individuals with AD. Transgenic strategies have begun to show great promise. The availability of transgenic mice with deposits of Aβ will allow strategies proven useful to examine the mechanisms of Aβ amyloidogenesis. These models can serve to examine therapeutic approaches that eventually may be useful for studying age-related behavioral deficits and to prevent amyloid deposits and other brain abnormalities that occur in humans with AD.

References

Abraham CR, Selkoe DJ, Potter H: Immunocytochemical identification of the serine protease inhibitor α_1-antichymotrypsin, in the brain amyloid deposits of Alzheimer's disease. Cell 52:487–501, 1988

Abraham CR, Selkoe DJ, Potter H, et al: α_1-antichymotrypsin is present together with the β-protein in monkey brain amyloid deposits. Neuroscience 32:715–720, 1989

Anderson JP, Esch FS, Keim PS, et al: Exact cleavage site of Alzheimer amyloid precursor in neuronal PC-12 cells. Neurosci Lett 128:126–128, 1991

Bachevalier J, Landis LS, Walker LC, et al: Aged monkeys exhibit behavioral deficits indicative of widespread cerebral dysfunction. Neurobiol Aging 12:99–111, 1991

Bartus RT, Fleming D, Johnson HR: Aging in the rhesus monkey: debilitating effects on short-term memory. J Gerontol 33:858–871, 1978

Bartus RT, Dean RL III, Fleming DL: Aging in the rhesus monkey: effects on visual discrimination learning and reversal learning. J Gerontol 34: 209–219, 1979

Bartus RT, Dean RL, Beer B: Memory deficits in aged Cebus monkeys and facilitation with central cholinomimetics. Neurobiol Aging 1:145–152, 1980

Bartus RT, Dean RL III, Beer B, Lippa AS: The cholinergic hypothesis of geriatric memory dysfunction. Science 217:408–417, 1982

Borchelt DR, Thinakaran G, Eckman CB, et al: Familial Alzheimer's disease-linked presenilin 1 variants elevate Aβ1–42/1–40 ratio in vitro and in vivo. Neuron 17:1005–1013, 1996

Brizzee KR, Ordy JM, Bartus RT: Localization of cellular changes within multimodal sensory regions in aged monkey brain: possible implications for age-related cognitive loss. Neurobiol Aging 1:45–52, 1980

Burdick D, Soreghan B, Kwon M, et al: Assembly and aggregation properties of synthetic Alzheimer's A4/β amyloid peptide analogs. J Biol Chem 267:546–554, 1992

Busciglio J, Gabuzda DH, Matsudaira P, Yankner BA: Generation of β-amyloid in the secretory pathway in neuronal and nonneuronal cells. Proc Natl Acad Sci U S A 90:2092–2096, 1993

Busciglio J, Lorenzo A, Yeh J, Yankner BA: β-amyloid fibrils induce tau phosphorylation and loss of microtubule binding. Neuron 14:879–888, 1995

Cai XD, Golde TE, Younkin SG: Release of excess amyloid β protein from a mutant amyloid β protein precursor. Science 259:514–516, 1993

Chartier-Harlin M-C, Crawford F, Houlden H, et al: Early-onset Alzheimer's disease caused by mutations at codon 717 of the β-amyloid precursor protein gene. Nature 353:844–846, 1991

Citron M, Oltersdorf T, Haass C, et al: Mutation of the β-amyloid precursor protein in familial Alzheimer's disease increases β-protein production. Nature 360:672–674, 1992

Cole GM, Huynh TV, Saitoh T: Evidence for lysosomal processing of amyloid β-protein precursor in cultured cells. Neurochem Res 14:933–939, 1989

Cork LC, Masters C, Beyreuther K, Price DL: Development of senile plaques. Relationships of neuronal abnormalities and amyloid deposits. Am J Pathol 137:1383–1392, 1990

Esch FS, Keim PS, Beattie EC, et al: Cleavage of amyloid β peptide during constitutive processing of its precursor. Science 248:1122–1124, 1990

Evans DA, Funkenstein HH, Albert MS, et al: Prevalence of Alzheimer's disease in a community population of older persons higher than previously reported. JAMA 262:2551–2556, 1989

Frackowiak J, Wisniewski HM, Wegiel J, et al: Ultrastructure of the microglia that phagocytose amyloid and the microglia that produce β-amyloid fibrils. Acta Neuropathol 84:225–233, 1992

Games D, Adams D, Alessandrini R, et al: Alzheimer-type neuropathology in transgenic mice overexpressing V717F β-amyloid precursor protein. Nature 373:523–527, 1995

Giaccone G, Tagliavini F, Linoli G, et al: Down patients: extracellular preamyloid deposits precede neuritic degeneration and senile plaques. Neurosci Lett 97:232–238, 1989

Glenner GG, Wong CW: Alzheimer's disease: initial report of the purification and characterization of a novel cerebrovascular amyloid protein. Biochem Biophys Res Commun 120:885–890, 1984

Goate A, Chartier-Harlin M-C, Mullan M, et al: Segregation of a missense mutation in the amyloid precursor protein gene with familial Alzheimer's disease. Nature 349:704–706, 1991

Golde TE, Estus S, Younkin LH, et al: Processing of the amyloid protein precursor to potentially amyloidogenic derivatives. Science 255:728–730, 1992

Gravina SA, Ho L, Eckman CB, et al: Amyloid β protein (Aβ) in Alzheimer's disease brain. J Biol Chem 270:7013–7016, 1995

Haass C: Presenile because of presenilin: the presenilin genes and early onset Alzheimer's disease. Curr Opin Neurol 9:254–259, 1996

Haass C, Koo EH, Mellon A, et al: Targeting of cell-surface β-amyloid precursor protein to lysosomes: alternative processing into amyloid-bearing fragments. Nature 357:500–503, 1992a

Haass C, Schlossmacher MG, Hung AY, et al: Amyloid β-peptide is produced by cultured cells during normal metabolism. Nature 359:322–325, 1992b

Haass C, Hung AY, Schlossmacher MG, et al: β-amyloid peptide and a 3-kDa fragment are derived by distinct cellular mechanisms. J Biol Chem 268:3021–3024, 1993

Haass C, Hung AY, Selkoe DJ, Teplow DB: Mutations associated with a locus for familial Alzheimer's disease result in alternative processing of amyloid β-protein precursor. J Biol Chem 269:17741–17748, 1994

Hendricks L, van Duijn CM, Cras P, et al: Presenile dementia and cerebral haemorrhage linked to a mutation at codon 692 of the β-amyloid precursor protein gene. Nat Genet 1:218–221, 1992

Hsiao KK, Borchelt DR, Olson K, et al: Age-related CNS disorder and early death in transgenic FVB/N mice overexpressing Alzheimer amyloid precursor proteins. Neuron 15:1203–1218, 1995

Hung AY, Selkoe DJ: Selective ectodomain phosphorylation and regulated cleavage of β-amyloid precursor protein. EMBO J 13:534–542, 1994

Iwatsubo T, Odaka A, Suzuki N, et al: Visualization of Aβ42(43)-positive and Aβ40-positive senile plaques with end-specific Aβ-monoclonal antibodies: evidence that an initially deposited Aβ species is Aβ1–42(43). Neuron 13:45–53, 1994

Jarrett JT, Lansbury PT Jr: Seeding "one-dimensional crystallization" of amyloid: a pathogenic mechanism in Alzheimer's disease and scrapie? Cell 73:1055–1058, 1993

Jarrett JT, Berger EP, Lansbury PT Jr: The carboxyl terminus of the β amyloid protein is critical for the seeding of amyloid formation: implications for the pathogenesis of Alzheimer's disease. Biochemistry 32:4693–4697, 1993

Kang J, Lemaire H-G, Unterbeck A, et al: The precursor of Alzheimer's disease amyloid A4 protein resembles a cell-surface receptor. Nature 325:733–736, 1987

Khachaturian Z: Diagnosis of Alzheimer's disease. Arch Neurol 42:1097–1105, 1985

Kirschner DA, Inouye H, Duffy LK, et al: Synthetic peptide homologous to β protein from Alzheimer disease forms amyloid-like fibrils *in vitro*. Proc Natl Acad Sci U S A 84:6953–6957, 1987

Kitaguchi N, Takahashi Y, Tokushima Y, et al: Novel precursor of Alzheimer's disease amyloid protein shows protease inhibitory activity. Nature 331:530–532, 1988

Kitt CA, Price DL, Struble RG, et al: Evidence for cholinergic neurites in senile plaques. Science 226:1443–1445, 1984

Kitt CA, Struble RG, Cork LC, et al: Catecholaminergic neurites in senile plaques in prefrontal cortex of aged nonhuman primates. Neuroscience 16:691–699, 1985

Kitt CA, Walker LC, Molliver ME, Price DL: Serotoninergic neurites in senile plaques in cingulate cortex of aged nonhuman primate. Synapse 3:12–18, 1989

Koo EH, Squazzo SL: Evidence that production and release of amyloid β-protein involves the endocytic pathway. J Biol Chem 269:17386–17389, 1994

Koo EH, Abraham CR, Potter H, et al: Developmental expression of

α_1-antichymotrypsin in brain may be related to astrogliosis. Neurobiol Aging 12:495–501, 1991

LaFerla FM, Tinkle BT, Bieberich CJ, et al: The Alzheimer's Aβ peptide induces neurodegeneration and apoptotic cell death in transgenic mice. Nat Genet 9:21–30, 1995

Lamb BT, Sisodia SS, Lawler AM, et al: Introduction and expression of the 400 kilobase *precursor amyloid protein* gene in transgenic mice. Nat Genet 5:22–30, 1993

Lemere CA, Blusztajn JK, Yamaguchi H, et al: Sequence of deposition of heterogeneous amyloid β-peptides and APO E in Down syndrome: implications for initial events in amyloid plaque formation. Neurobiology of Disease 3:16–32, 1996

Levy-Lahad E, Wasco W, Poorkaj P, et al: Candidate gene for the chromosome 1 familial Alzheimer's disease locus. Science 269:973–977, 1995a

Levy-Lahad E, Wijsman EM, Nemens E, et al: A familial Alzheimer's disease locus on chromosome 1. Science 269:970–973, 1995b

Martin LJ, Sisodia SS, Koo EH, et al: Amyloid precursor protein in aged nonhuman primates. Proc Natl Acad Sci U S A 88:1461–1465, 1991

Martin LJ, Pardo CA, Cork LC, Price DL: Synaptic pathology and glial responses to neuronal injury precede the formation of senile plaques and amyloid deposits in the aging cerebral cortex. Am J Pathol 145: 1358–1381, 1994

Masters CL, Multhaup G, Simms G, et al: Neuronal origin of a cerebral amyloid: neurofibrillary tangles of Alzheimer's disease contain the same protein as the amyloid of plaque cores and blood vessels. EMBO J 4:2757–2763, 1985a

Masters CL, Simms G, Weinman NA, et al: Amyloid plaque core protein in Alzheimer disease and Down syndrome. Proc Natl Acad Sci U S A 82:4245–4249, 1985b

May PC, Boggs LN, Fuson KS: Neurotoxicity of human amylin in rat primary hippocampal cultures: similarity to Alzheimer's disease amyloid-beta neurotoxicity. J Neurochem 61:2330–2333, 1993

McGeer PL, Kawamata T, Walker DG: Distribution of clusterin in Alzheimer brain tissue. Brain Res 579:337–341, 1992

McKhann G, Drachman D, Folstein M, et al: Clinical diagnosis of Alzheimer's disease: report of the NINCDS-ADRDA Work Group under the auspices of the Department of Health and Human Services Task Force on Alzheimer's Disease. Neurology 34:939–944, 1984

Miyakawa T, Katsuragi S, Yamashita K, Ohuchi K: Morphological study of amyloid fibrils and preamyloid deposits in the brain with Alzheimer's disease. Acta Neuropathol 83:340–346, 1992

Mullan M, Crawford F, Axelman K, et al: A pathogenic mutation for probable Alzheimer's disease in the APP gene at the N-terminus of β-amyloid. Nat Genet 1:345–347, 1992

Naruse S, Igarashi S, Kobayashi H, et al: Mis-sense mutation Val→Ile in exon 17 of amyloid precursor protein gene in Japanese familial Alzheimer's disease. Lancet 337:978–979, 1991

Oltersdorf T, Fritz LC, Schenk DB, et al: The secreted form of the Alzheimer's amyloid precursor protein with the Kunitz domain is protease nexin-II. Nature 341:144–147, 1989

Palmert MR, Podlisny MB, Witker DS, et al: The β-amyloid protein precursor of Alzheimer disease has soluble derivatives found in human brain and cerebrospinal fluid. Proc Natl Acad Sci U S A 86:6338–6342, 1989a

Palmert MR, Siedlak SL, Podlisny MB, et al: Soluble derivatives of the β amyloid protein precursor of Alzheimer's disease are labeled by antisera to the β amyloid protein. Biochem Biophys Res Commun 165:182–188, 1989b

Palmert MR, Usiak M, Mayeux R, et al: Soluble derivatives of the β amyloid protein precursor in cerebrospinal fluid: alterations in normal aging and in Alzheimer's disease. Neurology 40:1028–1034, 1990

Perez-Tur J, Froelich S, Prihar G, et al: A mutation in Alzheimer's disease destroying a splice acceptor site in the presenilin-1 gene. Neuroreport 7:297–301, 1995

Pike CJ, Burdick D, Walencewicz AJ, et al: Neurodegeneration induced by β-amyloid peptides *in vitro*: the role of peptide assembly state. J Neurosci 13:1676–1687, 1993

Ponte P, Gonzalez-DeWhitt P, Schilling J, et al: A new A4 amyloid mRNA contains a domain homologous to serine proteinase inhibitors. Nature 331:525–532, 1988

Presty SK, Bachevalier J, Walker LC, et al: Age differences in recognition memory of the rhesus monkey (Macaca mulatta). Neurobiol Aging 8:435–440, 1987

Price DL, Sisodia SS: Cellular and molecular biology of Alzheimer's disease and animal models. Annu Rev Med 45:435–446, 1994

Price DL, Borchelt DR, Walker LC, Sisodia SS: Toxicity of synthetic Aβ peptides and modeling of Alzheimer's disease. Neurobiol Aging 13:623–625, 1992

Rapp PR, Amaral DG: Evidence for task-dependent memory dysfunction in the aged monkey. J Neurosci 9:3568–3576, 1989

Rapp PR, Amaral DG: Individual differences in the cognitive and neurobiological consequences of normal aging. Trends Neurosci 15:340–345, 1992

Rogaev EI, Sherrington R, Rogaeva EA, et al: Familial Alzheimer's disease in kindreds with missense mutations in a gene on chromosome 1 related to the Alzheimer's disease type 3 gene. Nature 376:775–778, 1995

Rogers J, Luber-Narod J, Styren SC, Civin WH: Expression of immune system-associated antigens by cells of the human central nervous system: relationship to the pathology of Alzheimer's disease. Neurobiol Aging 9:339–349, 1988

Rumble B, Retallack R, Hilbich C, et al: Amyloid A4 protein and its precursor in Down's syndrome and Alzheimer's disease. N Engl J Med 320:1446–1452, 1989

Schellenberg GD: Genetic dissection of Alzheimer's disease, a heterogeneous disorder. Proc Natl Acad Sci U S A 92:8552–8559, 1995

Scheuner D, Eckman C, Jensen M, et al: Secreted amyloid β-protein similar to that in the senile plaques of Alzheimer's disease is increased *in vivo* by the presenilin 1 and 2 and *APP* mutations linked to familial Alzheimer's disease. Nat Med 2:864–852, 1996

Selkoe DJ, Bell DS, Podlisny MB, et al: Conservation of brain amyloid proteins in aged mammals and humans with Alzheimer's disease. Science 235:873–877, 1987

Seubert P, Vigo-Pelfrey C, Esch F, et al: Isolation and quantification of soluble Alzheimer's β-peptide from biological fluids. Nature 359:325–327, 1992

Seubert P, Oltersdorf T, Lee MG, et al: Secretion of β-amyloid precursor protein cleaved at the amino terminus of the β-amyloid peptide. Nature 361:260–263, 1993

Sherrington R, Rogaev EI, Liang Y, et al: Cloning of a gene bearing missense mutations in early-onset familial Alzheimer's disease. Nature 375:754–760, 1995

Shoji M, Golde TE, Ghiso J, et al: Production of the Alzheimer amyloid β protein by normal proteolytic processing. Science 258:126–129, 1992

Simmons LK, May PC, Tomaselli KJ, et al: Secondary structure of amyloid beta peptide correlates with neurotoxic activity in vitro. Mol Pharmacol 45:373–379, 1994

Sisodia SS: β-amyloid precursor protein cleavage by a membrane-bound protease. Proc Natl Acad Sci U S A 89:6075–6079, 1992

Sisodia SS, Price DL: Amyloidogenesis in Alzheimer's disease: basic biology and animal models. Curr Opin Neurobiol 2:648–652, 1992

Sisodia SS, Koo EH, Beyreuther K, et al: Evidence that β-amyloid protein in Alzheimer's disease is not derived by normal processing. Science 248:492–495, 1990

Slunt HH, Thinakaran G, Lee MK, Sisodia SS: Nucleotide sequence of the chromosome 14-encoded *S182* cDNA and revised secondary structure prediction. Amyloid: International Journal of Experimental and Clinical Investigations 2:188–190, 1995

Snow AD, Mar H, Nochlin D, et al: The presence of heparan sulfate proteoglycans in the neuritic plaques and congophilic angiopathy in Alzheimer's disease. Am J Pathol 133:456–463, 1988

St George-Hyslop PH, Haines P, Rogaev E, et al: Genetic evidence for a novel familial Alzheimer's disease locus on chromosome 14. Nat Genet 2:330–334, 1992

Struble RG, Cork LC, Whitehouse PJ, Price DL: Cholinergic innervation in neuritic plaques. Science 216:413–415, 1982

Struble RG, Hedreen JC, Cork LC, Price DL: Acetylcholinesterase activity in senile plaques of aged macaques. Neurobiol Aging 5:191–198, 1984

Struble RG, Price DL Jr, Cork LC, Price DL: Senile plaques in cortex of aged normal monkeys. Brain Res 361:267–275, 1985

Suzuki N, Cheung TT, Cai XD, et al: An increased percentage of long amyloid β protein secreted by familial amyloid β protein precursor (βAPP_{717}) mutants. Science 264:1336–1340, 1994

Tanzi RE, McClatchey AI, Lampert ED, et al: Protease inhibitor domain encoded by an amyloid protein precursor mRNA associated with Alzheimer's disease. Nature 331:528–530, 1988

Thinakaran G, Borchelt DR, Lee MK, et al: Endoproteolysis of presenilin 1 and accumulation of processed derivatives *in vivo*. Neuron 17:181–190, 1996

Tigges J, Gordon TP, McClure HM, et al: Survival rate and life span of rhesus monkeys at the Yerkes Regional Primate Research Center. Am J Primatol 15:263–273, 1988

Van Broeckhoven C: Presenilins and Alzheimer disease. Nat Genet 11:230–232, 1995

Walker LC, Kitt CA, Struble RG, et al: Glutamic acid decarboxylase-like immunoreactive neurites in senile plaques. Neurosci Lett 59:165–169, 1985

Walker LC, Kitt CA, Schwam E, et al: Senile plaques in aged squirrel monkeys. Neurobiol Aging 8:291–296, 1987

Walker LC, Kitt CA, Cork LC, et al: Multiple transmitter systems contribute neurites to individual senile plaques. J Neuropathol Exp Neurol 47:138–144, 1988a

Walker LC, Kitt CA, Struble RG, et al: The neural basis of memory decline in aged monkeys. Neurobiol Aging 9:657–666, 1988b

Wang R, Meschia JF, Cotter RJ, Sisodia SS: Secretion of the β/A4 amyloid precursor protein: identification of a cleavage site in cultured mammalian cells. J Biol Chem 266:16960–16964, 1991

Weidemann A, König G, Bunke D, et al: Identification, biogenesis, and localization of precursors of Alzheimer's disease A4 amyloid protein. Cell 57:115–126, 1989

Wisniewski HM, Terry RD: Morphology of the aging brain, human and animal. Prog Brain Res 40:167–186, 1973a

Wisniewski HM, Terry RD: Reexamination of the pathogeneisis of the senile plaque. Prog Neuropathol 1–26, 1973b

Wisniewski HM, Wegiel J, Wang KC, Lach B: Ultrastructural studies of the cells forming amyloid in the cortical vessel wall in Alzheimer's disease. Acta Neuropathol 84:117–127, 1992

CHAPTER

Dementia Associated With Poststroke Major Depression

Robert G. Robinson, M.D., and
Sergio Paradiso, M.D.

For many years, cognitive deficits, including dementia, have been a well-recognized consequence of cerebrovascular disease. Vascular dementia is a disorder characterized by a global decline of cognitive function in the face of clear consciousness resulting from the effects of cerebrovascular disease. Although the types of cerebrovascular disease that lead to vascular dementia are varied and include multi-infarct disease, strategic single infarcts, hypoperfusion of water shed regions, small dissel disease, hemorrhagic lesions, or embolic infarcts, the cognitive dysfunction is believed to be closely related to the size and location of the cerebral lesion (Damasio et al. 1985; Román et al. 1993). In fact, approximately 15%–25% of dementias in the elderly are attributed to vascular disease (Herskovits and Figueroa 1988). The relationship between cognitive im-

This work was supported by the following MH grants: Research Scientist Award MH00163 and MH40355.

141

pairment and neuropathology in vascular dementia, however, is not straightforward. For example, patients with similar size and location of lesions may show different severities of cognitive impairment (Starkstein et al. 1988), and patients with subcortical lesions may show the same degree of cognitive impairment or aphasia as patients with cortical infarcts (Basso et al. 1985). One reason why there may be a large degree of variability in the kinds and locations of lesions that produce dementia in patients with brain injury is the influence of depression. Numerous studies have identified that depression is a frequent consequence of ischemic brain infarction (Astrom et al. 1993; Eastwood et al. 1989; Morris et al. 1990; Robinson et al. 1983), and several studies have identified greater cognitive impairment in depressed compared with nondepressed patients with brain injury (House et al. 1990; Robinson et al. 1986a).

This chapter reviews evidence from our studies and those of other investigators that cognitive impairment is associated with major depression following stroke and that cognitive impairment associated with depression can be distinguished from intellectual disturbances associated with brain infarction. The first issue to be discussed, however, is the nature of cognitive impairments associated with depression.

Dementia of Depression

Clinicians have recognized for more than 40 years that patients with a variety of functional (i.e., no known neuropathology) psychiatric disorders, particularly depression, may show cognitive impairments (Kiloh 1961). Madden et al. (1952) reported that disorientation, as well as defects in recent memory, retention, calculation, and judgment, may appear in patients with psychiatric disorders. The main clinical features of dementia of depression as identified by Wells (1979) are the abrupt onset of intellectual impairment and rapid deterioration. The term *pseudodementia* was first used by Wernicke to refer to chronic hysterical states mimicking mental weakness (Bulbena and Berrios 1986). Madden et al.

(1952) used the term to describe improved cognitive performance after treatment in patients with conditions such as presenile depression, psychosis, and disorders associated with cerebrovascular diseases. Kiloh (1961) emphasized the clinical features of malingering and hysteria and a course characterized by abrupt onset and response to antidepressants as typical of pseudodementia.

Caine (1981) suggested that the diagnosis of pseudodementia or dementia of depression be based on four criteria: 1) intellectual impairment with primary psychiatric disorders; 2) features of neuropsychological abnormality resembling neuropathologically induced intellectual deficit; 3) reversibility of intellectual disorder; and 4) no apparent neurological process. While these criteria exclude a primary neuropathological process from the causes of dementia of depression, there is growing evidence that major depression associated with a variety of neuropathological disorders might lead to cognitive impairment (Starkstein et al. 1989). Furthermore, a number of parallels have been drawn between dementia associated with depression and dementia associated with subcortical neuropathology. Albert et al. (1974) and McHugh and Folstein (1985) reported that a particular type of cognitive impairment was associated with neurological diseases involving primarily subcortical neuropathology. These studies identified the presence of symptoms such as forgetfulness, slowness of thought processes, apathy or depression, generalized decrease in ability to integrate information, and improvement with stimulation as characteristics of the subcortical dementia. These disorders, however, did not include the prominent symptoms of aphasia, alexia, agnosia, and amnesia seen in patients with cortical dementias, such as Alzheimer's disease (AD) and Creutzfeldt-Jakob disease. Although there is debate about the extent to which cortical and subcortical dementias may be distinguished from one another (Cummings et al. 1984), the concept of a subcortical dementia emphasizes that neuropathological conditions may be associated with a type of cognitive impairment that is phenomenologically distinct from AD. Furthermore, these subcortical dementias are characterized by many of the clinical features seen in patients with dementia of depression. The characteristic symptoms of dementia associated with depression include improvement with organization, repetition errors in learning, intact recognition memory, abrupt onset, preserved attention and concentration, and the greatest number of errors in effort-demanding cognitive tasks (Goodnick 1985; Roy-Byrne et al. 1986).

Frequency of Poststroke Depression

Although the frequency of depression following stroke has varied from study to study depending on the population examined, the mean frequency of major depression during the acute poststroke period across all studies has been about 20% (Astrom et al. 1993; Eastwood et al. 1989; Morris et al. 1990; Robinson et al. 1983). This has included patients in rehabilitation hospitals, acute stroke hospitals, community samples, and outpatient clinics. Depression, including both major and minor types, is probably the most frequent emotional disorder occurring in this population.

Major and Minor Poststroke Depression

To examine patients with different severities of depression, we have divided patients into those meeting DSM-III criteria (American Psychiatric Association 1980) for either major or dysthymic (minor) depression. Under the American Psychiatric Association DSM-IV classification (American Psychiatric Association 1994), patients who meet criteria for major depression are diagnosed as having "depression due to stroke, major depression like episode." This utilizes the standard diagnostic criteria for major depressive disorder but identifies the depression as being associated with a particular medical condition (i.e., stroke). Dysthymic disorder is a milder form of depression and is diagnosed only if the duration of depression is greater than 2 years (and depression is present most of the time). To differentiate our depressed poststroke patients from those with long-term depressive disorders, we have utilized the term *minor de-*

pression from Research Diagnostic Criteria. Thus, the depressive disorder is defined by the symptom criteria for dysthymic disorder but does not require that the disorder be present for 2 years.

This classification of depressed patients into major and minor depression has been partially validated by finding several clinically significant differences between these two types of depression. While major depression has consistently been associated with cortical (dorsal lateral frontal cortex) or subcortical (basal ganglia) lesions of the left hemisphere, we have not been able to find a statistically significant relationship between minor depression and lesion location (Starkstein et al. 1987). However, other authors have replicated our finding of a strong association between major depression and left anterior lesion location (Astrom et al. 1993; Herrmann et al. 1993). Another significant difference between major and minor poststroke depression was the longitudinal evolution of these disorders. Without treatment, major depression lasted a mean duration of 9 months, whereas minor depression was more persistent in 70% of our cases and lasted for more than 2 years (Robinson et al. 1987). A third significant difference between major and minor depression was that major but not minor depression was associated with nonsuppression on the dexamethasone suppression test (Lipsey et al. 1985). Finally, the difference between major and minor poststroke depression most relevant to this chapter was that major depression but not minor depression was associated with greater cognitive impairment than that in controls (Robinson et al. 1986b).

Cognitive Impairment Associated With Major Versus Minor Depression

We have recently examined cognitive impairment in a large group of patients ($N = 309$) whom we have examined following an acute stroke (Downhill and Robinson 1994). The mean age ($\pm$ SD) for the group was 58.9 $\pm$ 13.4 years. The patients were 56.2% male, 43.2% married, 66.0% black, and 74.0% Hollingshead Social Class

IV–V. The mean number of days between stroke and cognitive examination was 11.2 ± 3.9 days.

Based on symptoms elicited from the structured interview of the Present State Examination (Wing et al. 1974), patients were given a DSM-III diagnosis of major depression, minor depression, or no depression. Mean scores on the Mini-Mental State Examination (MMSE) for patients with major depression, minor depression, and no depression are shown in Figure 7–1. Patients with major depression had significantly lower (i.e., more impaired) MMSE scores than patients with minor depression ($P = .02$) or nondepressed patients ($P = .002$). Patients with minor depression were not significantly different in their MMSE scores than nondepressed

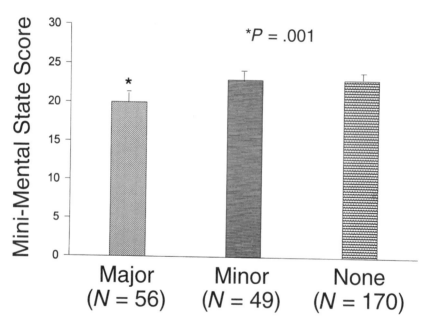

Figure 7–1. Mean Mini-Mental State Exam (MMSE) scores of patients hospitalized with acute stroke divided in groups based on the existence of DSM-III major depression, minor (dysthymic) depression, or no mood disorder. Patients with major depression had significantly lower (more impaired) scores than the other two groups. Bars indicate standard errors of the mean.

patients. Thus, cognitive impairment was associated with only one kind of depression, that is, major depression.

Patients were also divided into cognitively impaired and non–cognitively impaired groups based on their MMSE scores. Patients with MMSE scores ≥24 were considered not cognitively impaired, whereas those with MMSE scores <24 were cognitively impaired. In the nondepressed group, 73 of 170 patients (43%) were cognitively impaired. In the minor depression group, 21 of 49 patients (43%) were also cognitively impaired. In the major depression group, however, 39 of 56 patients (70%) were cognitively impaired (P = .0017). Individual group comparisons demonstrated that the frequency of cognitive impairment was significantly greater in patients with major depression compared to either the minor depression patients (P = .006) or the nondepressed patients (P = .0005). This finding also supports the conclusion that a greater degree and frequency of cognitive impairment is a phenomenon that distinguishes major depression but not minor depression patients from nondepressed patients with acute stroke.

Clinical Variables Associated With Poststroke Cognitive Impairment

We divided our acute stroke group into patients with or without major depression and with or without cognitive impairment (i.e., MMSE scores <24) (Table 7–1). Using a two-way analysis of variance (examining the factors of presence or absence of major depression and presence or absence of cognitive impairment), both major depression (P = .0018) and cognitive impairment (P = .002) were found to be significantly related to age but without significant interaction. Patients with major depression, however, were *younger* than nondepressed patients, whereas patients with cognitive impairment were significantly *older* than the non–cognitively impaired patients. Cognitive impairment but not depression was significantly related to the number of years of education (P = .0003).

Table 7-1. Demographic information

| | In-hospital evaluation | | | |
| | No cognitive impairment | | Cognitive impairment | |
	Nondepressed (N = 122)	Depressed (N = 18)	Nondepressed (N = 94)	Depressed (N = 39)
Age (years ± SD)	57.47 ± 13.5	49.9 ± 14.8[†]	63.6 ± 11.6*	57.3 ± 15.48*[†]
Education (years ± SD)	10.3 ± 3.8	11.3 ± 3.3	8.3 ± 4.3*	8.7 ± 3.2*
Socioeconomic status, Hollingshead class III–IV (%)	93 (83)	15 (83)	79 (93)	34 (97)

[†]Depressed versus nondepressed, $P < .05$.
*Cognitive versus noncognitive impairment, $P < .05$.

The patients with cognitive impairment had significantly fewer years of education than non–cognitively impaired patients.

A stepwise regression analysis to examine the influence of major depression, ethanol abuse, gender, age, and education on cognitive impairment as measured by MMSE showed that the greatest contribution to the variance was given by depression (F = 23.5, P = .00002) and age (F = 12.7, P = .0004).

Two-way analysis of variance (ANOVA) examining the factors of presence or absence of major depression and presence or absence of cognitive impairment on the Hamilton Depression score demonstrated an effect of depression (P = .0001) but no effect of cognitive impairment and no interaction. This result indicates that cognitively impaired patients were no more severely depressed than patients with depression and no cognitive impairment. Thus, although cognitive impairment was linked to major depression, it was not associated with a more severe form of major depression than that found in non–cognitively impaired patients.

Relationship to Lesion Location

Since brain lesions can affect cognitive function independent of depression, we have examined the separate effects of lesion location and depression. Using our overall group of patients with acute stroke (Downhill and Robinson 1994), patients were divided into those with right- or left-hemisphere lesions based on computed tomography (CT) or magnetic resonance imaging (MRI) scan visualization (60%) or clinical diagnosis (40%). A two-factor ANOVA of MMSE scores (right- or left-hemisphere lesion was one factor and presence or absence of major depression was the other factor) demonstrated significant effects of depressive diagnosis ($P = .0001$) and site of injury ($P = .0017$) but no interaction ($P = .18$). Individual comparisons demonstrated that patients with major depression and left-hemisphere lesions were significantly more cognitively impaired than nondepressed patients with left-hemisphere lesions (Figure 7–2) ($P = .001$). On the other hand, patients with right-hemisphere lesions showed only a trend for significantly greater impairment associated with depression (Figure 7–2) ($P = .0502$).

This finding that cognitive impairment and major depression occurred predominantly in patients with left-hemisphere lesions raised two fundamental questions. First, previous studies have demonstrated that the lesion locations most frequently associated with major depression were left basal ganglia and left dorsal lateral frontal cortex (Starkstein et al. 1987). Therefore, lesions associated with major depression may be in a different location than lesions not associated with depression. This finding might explain the association of depression with cognitive impairment. The second question that might be raised is whether the MMSE, which is primarily a verbal examination, might be more effective at demonstrating cognitive impairments associated with left-hemisphere lesions (i.e., language-related impairments) than cognitive impairments associated with right-hemisphere lesions.

To determine whether differences in lesion location may explain why patients with major depression had greater cognitive impairment than patients with no depression, we examined patients with and without major depression who were matched for lesion size and location (Starkstein et al. 1988). The study population consisted of 13 pairs of patients who were matched for lesion size, location, and hemisphere of injury; one patient of each pair had

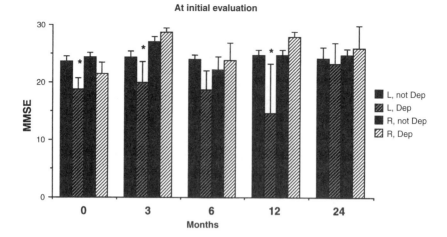

At initial evaluation

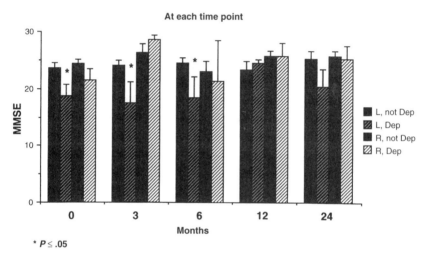

At each time point

* $P \leq .05$

Figure 7–2. MMSE scores of patients divided by hemisphere of stroke (L or R) with major depression (Dep) or no mood disorder (not dep—excluding patients with minor depression) in-hospital and over 2-year follow-up. The *top panel* shows scores of patients who were depressed in-hospital and the scores of those same patients (independent of whether they remained depressed) at each follow-up. The *bottom panel* shows scores of patients with major depression or no mood disorder at each follow-up time point (depressed group changes composition at each follow-up). Note that cognitive function is significantly more impaired in patients with major depression compared to nondepressed patients following left- but not right-hemisphere stroke. The association of major depression and left-hemisphere lesion location with cognitive impairment lasted about 1 year. At the 2-year follow-up, major depression was no longer associated with cognitive impairment. *Source.* Reprinted from Downhill JE Jr and Robinson RG: "Longitudinal Assessment of Depression and Cognitive Impairment Following Stroke." Journal of Nervous and Mental Disease 182:425–431, 1994. Used with permission. Copyright 1994 Williams & Wilkins.

major depression while the other was not depressed. Patients were matched for location based on the existence of a brain lesion that involved the same brain regions (i.e., regions defined by Levine and Grek [1984]). This classification distinguished groups as well as locations.

Although no significant between-group differences were found in background characteristics, such as age, gender, years of education, and socioeconomic status, patients with major depression had significantly lower MMSE scores than nondepressed patients (Figure 7–3). Of the 13 patients with major depression, 10 had lower MMSE scores than their respective lesion-matched controls, 2 had the same score, and only 1 nondepressed patient had a lower score than the lesion-matched patient with major depression ($P <$ .05). We concluded from this study that, although brain lesions frequently produce cognitive impairment as measured by the MMSE state examination, patients with major depression have a degree of cognitive impairment that cannot be explained based on the lesion alone.

The second question raised about the initial finding of greater cognitive impairment in patients with major depression following left-hemisphere lesions compared to nondepressed patients with left-hemisphere lesions is whether the MMSE is more effective at demonstrating language-related impairment (associated with dominant left-hemisphere injury) than visual spatial impairment (associated with right-hemisphere lesions). To examine this question, we evaluated the pattern of cognitive deficits in patients with major depression following stroke compared with nondepressed patients using a detailed neuropsychological evaluation. The neuropsychological examination assessed the following cognitive domains: 1) orientation, 2) language, 3) remote memory, 4) verbal memory, 5) visual memory, 6) recognition memory, 7) visual perception–visual construction, 8) executive motor functions, and 9) frontal lobe functions (Bolla-Wilson et al. 1989).

The study population consisted of a consecutive series of patients with acute stroke with either no depression or major depression and single stroke lesions involving either the right or left hemisphere. Patients with aphasia, other than anomia, were ex-

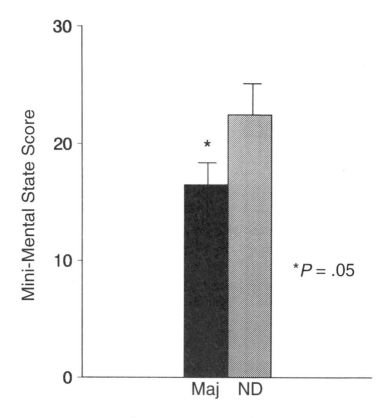

Figure 7–3. Mini-Mental State Exam scores for 13 pairs of patients who were matched for lesion size and location. Patients with major depression (Maj) were significantly more cognitively impaired than nondepressed (ND) patients. The groups were comparable in age and education as well as lesion characteristics. Bars indicate standard errors of the mean. Data from Starkstein et al. (1988).

cluded. There were no significant differences between depressed and nondepressed patients with left-hemisphere lesions in their age or years of education. The mean $\pm$ SD ages for the depressed ($N = 10$) and nondepressed ($N = 16$) left-hemisphere stroke patients were 57 ± 11 and 61 ± 13 years, respectively. The corresponding ages for the depressed ($N = 8$) and nondepressed ($N = 19$) patients with right-hemisphere lesions were 54 ± 16 and 62 ± 10 years, respectively. The years of education for the depressed and nondepressed left-hemisphere patients were 8 ± 4 and 10 ± 3 years, respectively. The years of education for the corresponding groups of right-hemisphere lesions were 10 ± 1 and 8 ± 4 years, respectively.

Direct measurements of lesions from CT scans were obtained in 37 of the 53 patients. There were no significant differences in the number of patients with purely cortical or subcortical lesions between the depressed and nondepressed groups with left-hemisphere lesions ($P = .58$) or the depressed and nondepressed patients with right-hemisphere lesions. The anterior border of the lesion (expressed as mean ± SD percentage of the anterior-posterior measurement of the brain) for depressed and nondepressed left-hemisphere stroke patients was 30.4% ± 6.0% and 37.9% ± 20.0% ($P = $ NS). The anterior border of the lesion in the right hemisphere for depressed and nondepressed patients was 45.9% ± 17.0% and 40.5% ± 22.0%, respectively ($P = $ NS). The mean ± SD lesion volume measurements for the depressed and nondepressed left-hemisphere lesion group and depressed and nondepressed right-hemisphere lesion group were 2.0% ± 2.0%, 5.3% ± 4.0%, 3.5% ± 2.0%, and 6.8% ± 6.0%, respectively. There were no significant intergroup differences in lesion volume or location.

The degree of impairment in each of the cognitive domains examined for depressed and nondepressed patients with left- or right-hemisphere lesions are shown in Figure 7–4. Data analysis included a two-way ANOVA of Z scores (scores in each cognitive domain were transformed to Z scores to allow comparison between domains; factors in the ANOVA were presence or absence of depression and existence of right- or left-hemisphere lesions). Although there was no main effect of hemisphere ($P = .07$) or depression ($P = .20$) on total Z score (i.e., summed across all domains), there was a significant depression by side interaction ($P = .01$). The left-hemisphere depressed group performed significantly below the left-hemisphere nondepressed group ($P = .01$), the right-hemisphere depressed group ($P = .01$), and the right-hemisphere nondepressed group ($P = .01$). There were no significant differences among the depressed and nondepressed patients with right-hemisphere lesions or among the patients with left-

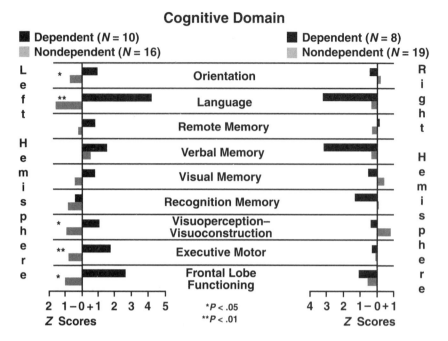

Figure 7–4. Performance on nine cognitive domains taken from a comprehensive neuropsychological test battery. Patients with acute stroke but without aphasia were divided into those with major depression or no mood disorder and right- or left-hemisphere injury. The groups were comparable in age, education, and lesion size and location. Performance test scores were converted to Z scores so that comparisons could be made between different domains with differing numbers of questions. Positive scores indicate greater impairment. Note that patients with left-hemisphere lesions and major depression were more impaired on every cognitive domain compared to patients with left-hemisphere lesions who were nondepressed. These differences reached statistical significance for orientation, language, visuoperceptional–visuoconstruction, executive motor, and frontal lobe functions. There were no significant differences in cognitive function between depressed and nondepressed patients with right-hemisphere lesions. Data taken from Bolla-Wilson et al. (1989).

hemisphere lesions, who were nondepressed or depressed, or non depressed patients with right-hemisphere lesions ($P = .3$ to $.7$). Within the left-hemisphere lesion group, the presence of depression was associated with significantly lower scores in orientation ($P = .02$), language ($P = .01$), executive motor function ($P = .01$), frontal lobe function ($P = .01$), and visual construction–visual perceptual ability ($P < .05$). In the right-hemisphere lesion group, there were no significant differences between the depressed and nondepressed groups in any of the nine cognitive domains.

We concluded from this study that, using a detailed neuropsychological battery that examined both right- and left-hemisphere cognitive functions, major depression was associated with cognitive impairment only following left-hemisphere lesions. In addition, the cognitive impairment involved a range of neuropsychological tasks generally associated with left- and right-parietal as well as frontal lobe function. Major depression following right-hemisphere lesions, on the other hand, did not produce any greater cognitive impairment than right-hemisphere lesions without major depression.

It is interesting to note similarities between the pattern of cognitive impairment found in patients with major depression following stroke and the pattern of cognitive deficits described in patients with functional (i.e., no known neuropathology) depression. For example, patients with major depression following left-hemisphere lesions showed significant deficits in naming and repetition, which has also been reported by Speedie et al. (1990) in patients with functional depression. Our study also found that patients with left-hemisphere lesions and major depression performed significantly worse than nondepressed patients on the logical memory task, both immediate- and delayed-recall tasks. Memory impairment constitutes one of the most conspicuous cognitive deficits in patients with functional depression (Caine 1981) and is manifested by both verbal and visuospatial memory impairment (Calev et al. 1986; Miller and Lewis 1977; Weingartner et al. 1981). We also examined learning curves as determined by performance on the Rey Auditory Verbal Learning Test. We found that the depressed group with left-hemisphere lesions showed the least amount of learning over trials.

By trial five (a measure of overall learning), the depressed patients had learned significantly fewer words than the nondepressed patients ($P < .05$) with left-hemisphere lesions. This finding suggests that depressed patients with left-hemisphere lesions may have poor sequential learning. Functional depression has also been shown to be associated with poor sequence learning (Weingartner et al. 1981). These impairments have been attributed to deficits in the use of encoding strategies and in the organization of inputs for subsequent facilitation of recall (Weingartner et al. 1981).

Longitudinal Course of Cognitive Impairment

Of the patients evaluated with acute stroke, 140 patients were reexamined at 3, 6, 12, or 24 months following stroke. One-way ANOVA comparing MMSE scores between patients with major depression and nondepressed patients at each follow-up interval (i.e., all patients with major depression at each time point regardless of whether they were depressed in-hospital) demonstrated a significant effect of depression only at the initial evaluation ($P = .005$).

Because the failure to find an effect of depression could be attributed to a change in patient population at each follow-up time point (i.e., some patients had remission of their depression and therefore joined the nondepressed group, while some nondepressed patients had developed depression and therefore joined the depressed group), we examined the longitudinal course of patients with in-hospital major depression regardless of their diagnosis at follow-up. Repeated-measures ANOVA of patients with in-hospital major depression versus nondepressed patients showed a significant effect of depression in-hospital ($P = .01$) and at 3 months ($P = .02$) but not at 6, 12, or 24 months.

Since our previous data demonstrated that cognitive impairment was associated with major depression following a left-hemisphere lesion, we examined the effect of lesion location on follow-up cognitive status. The MMSE scores for patients with left-hemisphere stroke and in-hospital major depression (regardless of their diagnosis at follow-up) were compared to those of patients with left-hemisphere stroke but without in-hospital depression (regardless of their diagnoses at follow-up). There was a significant effect of depression on MMSE scores in-hospital, at 6 months ($P = .03$), and at 1-year follow-up ($P = .019$) (Figure. 7–2). We also examined patients who had major depression at each time point (regardless of whether they had major depression at the initial evaluation). Patients with major depression and left-hemisphere lesion had significantly lower MMSE scores at 3 and 6 months follow-up compared to patients who were nondepressed at each time point (3 months [$P = .007$], 6 months [$P = .03$]). There were no significant effects at 1 and 2 years following stroke.

These findings indicate that the association of depression with cognitive impairment is strongest during the acute stroke period, but there is some effect for up to 1 year. At 2 years following stroke, however, major depression, even after a left-hemisphere stroke, is no longer associated with cognitive impairment.

Relationship of Cognitive Impairment to Duration of Depression

The duration of depression was examined in patients with or without cognitive impairment and with or without major depression. At 3 months follow-up, 6 of 10 patients (60%) who had depression and cognitive impairment at the initial evaluation remained depressed compared with 0 of 3 who had major depression without cognitive impairment ($P = .003$). At 6 months follow-up, patients with major depression and cognitive impairment in-hospital again were more likely to remain depressed (6 of 11 patients, 54%) compared to non–cognitively impaired depressed patients (0 of 3) ($P = .03$). At the 1- and 2-year follow-up evaluation, there was no longer a significant relationship between in-hospital cognitive status and the likelihood of remaining depressed (12 months [$P = .12$], 24 months [$P = .48$]).

We also examined whether the existence of cognitive impairment might predict the development of depression. The frequency of new onset depression beginning between the in-hospital evaluation and 3- or 6-month follow-up evaluation was not significantly different between in-hospital cognitively impaired and nonimpaired patients. Of 26 patients with cognitive impairment, 2% developed depression at 3 months compared to 6 of 36 (7%) without cognitive impairment; at 6 months 4 of 25 (16%) cognitively impaired patients developed depression compared with 7 of 40 (17%) without cognitive impairment. Thus, the existence of cognitive impairment did not predict the development of depression at either 3 or 6 months follow-up.

Mechanism of Cognitive Impairment Associated With Depression

Folstein and McHugh (1978) pointed out similarities between dementia of depression and subcortical dementia and suggested that dementia of depression may be a consequence of pathological changes in subcortical biogenic amine–containing neural pathways. This suggestion was later supported by the finding that the depressed patients improved their performances on effort-demanding motor and cognitive tasks when they were treated with levodopa (Roy-Byrne et al. 1986) or amphetamine (Reus et al. 1979).

In a previous publication (Robinson et al. 1987), we have suggested that patients with major depression and cognitive impairment following stroke may have dysfunction of the brain's biogenic amine pathways. This suggestion was based in part on our findings using a rat model of stroke (Robinson and Coyle 1979) in which right- but not left-hemisphere cerebral infarction produced significant depletions of norepinephrine and dopamine concentrations in uninjured areas of cortical and subcortical brain tissue. Thus different degrees of biogenic amine depletion based on the side of injury could explain why left- but not right-hemisphere stroke is associated with both cognitive impairment and depression.

We have conducted two studies examining the binding of (11-

C)N-methylspiperone (NMSP) in patients with unilateral stroke. Cortical binding of N-methylspiperone has been demonstrated to be predominantly serotonin S_2-receptor binding (Mayberg et al. 1990). The first study examined nine patients with single lesions of the right hemisphere and eight patients with single lesions of the left hemisphere (Mayberg et al. 1988). Among patients with left-hemisphere stroke, there was a significant negative correlation ($r = -.93, P < .05$) between the severity of depressive symptoms measured by the Zung Depression Rating Scale and the amount of serotonin S_2-receptor binding (i.e., the amount of S_2-receptor binding in an ipsilateral region of interest in the left temporal cortex compared to the binding in the identical contralateral region of interest in the left temporal cortex). This finding suggested that patients with left-hemisphere stroke and more severe depressive symptoms had less serotonin S_2-receptor binding in the left temporal cortex compared to those with fewer depressive symptoms. This study was also consistent with the finding in rats that injury to the left hemisphere produces a different biochemical response (as measured by serotonin S_2-receptor binding) than right-hemisphere lesions (i.e., depression was not significantly correlated with S_2-receptor binding in the right temporal cortex).

We have also recently examined the relationship between cortical serotonin S_2-receptor binding and cognitive function (Morris et al. 1993). The study included 26 patients with single stroke lesions of the right or left hemisphere. The amount of serotonin S_2-receptor binding as measured by cortical to cerebellar positron counts was significantly correlated with the MMSE score in the left frontal cortex, left temporal cortex, left parietal cortex, and right frontal cortex. The strongest correlation, however, was between S_2-receptor binding ratio and MMSE score in the left frontal cortex ($r = .50, P = .009$) (Figure 7–5). This finding suggests that serotonin function in several regions of the left hemisphere, but particularly left frontal cortex, may play a role in cognitive processes. As indicated previously, however, serotonergic function in the left temporal cortex may play a role in depressive disorder.

Based on these findings, we have proposed the hypothesis that stroke lesions of the left hemisphere that disrupt serotonergic function in the left temporal cortex will produce depressive disorder

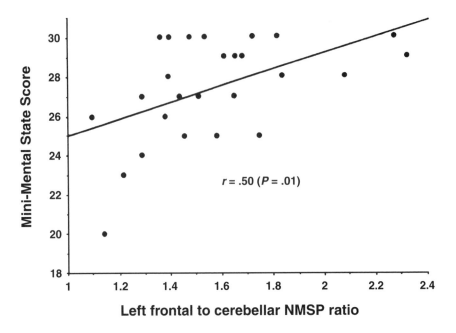

Figure 7–5. Relationship between left frontal to cerebellar [11-C] *N*-methylspiperone (NMSP) binding ratio and Mini-Mental State Exam score (MMSE) (*N* = 26). Patients with a single stroke lesion underwent positron emission tomography (PET) imaging following injection of NMSP. Prior work has shown that NMSP binds primarily to serotonin S_2 receptors in the cerebral cortex, whereas cerebellar binding is nonspecific. This finding demonstrates that cognitive function improves with increased amount of serotonin receptor binding in the left frontal cortex.
Source. Reprinted from Morris PLP, Mayberg H, Bolla K, et al.: "A Preliminary Study of Cortical S_2 Serotonin Receptors and Cognitive Performance Following Stroke." Journal of Neuropsychiatry and Clinical Neurosciences 5:395–400, 1993. Used with permission. Copyright 1993 American Psychiatric Press, Inc.

whereas disruption of serotonergic receptor function in the left frontal cortex (and perhaps right frontal cortex) will produce cognitive impairment. In our study of cognitive impairment associated with *N*-methylspiperone binding (Morris et al. 1993), a subset of patients with detailed neuropsychological testing revealed there were significant correlations between NMSP binding and performance on orientation, repetition, and naming. These impairments in cognitive function were also found in patients with major depression following left-hemisphere stroke (Bolla-Wilson et al. 1989). Thus, if both frontal and temporal serotonergic function is disrupted, both major depression and cognitive impairment may occur. In the instances where only temporal lobe dysfunction is produced, major depression may occur without cognitive impairment. Similarly, frontal dysfunction may produce cognitive impairment without accompanying depression. This hypothesis will require further investigation but represents a testable hypothesis that could explain why cognitive dysfunction and major depression are frequently but not always associated.

Treatment

Based on the findings that treatment of depression significantly improves cognitive function in patients with functional depressive disorders (Caine 1981; Folstein and McHugh 1978), it would be predicted that treatment of depression should improve cognitive function in patients with stroke. Although this finding has been demonstrated in anecdotal cases (Fogel and Sparadeo 1985), it has not been confirmed in a controlled treatment trial. Several double-blind, randomized treatment trials have demonstrated the effectiveness of antidepressant treatment for poststroke depression (Andersen et al. 1994; Lipsey et al. 1984; Reding et al. 1985). These trials, however, either have not examined the effect of treatment of depression on cognitive function (Andersen et al. 1994; Reding et al. 1985) or have failed to show a significant improvement in MMSE scores associated with active treatment (Lipsey et al. 1985). Our failure to find a significant effect of nortriptyline treatment of depression on cognitive function may be related to the time since injury (patients were treated on an average of 4 to 6 months following stroke) or the fact that both major and minor depressive disorder were included in the study. Both anecdotal reports (Fogel and Sparadeo 1985) and systematic (open trial) studies (González-Torrecillas et al. 1996) have demonstrated significant improvement in cognitive function associated with treatment of poststroke depression. Based on the data presented here, however, only patients with major depression during the first year following stroke would be expected to show improvement in cognitive function associated with treatment. In any event, additional controlled, double-blind studies will be needed to determine whether cognitive dysfunction associated with major depression responds to the treatment of depression.

Conclusion

We have demonstrated that cognitive impairment associated with depression is a very specific phenomenon in patients with stroke. Cognitive impairment associated with depression occurs only in patients with major depression and only in patients with left-hemisphere lesions. The phenomenon cannot be explained based on differences in lesion location between depressed and nondepressed patients or as a result of the cognitive measurement instrument. The association of major depression with cognitive impairment is most pronounced during the acute poststroke period but has a significant effect over the first year following stroke. Major depression, however, at 2 years following stroke, does not have an associated cognitive impairment, even among patients with left-hemisphere lesions.

Studies of serotonin S_2-receptor binding suggest that left- and right-hemisphere lesions produce differential effects on serotonin receptors. Among patients with left-hemisphere lesions, S_2-receptor binding in the left temporal cortex is associated with severity of depressive symptoms. As S_2-receptor binding decreases, severity of depressive symptoms increases. In addition, there is a significant correlation between decreased serotonin S_2-receptor binding in the frontal cortex and greater cognitive impairment. Furthermore, the kinds of cognitive impairments (i.e., orientation and language function) that correlate significantly with frontal serotonergic function are the same as the impairments associated with major depression. Thus, we have proposed the hypothesis that left-hemisphere stroke lesions that produce serotonergic dysfunction in both left frontal and left temporal cortex may produce both cognitive impairment and major depression, whereas serotonergic dysfunction within the left temporal lobe alone may produce major depression without cognitive disturbance.

Further studies are needed to examine the effect of treatment of depression on cognitive function in patients with acute stroke. Currently, only anecdotal reports and open treatment trials have demonstrated significant improvements in cognitive function associated with the treatment of depression. There are sufficient data, however, to support the recommendation that any patient being evaluated for a vascular dementia be carefully examined for major depression following left-hemisphere stroke because the treatment of depression within the first year may significantly improve the patient's cognitive function.

In conclusion, cognitive dysfunction associated with poststroke depression is a specific phenomenon related to type of depression, lesion location, and time since stroke. This suggests that a specific pathophysiological mechanism (perhaps mediated by serotonergic dysfunction) produces the clinical syndromes of major depression and cognitive dysfunction. Future studies identifying the mechanism of this cognitive dysfunction may lead to the development of specific and rational treatments targeted at the pathophysiological processes disrupted by left-hemisphere stroke.

References

Albert ML, Feldman RG, Willis AL: "Subcortical dementia" of progressive nuclear palsy. J Neurol Neurosurg Psychiatry 37:121–130, 1974

American Psychiatric Association: Diagnostic and Statistical Manual of Mental Disorders, 3rd Edition. Washington, DC, American Psychiatric Association, 1980

American Psychiatric Association: Diagnostic and Statistical Manual of Mental Disorders, 4th Edition. Washington, DC, American Psychiatric Association, 1994

Andersen G, Vestergaard K, Lauritzen L: Effective treatment of poststroke depression with the selective serotonin reuptake inhibitor citalopram. Stroke 25:1099–1104, 1994

Astrom M, Adolfsson R, Asplund K: Major depression in stroke patients: a 3-year longitudinal study. Stroke 24:976–982, 1993

Basso A, Lecours AR, Moraschini S, et al: Anatomoclinical correlations of the aphasias as defined through the computerized tomography: exceptions. Brain and Language 26:201–229, 1985

Bolla-Wilson K, Robinson RG, Starkstein SE, et al: Lateralization of dementia of depression in stroke patients. Am J Psychiatry 146:627–634, 1989

Bulbena A, Berrios GE: Pseudodementia: facts and figures. Br J Psychiatry 148:87–94, 1986

Caine ED: Pseudodementia. Arch Gen Psychiatry 38:1359–1364, 1981

Calev A, Korin Y, Shapira B, et al: Verbal and non-verbal recall by depressed and euthymic affective patients. Psychol Med 16:789–794, 1986

Cummings JL, Benson DF: Subcortical dementia: review of an emerging concept. Arch Neurol 41:874–879, 1984

Damasio AR, Geschwind N: Anatomical Localization in Clinical Neuropsychology, Vol. 1. Amsterdam, Elsevier, 1985

Downhill JE Jr, Robinson RG: Longitudinal assessment of depression and cognitive impairment following stroke. J Nerv Ment Dis 182:425–431, 1994

Eastwood MR, Rifat SL, Nobbs H, et al: Mood disorder following cerebrovascular accident. Br J Psychiatry 154:195–200, 1989

Fogel BS, Sparadeo FR: Focal cognitive deficits accentuated by depression. J Nerv Ment Dis 173:129–134, 1985

Folstein MF, McHugh PR: Dementia syndrome of depression, in Aging, Vol. 7: Alzheimer's Disease: Senile Dementia. Edited by Katzman R, Terry RD, Bick KL. New York, Raven, 1978, pp 87–93

González-Torrecillas JL, Mendlewicz J, Lobo A: Effects of early treatment of post-stroke depression on neuropsychological rehabilitation. Int Psychogeriatr 7:547–560, 1996

Goodnick PJ: Pseudomentia. Geriatric Medicine Today 4:31–40, 1985

Herrmann M, Bartles C, Wallesch C-W: Depression in acute and chronic aphasia: symptoms, pathoanatomical-clinical correlations and functional implications. J Neurol Neurosurg Psychiatry 56:672–678, 1993

Herskovits E, Figueroa E: Planning clinical trials of treatment for vascular and multi-infarct dementia. Mount Kisco, NY, Futura, 1988

House A, Dennis M, Warlow C, et al: The relationship between intellectual impairment and mood disorder in the first year after stroke. Psychol Med 20:805–814, 1990

Kiloh LG: Pseudo-dementia. Acta Psychiatr Scand 37:336–351, 1961

Levine DN, Grek A: The anatomic basis of delusions after right cerebral infarction. Neurology 34:577–582, 1984

Lipsey JR, Robinson RG, Pearlson GD, et al: Nortriptyline treatment of post-stroke depression: a double-blind treatment trial. Lancet 1:297–300, 1984

Lipsey JR, Robinson RG, Pearlson GD, et al: Dexamethasone suppression test and mood following stroke. Am J Psychiatry 142:318–323, 1985

Madden JJ, Luhan JA, Kaplan LA, et al: Nondementing psychoses in older persons. JAMA 150:1567–1570, 1952

Mayberg HS, Robinson RG, Wong DF, et al: PET imaging of cortical S_2-serotonin receptors after stroke: lateralized changes and relationship to depression. Am J Psychiatry 145:937–943, 1988

Mayberg HS, Moran TH, Robinson RG: Remote lateralized changes in cortical ^{3}H-spiperone binding following focal frontal cortex lesions in the rat. Brain Res 516:127–131, 1990

McHugh PR, Folstein MF: Organic Mental Disorders. Philadelphia, JB Lippincott, 1985

Miller E, Lewis P: Recognition memory in elderly patients and depression and dementia: a signal detection analysis. J Abnorm Psychol 86:84–86, 1977

Morris PLP, Robinson RG, Raphael B: Prevalence and course of depressive disorders in hospitalized stroke patients. Int J Psychiatry Med 20:349–364, 1990

Morris PLP, Mayberg H, Bolla K, et al: A preliminary study of cortical S_2 serotonin receptors and cognitive performance following stroke. J Neuropsych Clin Neurosci 5:395–400, 1993

Reding M, Orto L, Willensky P, et al: The dexamethasone suppression test: an indicator of depression in stroke but not a predictor of rehabilitation outcome. Arch Neurol 42:209–212, 1985

Reus VI, Silberman E, Post RM, et al: d-Amphetamine effects on memory in a depressed population. Biol Psychiatry 14:345–356, 1979

Robinson RG, Coyle JT: Lateralization of catecholaminergic and behavioral response to cerebral infarction in the rat. Life Sci 24:943–950, 1979

Robinson RG, Starr LB, Kubos KL, et al: A two year longitudinal study of post-stroke mood disorders: findings during the initial evaluation. Stroke 14:736–744, 1983

Robinson RG, Bolla-Wilson K, Kaplan E, et al: Depression influences intellectual impairment in stroke patients. Br J Psychiatry 148:541–547, 1986a

Robinson RG, Lipsey JR, Rao K, et al: Two-year longitudinal study of post-stroke mood disorders: comparison of acute-onset with delayed-onset depression. Am J Psychiatry 143:1238–1244, 1986b

Robinson RG, Bolduc P, Price TR: A two year longitudinal study of post-stroke depression: diagnosis and outcome at one and two year follow-up. Stroke 18:837–843, 1987

Román GC, Tatemichi TK, Ekinjuntti T, et al: Vascular dementia: diagnostic criteria for research studies. Report of the NINDS-AIREN International Workshop. Neurology 43:250–260, 1993

Roy-Byrne RP, Weingartner H, Bierer LM, et al: Effortful and automatic processes in depression. Arch Gen Psychiatry 43:265–267, 1986

Speedie L, Rabins P, Pearlson G, et al: Confrontation naming deficit in dementia of depression. J Neuropsych Clin Neurosci 2:59–63, 1990

Starkstein SE, Robinson RG, Price TR: Comparison of cortical and subcortical lesions in the production of post-stroke mood disorders. Brain 110:1045–1059, 1987

Starkstein SE, Robinson RG, Price TR: Comparison of patients with and without post-stroke major depression matched for size and location of lesion. Arch Gen Psychiatry 45:247–252, 1988

Starkstein SE, Rabins PV, Berthier ML, et al: Dementia of depression: evidence from neurological disorders and functional depression. J Neuropsych Clin Neurosci 1:263–268, 1989

Weingartner H, Cohen RM, Murphy DL, et al: Cognitive processes in depression. Arch Gen Psychiatry 38:42–47, 1981

Wells CE: Pseudodementia. Am J Psychiatry 136:895–900, 1979

Wing JK, Cooper JE, Sartorius N: The Measurement and Classification of Psychiatric Symptoms: An Instructional Manual for the PSE and CATEGO Programs. New York, Cambridge University Press, 1974

CHAPTER

8

Vascular Dementia

David W. Desmond, Ph.D., and
Thomas K. Tatemichi, M.D.

Background

Vascular dementia may be defined as a clinical syndrome of acquired intellectual impairment resulting from brain injury due to a cerebrovascular disorder (Tatemichi et al. 1994d). While research into cerebrovascular disease as a basis for dementia has a long history, use of the term *vascular dementia* is relatively recent. In early work, cerebral arteriosclerosis was a central thesis, as reflected in the concept of *arteriosclerotic brain degeneration*. It was proposed by Binswanger (1894) and Alzheimer (1895), both of whom studied and lectured on the topic in the late nineteenth century, several years before Alzheimer described the primary degenerative dementia that bears his name. Many years later, Hachinski and colleagues (1974) proposed the term *multi-infarct dementia,*

This work was supported by Grant R01-NS26179 and Contract N01-NS92334 from the National Institutes of Health. Joan Moroney, M.D., provided critical comments on this manuscript. Dr. Tatemichi passed away on April 22, 1995.

reflecting the greater importance placed on the multiplicity of frank infarctions. It was not until the late 1980s that the term *vascular dementia* became officially sanctioned as a subject heading in the *Index Medicus* (National Library of Medicine 1989), and it has since been incorporated into the fourth edition of the *Diagnostic and Statistical Manual of Mental Disorders* (American Psychiatric Association 1994).

Despite 100 years of research, the concept of a vascular dementia—indeed, the actual existence of the entity—continues to be challenged. Among the several issues that fuel this controversy is the question of whether cerebrovascular disease can produce progressive mental deterioration, mimicking Alzheimer's disease (AD), as a result of vascular insufficiency and in the absence of clinically obvious stroke. That is, if AD can be considered a primary dementia resulting from neuronal failure, is there a primary vascular dementia resulting from supply failure? In particular, this controversy has focused on the role of white matter disease, also termed leukoaraiosis (Hachinski et al. 1987), which is commonly found on brain imaging in elderly with and without dementia and thought to be ischemic in origin. Based on pathologic studies, Alzheimer (1895) himself foresaw this issue with his contention that disease of the small arteries due to arteriosclerosis resulted in "incomplete softening" and atrophy of the white matter, in contrast to thromboembolic disease of the large arteries, which led to "acute colliquation necrosis." According to Alzheimer (1895), the clinical consequences differed: small-artery disease produced dementia, while large-artery disease resulted in stroke.

An affirmative response to the question of whether cerebrovascular disease can produce progressive mental deterioration, which we will attempt to develop in the discussion to follow, has important implications. If vascular dementia is merely a matter of several strokes (i.e., multiple infarcts leading to mental decline, as in multi-infarct dementia), then preventing it is merely a matter of preventing clinically obvious stroke. On the other hand, if some forms of vascular dementia are the result of white matter ischemic damage, then preventive strategies may be different, depending on what is understood about its pathogenesis. Our argument will be developed based on a series of questions:

1. How does cerebrovascular disease cause dementia?
2. Can cerebrovascular disease cause cognitive impairment in the absence of clinically evident stroke?
3. Does progressive cognitive decline occur due to cerebrovascular disease?

How Does Cerebrovascular Disease Cause Dementia?

Estimates of the prevalence of vascular dementia have varied widely due to differences in sampling methods, assessment techniques, and diagnostic paradigms, as well as true differences among populations. In community-based studies, the proportions of dementia patients considered to have vascular dementia have ranged from 9.0% in the Framingham study (Kase et al. 1989a) to greater than 50% in studies conducted in Japan (Ueda et al. 1992) and China (Li et al. 1989). Among the few hospital-based studies of dementia in patients presenting with stroke, the frequencies of dementia reported have ranged from 16.0% in the Stroke Data Bank cohort, in which the diagnosis of dementia was based solely on clinical information and the judgment of neurologists (Tatemichi et al. 1990a), to 56.3% in a study performed by Ladurner et al. (1982), in which the diagnosis of dementia was based on clinical information, the judgment of neurologists, and the results of psychological testing. In autopsy series, Tomlinson et al. (1970) reported that AD was the primary basis for dementia in 25% of their cases, while "arteriosclerosis" was the primary basis in 18%. Similar proportions have been reported in other autopsy studies (Chui 1989), leading to the inference that AD is the most common cause of dementia, followed by cerebrovascular disease. O'Brien (1988,

p. 798) has concluded that "at least one-third of all patients with dementia have a significant vascular component," while Katzman (1983, p. 155) has suggested that "25% of persons with dementia either have vascular disease as the primary cause or as an etiology accompanied by or adding to an Alzheimer process."

In attempting to address the question of how cerebrovascular disease causes cognitive impairment, we have taken the approach of studying poststroke dementia. We assembled a group of 251 patients consecutively hospitalized with acute ischemic stroke at Columbia-Presbyterian Medical Center and examined them with neuropsychological tests tapping multiple cognitive domains as well as a measure of functional capacity. We diagnosed dementia based on criteria modified from DSM-III-R (American Psychiatric Association 1987), requiring that subjects exhibit deficits in memory and two or more additional cognitive domains as well as functional impairment. We attempted to minimize the potential for aphasia to confound our diagnosis of dementia by excluding from the study patients with Boston Diagnostic Aphasia Examination (Goodglass and Kaplan 1983) severity ratings of 0 or 1 and requiring evidence of nonverbal memory impairment to support the diagnosis of dementia in enrolled patients with less-severe aphasias. Our method for determining whether vascular dementia was present was consistent with guidelines later developed by Román et al. (1993), which are presented in Table 8–1. In addition to the presence of cognitive and functional impairment consistent with dementia, we required that significant cerebrovascular disease be evident based on brain imaging, clinical history, or neurologic examination, and that there be a meaningful relationship between the dementia syndrome and cerebrovascular disease.

We found that 66 patients, or 26.3% of the cohort, had dementia 3 months after stroke, compared to 3.2% of controls, resulting in an odds ratio of 9.4 (95% confidence interval, 4.2 to 21.1), adjusted for demographic variables (Tatemichi et al. 1992a). Within the sample of 66 patients with dementia, 56.1% had dementia that was directly attributable to stroke, or vascular dementia; 36.4% had dementia due to the combined effects of stroke and AD, the diagnosis of which was suggested by a prestroke history of functional im-

Table 8–1. NINDS-AIREN criteria for the diagnosis of vascular dementia

Required elements

1. Dementia involving deficits in memory and two or more other cognitive domains with concomitant impairment of functional capabilities.
2. Cerebrovascular disease, with evidence provided by patient history, examination findings, and/or the results of brain imaging.
3. A causal relationship between elements 1 and 2, as determined based on a temporal relationship between stroke and dementia, abrupt or stepwise decline in cognitive function or a fluctuating course, and/or brain imaging findings documenting damage to brain structures relevant to cognitive function.

Supportive information

1. History of risk factors for cerebrovascular disease (e.g., hypertension, diabetes).
2. Presence of a gait disturbance or a history of falls.
3. Early appearance of urinary incontinence not explained by urologic disease.
4. Frontal lobe or extrapyramidal features.
5. Pseudobulbar features.

Source. Adapted from Román et al. 1993.

pairment; and 7.5% had dementia for other reasons, such as alcohol abuse.

We have also observed that cognitive impairment, independent of dementia status, is quite common following stroke (Desmond et al. 1992b). As shown in Figure 8–1, among 148 stroke patients without a history of prior stroke, we recognized deficits in one cognitive domain in 19.7%, in two cognitive domains in 17.0%, and in three or more cognitive domains in 15.7%, with 47.6% exhibiting no deficits. That is, more than half of the patients in our cohort who had never experienced a clinically evident prior stroke exhibited signs of significant cognitive impairment. In contrast, 81.6% of our stroke-free control group exhibited no deficits.

To investigate the determinants of dementia in our cohort, we compared the 66 patients with dementia to the remaining 185 patients without dementia regarding all available clinical information and computed tomography (CT) scan findings (Tatemichi et al. 1993). As shown in Table 8–2, significant correlates of dementia can be grouped into three broad categories: lesion characteristics, vascular risk factors, and host susceptibility factors. The relevant

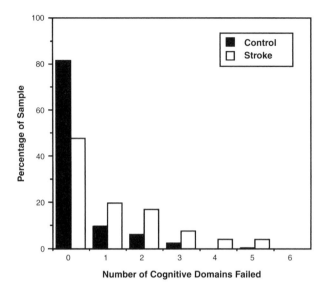

Figure 8–1. Neuropsychological test performance of patients with first stroke and stroke-free control subjects.
Source. Adapted from Desmond et al. 1992b.

Table 8–2. Clinical determinants of dementia diagnosed 3 months after stroke

Variable	Odds ratio	95% confidence interval
Age (vs. 60 to 69 years)		
≥80 years	14.5	5.4–38.9
70–79 years	2.9	1.3–6.4
Race (nonwhite vs. white)	2.4	1.0–5.6
Education (vs. 13+ years)		
≤8 years	2.9	0.9–8.7
9–12 years	3.4	1.2–9.6
Diabetes mellitus	2.6	1.3–5.3
Prior stroke	2.7	1.3–5.9
Lacunar infarction (vs. others)	2.7	1.2–6.0
Hemispheral side (vs. vertebrobasilar)		
Left	4.7	1.7–12.9
Right	3.3	1.2–9.0
Major dominant hemispheral syndrome	3.9	1.3–11.3

Source. Adapted from Tatemichi et al. 1993.

brain lesions appeared to be large infarcts, particularly those involving the left hemisphere; cortical lesions in the anterior cerebral artery (i.e., medial frontal lobe) and posterior cerebral artery (i.e., medial temporal lobe) territories; and lacunar infarcts. Atrophy was also associated with dementia status (Figueroa et al. 1992a). Regarding vascular risk factors, diabetes mellitus and prior stroke significantly increased the risk of dementia. Factors related to host susceptibility, including age, education, and race, were as important as brain lesion features. The contribution of education may be related to its influence on the functional reserve of the brain, consistent with the findings of prior studies of patients with AD (Katzman 1993). Aphasia was not related to dementia status in our cohort.

These findings confirm previous ideas about the mechanisms of dementia resulting from cerebrovascular disease, but they also suggest newer concepts. Increasing volume of infarction was found to be associated with dementia in the pathologic studies of Tomlinson et al. (1970), but the observed volumes were much larger than those recognized in more recent pathologic (del Ser et al. 1990; Erkinjuntti et al. 1988) or clinical CT (Gorelick et al. 1992; Loeb et al. 1988) series, including our own (Figueroa et al. 1992a). Clearly, there is an overlap in volumes between patients with and without dementia, with small infarcts occasionally responsible for dementia and large infarcts sparing mental functions.

In our own work, we have found that certain small, deep infarcts, depending on their location (e.g., the thalamus and anterior limb or genu of the internal capsule), may cause significant cognitive impairment (Desmond et al. 1992a, 1994; Figueroa et al. 1992b, 1993). We have identified the syndrome of *strategic infarct dementia* as a result of our observations of a case series of patients with lacunar infarctions involving the capsular genu (Tatemichi et al. 1992b). We recognized a striking syndrome of confusion and memory loss with frontal lobe features in those patients, and functional brain imaging demonstrated ipsilateral reductions in cortical perfusion, maximal in the frontal and temporal lobes, suggesting disconnection or diaschisis as possible mechanisms for their cognitive impairment. Other functional imaging studies of subjects with cognitive impairment or dementia due to white matter lesions have also indicated that the frontal cortex tends to be most severely involved (De Reuck et al. 1992; Tohgi et al. 1991; Ujike et al. 1985). An emerging view from those studies is that the occurrence and severity of mental changes are correlated with decreased cerebral blood flow and oxygen metabolism in cortical regions, especially the frontal lobes (De Reuck et al. 1992; Yao et al. 1990), consistent with the suggestion that disconnection between cortical and subcortical structures from intervening ischemic white matter damage accounts for the dementia (Kawamura et al. 1991; Román 1985; Tatemichi 1990b; Yao et al. 1990).

Can Cerebrovascular Disease Cause Cognitive Impairment in the Absence of Clinically Evident Stroke?

While vascular dementia typically follows one or more clinically obvious brain infarctions, the results of two recent studies suggest that it can also be present in subjects without a history of stroke. With the assistance of a number of investigators throughout the world, we pooled all available clinical and pathologic data to investigate the utility of the Hachinski Ischemic Score in distinguishing among patients with multi-infarct dementia, AD, and mixed dementia (Tatemichi et al. 1995b). Although our primary finding, that the Hachinski Ischemic Score is a sensitive and specific scale for use in distinguishing between patients with multi-infarct dementia and AD, may be of interest, it is perhaps of greater importance to the present discussion to note that 35% of subjects meeting pathologic criteria for multi-infarct dementia had no history of clinically evident stroke. Additionally, in a population-based study of the incidence of dementia in which 828 subjects without dementia age 65 and older were followed for 7 years (Yoshitake et al. 1995), multiple lacunar infarcts were recognized at autopsy in 41.9% of the patients who developed vascular dementia. Similar to the findings of our meta-analysis, half of those patients had no history of prior clinically evident stroke.

White matter disease, or leukoaraiosis, is a common finding on brain imaging in the clinically stroke-free elderly, but its importance as a basis for cognitive impairment remains unclear. The results of studies focusing on this issue have been inconsistent due to differences in brain imaging techniques; the definition of lesions and method for characterizing their severity; neuropsychological assessment procedures, including whether subcortical or executive functions were examined; the selection of subjects, including whether healthy elderly or stroke patients were examined; and problems with sample size. Quantitative lesion analyses using magnetic resonance imaging (MRI) have suggested that correlations with cognitive impairment may in part depend on the extent of white matter changes as measured by area (Boone et al. 1992; Liu et al. 1992), a severity rating (Bowen et al. 1990), or a lesion-to-brain ratio (Bondareff et al. 1990). In one study of healthy elderly subjects (Boone et al. 1992), the threshold area for cognitive impairment was large (i.e., >10 cm^2), consistent with the results of Liu et al. (1992), who studied stroke patients and found that the mean area of white matter lesion in those with dementia was 26.7 cm^2 compared to 2.5 cm^2 in patients without dementia. It should be emphasized, however, that when white matter disease affects cognitive function, the effects tend to be subtle (Boone et al. 1992). Typically, deficits in executive function (Boone et al. 1992; Gupta et al. 1988) or speed of mental processing (Junqué et al. 1990) have been found, suggesting subcortical dysfunction.

Other studies have examined risk factors for cerebrovascular disease as determinants of cognitive function in the clinically stroke-free elderly in order to identify the earliest neurologic consequences of exposure (Bornstein and Kelly 1991). In our own work, we have investigated the effects of a variety of risk factors for cerebrovascular disease (i.e., hypertension, diabetes mellitus, myocardial infarction, angina, hypercholesterolemia, and cigarette smoking) on cognitive function in our clinically stroke-free control cohort of 249 subjects, who were given tests of memory, orientation, language, visuospatial function, abstract reasoning, and attentional skills (Desmond et al. 1993). We found that diabetes mellitus was independently associated with deficits in abstract reasoning (odds ratio, 10.9; 95% confidence interval, 2.2 to 54.9) and visuospatial function (odds ratio, 3.5; 95% confidence interval, 1.2 to 10.7), while hypercholesterolemia was associated with deficits in memory function (odds ratio, 3.0; 95% confidence interval, 1.4 to 6.6).

One possible explanation for the cognitive dysfunction that we recognized in our control cohort is the presence of clinically silent brain lesions resulting from chronic exposure to risk factors for cerebrovascular disease (Matsubayashi et al. 1992). Elevated levels of plasma lipids and diabetes mellitus have been reported to be associated with microcirculatory disturbances; microangiopathy, sometimes resulting in lacunar infarction; and, in severe cases, subcortical arteriosclerotic encephalopathy (Schneider and Kiesewetter 1988). In an imaging study of 246 neurologically normal adults, silent lacunar infarctions were noted in 13% of the subjects, with a history of hypertension, mean arterial blood pressure, retinal artery sclerosis, and demographic factors significantly related to presence of the lesions (Kobayashi et al. 1991). In the Framingham study, glucose intolerance was the only significant correlate of imaged but clinically silent lesions in patients with first stroke (Kase et al. 1989b). In other studies of subjects with (Awad et al. 1987) and without (Lechner et al. 1988) symptoms of cerebrovascular disease, a significant relationship has been noted between number of risk factors and number of silent or incidental infarctions noted on brain imaging, but the role of specific risk factors in producing those lesions was not investigated.

Does Progressive Cognitive Decline Occur Due to Cerebrovascular Disease?

Given that patients with vascular dementia are at significantly increased risk of early death relative to stroke patients without dementia (Tatemichi et al. 1994a) and patients with AD (Barclay et al. 1985; Katzman et al. 1994; Mölsä et al. 1995), community-based studies of the prevalence of vascular dementia may tend to underestimate the magnitude of the risk imposed by cerebrovascular disease. Although studies of the incidence of vascular dementia can provide a more accurate estimate of that risk, few such studies have been conducted. We have prospectively examined the 185 patients in our baseline cohort who were found to be free of dementia 3 months after stroke and compared them with 241 stroke-free control subjects who were also free of dementia with regard to new dementia recognized at subsequent annual examinations (Tatemichi et al. 1994b). We found that the incidence of dementia was 8.4 per 100 person-years in the stroke group and 1.3 per 100 person-years in the control group. The cumulative proportion ($\pm$SE) surviving without dementia after 52 or fewer months of follow-up was 66.3% $\pm$ 5.5% for the stroke sample and 90.3% $\pm$ 4.3% for the control sample. These results are illustrated graphically with survival curves, which are significantly different by the log rank test ($P < .001$), in Figure 8–2. In a Cox proportional hazards analysis, the relative risk of dementia associated with stroke compared to controls was 5.5

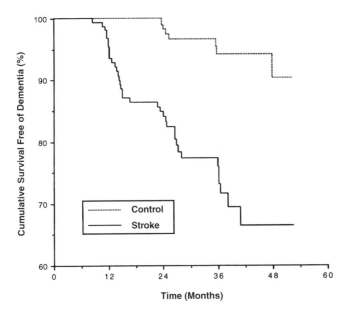

Figure 8–2. Cumulative proportions of stroke and control subjects surviving free of dementia during follow-up of ≤52 months.
Source. Reprinted from Tatemichi TK, Paik M, Bagiella E, et al.: "Risk of Dementia After Stroke in a Hospitalized Cohort: Results of a Longitudinal Study." Neurology 44:1885–1891, 1994. Used with permission.

(95% confidence interval, 2.5 to 11.1), while adjusting for demographic factors.

Although studies performed by other investigators have utilized methods different from our own, their results serve as additional evidence for an elevated risk of delayed dementia associated with cerebrovascular disease. Among studies that have prospectively examined stroke cohorts without stroke-free reference groups, Kotila et al. (1986) recognized new dementia in 5.8% of a sample of patients under the age of 65 who were followed for 4 years after stroke, while Aronovich et al. (1992) recognized new dementia in 24.0% of a sample of stroke patients initially free of dementia followed for 3 years after their first strokes. In the Stroke Data Bank Cohort, the probability of new dementia at 1 year was 5.4% and 10.4% for patients ages 60 and 90, respectively, adjusted for the significant effects of prior stroke, cortical atrophy, and atherothrombotic stroke subtype (Tatemichi et al. 1990a).

Other incidence studies have used varied definitions of cerebrovascular disease as an exposure. An elevated risk of dementia has been recognized in patients with only risk factors for stroke (Rogers et al. 1986), for example, while a further increase in risk has been reported in patients with a history of stroke in a community-based study (Katzman et al. 1989), suggesting that increasing levels of cerebrovascular disease may be associated with a corresponding increase in the risk of dementia. In a population-based incidence study performed in Rochester, Minnesota, using the medical records of 971 patients seen from 1960 to 1984 who had been free of dementia before their first cerebral infarction, Kokmen et al. (1996) found that the standardized morbidity ratio for new dementia was 8.6 (95% confidence interval, 6.6 to 10.7) for patients in the first year after first infarction, with the rate of new dementia approximately doubled during up to 24 years of subsequent follow-up. They also reported that the incidence of clinically diagnosed AD was approximately 50% greater in this cohort than would have been expected in the population as a whole, suggesting that stroke may have acted as a catalyst for the earlier expression of AD or, alternatively, that a bias favoring the detection of AD in patients with stroke may have been present.

Certain subgroups of stroke patients may be at particularly high risk of cognitive decline; potential mechanisms are listed in Table 8–3. While it is likely that patients with clinically evident recurrent strokes most frequently exhibit the stereotypic pattern of stepwise progression of vascular dementia (Loeb et al. 1992), it is also possible for clinically silent recurrent brain infarction to serve as a basis for cognitive decline. Meyer et al. (1995) followed a sample of 24 patients for a mean duration of 42 months following stroke. Although none of those patients had experienced a clinically evident recurrent stroke, follow-up CT scans revealed that four of them (16.7%) had experienced clinically silent recurrent brain infarctions, with cognitive decline observed in all of those patients in association with new lesions involving the frontal white matter and thalamus. In contrast, among patients receiving treatment for the prevention of recurrent stroke, 67.0% exhibited improvement or stability of cognitive function as assessed with a mental status test while 33.0% declined. Improvement or decline on that mental status test was associated with comparable changes in perfusion within the frontal white matter, thalamus, and internal capsule. These interesting and important findings suggest that patients may exhibit gradually progressive cognitive decline in association with clinically silent recurrent stroke, mimicking the stereotypic course of AD, and that decline may be arrested or prevented in such patients by the initiation of stroke prophylaxis. It is also worthy of note that cognitive impairment may be a significant risk factor for recurrent stroke (Moroney et al. 1995b), however, suggesting that a bidirectional pathway may exist in which recurrent stroke, whether clinically evident or clinically silent, may result in cogni-

---

Table 8–3.   Potential mechanisms of progressive cognitive decline in patients with cerebrovascular disease

---

▮ Clinically evident recurrent stroke
▮ Progressive but silent cerebrovascular disease
▮ Events or disorders causing global cerebral hypoxia or ischemia
▮ Stroke as a catalyst for the expression of Alzheimer's disease
▮ Borderline intellectual function leading to crossover

---

tive decline and delayed dementia, which may then lead to further recurrences.

We would also like to highlight an additional potential mechanism of cognitive decline in patients with stroke, that of supply failure. First, we have investigated the hypothesis that events or conditions that may cause global cerebral hypoxia or ischemia (e.g., seizures, cardiac arrhythmias, congestive heart failure, pneumonia) place stroke patients at elevated risk of delayed dementia (Moroney et al. 1995a). After adjusting for demographic factors, recurrent stroke, and baseline cognitive function in a Cox proportional hazards analysis, we identified a significant association between those events or conditions and new dementia, with a relative risk of 4.3 (95% confidence interval, 1.9 to 9.6). We have also specifically examined ischemic cardiac disease as a potential correlate of cognitive decline, as assessed with the Mini-Mental State Examination (MMSE), in our stroke cohort (Tatemichi et al. 1994c). Using random effects analysis, we found that a history of ischemic cardiac disease was significantly associated with a more rapid decline in performance on that mental status test. Consistent with our findings and the concept of a cardiogenic or hypoperfusion dementia, Sulkava and Erkinjuntti (1987) have reported that 4.5% of patients with a clinical diagnosis of vascular dementia had cerebral hypoperfusion resulting from cardiac arrhythmias or systemic hypotension. Similarly, Skoog et al. (1993) have reported that among 147 85-year-old subjects with dementia, 4.1% had cerebral hypoperfusion as the primary basis for their dementia syndrome. Among 175 consecutively examined patients with dementia in a study conducted by Brun (1994), 21.7% had dementia associated with hypoperfusion due to either selective incomplete white matter infarction or borderzone infarction.

Although it is understood that dementia may result from occlusion of the internal carotid arteries through the mechanism of multifocal infarction in the borderzone territories, a less commonly recognized basis for intellectual decline from internal carotid artery occlusion is chronic ischemia due to hemodynamic insufficiency (Ferguson and Peerless 1976; Fisher 1951; Leblanc et al. 1987; Paulson et al. 1966; Tsuda et al. 1994; Yanagihara et al. 1990).

A patient whom we have studied (Tatemichi et al. 1995a) will serve to illustrate this additional potential basis for dementia resulting from supply failure. A 55-year-old man with bilateral internal carotid and unilateral vertebral artery occlusions presented subacutely with profound behavioral and personality changes featuring frontal lobe deficits. While structural brain imaging demonstrated only a small right superior frontal infarction, neuropsychological testing revealed severe cognitive impairment consistent with dementia. Cerebral blood flow was severely reduced, with profound hypofrontality and limited hypercapnic reactivity. Positron emission tomography (PET) revealed that cerebral metabolism was also reduced, primarily in the medial frontal lobes bilaterally. Following right-sided extracranial-to-intracranial bypass surgery, both cerebral blood flow and metabolism improved, as did the patient's behavioral and neuropsychological deficits. The magnitude of the changes was striking and exceeded the improvement expected as part of the natural history of acute cerebral infarction. Thus, perfusion insufficiency from bilateral carotid occlusions, with secondarily reduced metabolism in the frontal lobes bilaterally, may have been an unusual cause of a reversible dementia syndrome in our patient.

No discussion of progressive forms of vascular dementia would be complete without a mention of Binswanger's disease. In a review of all cases published in the international literature between 1912 and 1986, Babikian and Ropper (1987) identified only 47 patients with pathologically verified Binswanger's disease, suggesting that it is a rare disorder. They noted that patients tended to be elderly and hypertensive and typically exhibited a syndrome that included cognitive dysfunction, focal motor signs, and pseudobulbar characteristics such as gait difficulty and incontinence. Brain imaging studies typically revealed multiple lacunar infarctions and leukoaraiosis. The clinical course of these patients tended to be slowly progressive, although it may sometimes have been interrupted by strokes followed by partial recovery. Given that patients with this disorder exhibit a characteristic syndrome with coexistent lacunar infarctions and leukoaraiosis, Binswanger's disease should be considered to be distinct from multi-infarct dementia and an important, although uncommon, basis for progressive cognitive decline in patients with cerebrovascular disease.

Finally, we would like to comment on certain contributions of genetics research to the study of vascular dementia. Recently, a progressive syndrome of cerebral autosomal dominant arteriopathy with subcortical infarcts and leukoencephalopathy (CADASIL) mapping to chromosome 19 (Tournier-Lasserve et al. 1993) has been reported. Tournier-Lasserve et al. (1991) studied 45 members of a single family both clinically and with brain imaging. They found that nine members of that family had a history of strokelike episodes or stroke beginning between the ages of 30 and 60, with MRI evidence of small, deep infarcts and widespread white matter disease. In addition to other clinical problems, two of those individuals had dementia. Although eight other family members were clinically normal, they were also found to have widespread white matter disease. Pathologic studies based on one family member noted that the underlying lesions in this disorder tended to involve the small cerebral arteries and appeared to be similar to those described in some cases of hereditary multi-infarct dementia (Baudrimont et al. 1993). In a study of 148 members of seven families in France, Chabriat et al. (1995) found that 45 subjects were clinically affected, with recurrent subcortical ischemic events in 84%, progressive subcortical dementia with pseudobulbar features in 31%, migraine with aura in 22%, and mood disorders with severe depressive episodes in 20%. All symptomatic subjects and 19 asymptomatic subjects had hyperintense lesions in the subcortical white matter and basal ganglia on MRI.

Other genetics studies have focused on the role of the apolipoprotein E polymorphism, which has also been examined as a potential marker for AD (Mayeux et al. 1993; Saunders et al. 1993). It has been reported that the ε4 allele may be associated with a predisposition toward atherosclerosis and ischemic cerebrovascular disease (Pedro-Botet et al. 1992) and that the frequency of the ε4 allele may be greater in patients with vascular dementia relative to control subjects (Frisoni et al. 1994a,b; Noguchi et al. 1993; Shimano et al. 1989) and comparable in vascular dementia and AD (Frisoni et al. 1994a,b; Noguchi et al. 1993). Other studies have found no association (Kawamata et al. 1994; Lucotte et al. 1995), however, suggesting that more work will need to be done before definitive conclusions might be drawn.

Summary and Conclusions

When dementia results from cerebrovascular disease, cognitive decline usually follows one or more clinically obvious strokes. Specific brain lesions are probably necessary for dementia to occur, such as those exceeding a volume threshold or those located in specific regions important for mental function, but they are not sufficient. The host must be susceptible, and other risk factors may be involved. Small, deep infarcts may produce a *strategic infarct dementia* due to cortical deactivation resulting from disconnection or diaschisis. White matter lesions or leukoaraiosis may also cause cognitive impairment, but the mental changes are often subtle.

Although the course of dementia after stroke is generally stable, and in some cases remitting, certain patients are at risk of developing delayed dementia following a clinically obvious stroke. Potential correlates of cognitive decline include recurrent stroke, whether clinically evident or silent; events or conditions associated with global cerebral hypoxia or ischemia; and borderline intellectual function, with stroke facilitating crossover into dementia. Stroke may also accelerate the clinical expression of AD.

There is increasing evidence that vascular dementia is not a unitary phenomenon, and research efforts should continue to be directed toward the description of subtypes of that disorder. The findings of such investigations could have important implications for interventional studies, because it is likely that treatments would need to be targeted to specific subtypes of vascular dementia to be effective. Several future approaches should be considered, including a more detailed analysis of risk factors for early versus delayed dementia after stroke; the role of single small infarcts, both clinically evident and clinically silent, in causing dementia; and the possibility that some dementia syndromes are reversible. Further investigation of the concept of supply failure as a basis for vascular dementia, as well as the role of genetic factors, should also be pursued.

References

Alzheimer A: Die arteriosklertische Atrophie des Gehirns. Allgemeine Zeitschrift für Psychiatrie 51:809–812, 1895

American Psychiatric Association: Diagnostic and Statistical Manual of Mental Disorders, 3rd Edition, Revised. Washington, DC, American Psychiatric Association, 1987

American Psychiatric Association: Diagnostic and Statistical Manual of Mental Disorders, 4th Edition. Washington, DC, American Psychiatric Association, 1994

Aronovich BD, Treves TA, Bornstein NM, Korczyn AD: Dementia after first stroke: 3-years survival analysis. Cerebrovascular Diseases 2:216, 1992

Awad IA, Spetzler RF, Hodak JA, et al: Incidental lesions noted on magnetic resonance imaging of the brain: prevalence and clinical significance in various age groups. Neurosurgery 20:222–227, 1987

Babikian V, Ropper AH: Binswanger's disease: a review. Stroke 18:2–12, 1987

Barclay LL, Zemcov A, Blass JP, Sansone J: Survival in Alzheimer's disease and vascular dementias. Neurology 35:834–840, 1985

Baudrimont M, Dubas F, Joutel A, et al: Autosomal dominant leukoencephalopathy and subcortical ischemic stroke: a clinicopathological study. Stroke 24:122–125, 1993

Binswanger O: Die Abgrenzung der allgemeinen progressiven Paralyse. Berliner Klinische Wochenschrift 31:1103–1105, 1137–1139, 1180–1186, 1894

Bondareff W, Raval J, Woo B, et al: Magnetic resonance imaging and the severity of dementia in older adults. Arch Gen Psychiatry 47:47–51, 1990

Boone KB, Miller BL, Lasser IM, et al: Neuropsychological correlates of white-matter lesions in healthy elderly subjects: a threshold effect. Arch Neurol 49:549–554, 1992

Bornstein RA, Kelly MP: Risk factors for stroke and neuropsychological performance, in Neurobehavioral Aspects of Cerebrovascular Disease.

Edited by Bornstein RA, Brown GG. New York, Oxford University Press, 1991, pp 182–201

Bowen BC, Barker WW, Loewenstein DA, et al: MR signal abnormalities in memory disorder and dementia. AJNR Am J Neuroradiol 11:283–290, 1990

Brun A: Pathology and pathophysiology of cerebrovascular dementia: pure subgroups of obstructive and hypoperfusive etiology. Dementia 5: 145–147, 1994

Chabriat H, Vahedi K, Iba-Zizen MT, et al: Clinical spectrum of CADASIL: a study of 7 families. Lancet 346:934–939, 1995

Chui HC: Dementia: a review emphasizing clinicopathologic correlation and brain-behavior relationships. Arch Neurol 46:806–814, 1989

De Reuck J, Decoo D, Strijckmans K, Lemahieu I: Does the severity of leukoaraiosis contribute to senile dementia? a comparative computerized and positron emission tomographic study. Eur Neurol 32:199–205, 1992

del Ser T, Bermejo F, Portera A, et al: Vascular dementia: a clinicopathological study. J Neurol Sci 96:1–17, 1990

Desmond DW, Tatemichi TK, Figueroa M, et al: Cognitive dysfunction following lacunar infarction (abstract). Ann Neurol 32:240, 1992a

Desmond DW, Tatemichi TK, Stern Y, Sano M: Cognitive dysfunction following first stroke (abstract). Neurology 42(suppl 3):426, 1992b

Desmond DW, Tatemichi TK, Paik M, Stern Y: Risk factors for cerebrovascular disease as correlates of cognitive function in a stroke-free cohort. Arch Neurol 50:162–166, 1993

Desmond DW, Tatemichi TK, Mohr JP. Clinical and neuropsychological findings following anterior thalamic infarction (abstract). Ann Neurol 36:304, 1994

Erkinjuntti T, Haltia M, Palo J, et al: Accuracy of the clinical diagnosis of vascular dementia: a prospective clinical and post-mortem neuropathological study. J Neurol Neurosurg Psychiatry 51:1037–1044, 1988

Ferguson GG, Peerless SJ: Extracranial-intracranial arterial bypass in the treatment of dementia and multiple extracranial arterial occlusion (abstract). Stroke 7:13, 1976

Figueroa M, Tatemichi TK, Cross DT, Desmond DW: CT correlates of dementia after stroke (abstract). Neurology 42(suppl 3):176, 1992a

Figueroa M, Tatemichi TK, Desmond DW, Cross DT: CT correlates of dementia in lacunar infarction (abstract). Ann Neurol 32:266, 1992b

Figueroa M, Tatemichi TK, Desmond DW, et al: Dementia following subcortical stroke: the role of infarct location. Neurology 43(suppl 2): A244–A245, 1993

Fisher M: Senile dementia: a new explanation of its causation. Can Med Assoc J 65:1–7, 1951

Frisoni GB, Bianchetti A, Govoni S, et al: Association of apolipoprotein *E* e4 with vascular dementia (letter). JAMA 271:1317, 1994a

Frisoni GB, Calabresi L, Geroldi C, et al: Apolipoprotein E ε4 allele in Alzheimer's disease and vascular dementia. Dementia 5:240–242, 1994b

Goodglass H, Kaplan E: The Assessment of Aphasia and Related Disorders, 2nd Edition. Philadelphia, Lea & Febiger, 1983

Gorelick PB, Chatterjee A, Patel D, et al: Cranial computed tomographic observations in multi-infarct dementia: a controlled study. Stroke 23: 804–811, 1992

Gupta SR, Naheedy MH, Young JC, et al: Periventricular white matter changes and dementia: clinical, neuropsychological, radiological, and pathological correlation. Arch Neurol 45:637–641, 1988

Hachinski VC, Lassen NA, Marshall J: Multi-infarct dementia: a cause of mental deterioration in the elderly. Lancet 2:207–210, 1974

Hachinski VC, Potter P, Merskey H: Leuko-araiosis. Arch Neurol 44:21–23, 1987

Junqué C, Pujol J, Vendrell P, et al: Leuko-araiosis on magnetic resonance imaging and speed of mental processing. Arch Neurol 47:151–156, 1990

Kase CS, Wolf PA, Bachman DL, et al: Dementia and stroke: the Framingham study, in Cerebrovascular Diseases. Edited by Ginsberg MD, Dietrich WD. New York, Raven, 1989a, pp 193–198

Kase CS, Wolf PA, Chodosh EH, et al: Prevalence of silent stroke in patients presenting with initial stroke: the Framingham study. Stroke 20:850–852, 1989b

Katzman R: Vascular disease and dementia, in H. Houston Merritt Memorial Volume. Edited by Yahr MD. New York, Raven, 1983, pp 153–176

Katzman R: Education and the prevalence of dementia and Alzheimer's disease. Neurology 43:13–20, 1993

Katzman R, Aronson M, Fuld P, et al: Development of dementing illnesses in an 80-year-old volunteer cohort. Ann Neurol 25:317–324, 1989

Katzman R, Hill LR, Yu ESH, et al: The malignancy of dementia: predictors of mortality in clinically diagnosed dementia in a population survey of Shanghai, China. Arch Neurol 51:1220–1225, 1994

Kawamata J, Tanaka S, Shimohama S, et al: Apolipoprotein E polymorphism in Japanese patients with Alzheimer's disease or vascular dementia. J Neurol Neurosurg Psychiatry 57:1414–1416, 1994

Kawamura J, Meyer JS, Terayama Y, Weathers S: Leukoaraiosis correlates with cerebral hypoperfusion in vascular dementia. Stroke 22:609–614, 1991

Kobayashi S, Okada K, Yamashita K: Incidence of silent lacunar lesion in normal adults and its relation to cerebral blood flow and risk factors. Stroke 22:1379–1383, 1991

Kokmen E, Whisnant JP, O'Fallon WM, et al: Dementia after ischemic stroke: a population-based study in Rochester, Minnesota (1960–1984). Neurology 19:154–159, 1996

Kotila M, Waltimo O, Niemi ML, Laaksonen R: Dementia after stroke. Eur Neurol 25:134–140, 1986

Ladurner G, Iliff LD, Lechner H: Clinical factors associated with dementia in ischaemic stroke. J Neurol Neurosurg Psychiatry 45:97–101, 1982

Leblanc R, Tyler JL, Mohr G, et al: Hemodynamic and metabolic effects of cerebral revascularization. J Neurosurg 66:529–535, 1987

Lechner H, Schmidt R, Bertha G, et al: Nuclear magnetic resonance image white matter lesions and risk factors for stroke in normal individuals. Stroke 19:263–265, 1988

Li G, Shen YC, Chen CH, et al: An epidemiological survey of age-related dementia in an urban area of Beijing. Acta Psychiatr Scand 79:557–563, 1989

Liu CK, Miller BL, Cummings JL, et al: A quantitative MRI study of vascular dementia. Neurology 42:138–143, 1992

Loeb C, Gandolfo C, Bino G: Intellectual impairment and cerebral lesions in multiple cerebral infarcts: a clinico-computed tomography study. Stroke 19:560–565, 1988

Loeb C, Gandolfo C, Croce R, Conti M: Dementia associated with lacunar infarction. Stroke 23:1225–1229, 1992

Lucotte G, Turpin JC, Raisonnier A: Association of apolipoprotein e4 allele with late and early Alzheimer's disease, but not with vascular dementia or Parkinson's disease, in French patients. Alzheimer's Research 1:145–146, 1995

Matsubayashi K, Shimada K, Kawamoto A, Ozawa T: Incidental brain lesions on magnetic resonance imaging and neurobehavioral functions in the apparently healthy elderly. Stroke 23:175–180, 1992

Mayeux R, Stern Y, Ottman R, et al: The apolipoprotein ε4 allele in patients with Alzheimer's disease. Ann Neurol 34:752–754, 1993

Meyer JS, Muramatsu K, Mortel KF, et al: Prospective CT confirms differences between vascular and Alzheimer's dementia. Stroke 26:735–742, 1995

Mölsä PK, Marttila RJ, Rinne UK: Long-term survival and predictors of mortality in Alzheimer's disease and multi-infarct dementia. Acta Neurol Scand 91:159–164, 1995

Moroney JT, Bagiella E, Desmond DW, et al: Global hypoxic-ischemic events increase the risk of dementia after stroke. Ann Neurol 38:290–291, 1995a

Moroney JT, Bagiella E, Desmond DW, Tatemichi TK: Dementia is a predictor of long-term stroke recurrence. Neurology 45(suppl 4):A300–A301, 1995b

National Library of Medicine: Cumulated Index Medicus. Washington, DC, United States Government Printing Office, 1989

Noguchi S, Murakami K, Yamada N: Apolipoprotein E genotype and Alzheimer's disease (letter). Lancet 342:737, 1993

O'Brien MD: Vascular dementia is underdiagnosed. Arch Neurol 45:797–798, 1988

Paulson GW, Kapp J, Cook W: Dementia associated with bilateral carotid artery disease. Geriatrics 21:159–166, 1966

Pedro-Botet J, Sentí M, Nogués X, et al: Lipoprotein and apolipoprotein profile in men with ischemic stroke: role of lipoprotein(a), triglyceride-rich lipoproteins, and apolipoprotein E polymorphism. Stroke 23:1556–1562, 1992

Rogers RL, Meyer JS, Mortel KF, et al: Decreased cerebral blood flow precedes multi-infarct dementia, but follows senile dementia of Alzheimer type. Neurology 36:1–6, 1986

Román GC: The identity of lacunar dementia and Binswanger disease. Med Hypotheses 16:389–391, 1985

Román GC, Tatemichi TK, Erkinjuntti T, et al: Vascular dementia: diagnostic criteria for research studies. Report of the NINDS-AIREN International Workshop. Neurology 43:250–260, 1993

Saunders AM, Strittmatter WJ, Schmechel D, et al: Association of apolipoprotein E allele ε4 with late-onset familial and sporadic Alzheimer's disease. Neurology 43:1467–1472, 1993

Schneider R, Kiesewetter H: The significance of microcirculatory disturbances in the pathogenesis of vascular dementia. Pharmacopsychiatry 21(suppl 1):11–16, 1988

Shimano H, Ishibashi S, Murase T, et al: Plasma apolipoproteins in patients with multi-infarct dementia. Atherosclerosis 79:257–260, 1989

Skoog I, Nilsson L, Palmertz B, et al: A population-based study of dementia in 85-year-olds. New Engl J Med 328:153–158, 1993

Sulkava R, Erkinjuntti T: Vascular dementia due to cardiac arrhythmias and systemic hypotension. Acta Neurol Scand 76:123–128, 1987

Tatemichi TK: How acute brain failure becomes chronic: a view of the mechanisms of dementia related to stroke. Neurology 40:1652–1659, 1990

Tatemichi TK, Foulkes MA, Mohr JP, et al: Dementia in stroke survivors in the Stroke Data Bank cohort: prevalence, incidence, risk factors, and computed tomographic findings. Stroke 21:858–866, 1990

Tatemichi TK, Desmond DW, Mayeux R, et al: Dementia after stroke: baseline frequency, risks, and clinical features in a hospitalized cohort. Neurology 42:1185–1193, 1992a

Tatemichi TK, Desmond DW, Prohovnik I, et al: Confusion and memory loss from capsular genu infarction: a thalamocortical disconnection syndrome? Neurology 42:1966–1979, 1992b

Tatemichi TK, Desmond DW, Paik M, et al: Clinical determinants of dementia related to stroke. Ann Neurol 33:568–575, 1993

Tatemichi TK, Paik M, Bagiella E, et al: Dementia after stroke is a predictor of long-term survival. Stroke 25:1915–1919, 1994a

Tatemichi TK, Paik M, Bagiella E, et al: Risk of dementia after stroke in a hospitalized cohort: results of a longitudinal study. Neurology 44: 1885–1891, 1994b

Tatemichi TK, Paik M, Bagiella E, Desmond DW: Cardiac disease as a risk factor for cognitive decline after stroke (abstract). Neurology 44(suppl 2):A381, 1994c

Tatemichi TK, Sacktor N, Mayeux R: Dementia associated with cerebrovascular disease, other degenerative diseases, and metabolic disorders, in Alzheimer Disease. Edited by Terry RD, Katzman R, Bick KL. New York, Raven, 1994d, pp 123–164

Tatemichi TK, Desmond DW, Prohovnik I, Eidelberg D: Dementia associated with bilateral carotid occlusions: neuropsychological and haemodynamic course after extracranial to intracranial bypass surgery. J Neurol Neurosurg Psychiatry 58:633–636, 1995a

Tatemichi TK, Moroney J, Bagiella E, et al: Meta-analysis of the Hachinski Ischemic Score in pathologically verified dementias (abstract). Neurology 45(suppl 4):A239, 1995b

Tohgi H, Chiba K, Sasaki K, et al: Cerebral perfusion patterns in vascular dementia of Binswanger type compared with senile dementia of Alzheimer type: a SPECT study. J Neurol 238:365–370, 1991

Tomlinson BE, Blessed G, Roth M: Observations on the brains of demented old people. J Neurol Sci 11:205–242, 1970

Tournier-Lasserve E, Iba-Zizen MT, Romero N, Bousser MG: Autosomal dominant syndrome with strokelike episodes and leukoencephalopathy. Stroke 22:1297–1302, 1991

Tournier-Lasserve E, Joutel A, Melki J, et al: Cerebral autosomal dominant arteriopathy with subcortical infarcts and leukoencephalopathy maps to chromosome 19q12. Nat Genet 3:256–259, 1993

Tsuda Y, Yamada K, Hayakawa T, et al: Cortical blood flow and cognition after extracranial-intracranial bypass in a patient with severe carotid occlusive lesions: a three-year follow-up study. Acta Neurochir 129: 198–204, 1994

Ueda K, Kawano H, Hasuo Y, Fujishima M: Prevalence and etiology of dementia in a Japanese community. Stroke 23:798–803, 1992

Ujike T, Terashi A, Soeda T, et al: Cerebral blood flow and metabolism in multi-infarct dementia. J Cereb Blood Flow Metab 5(suppl 1):S149–S150, 1985

Yanagihara T, Marsh WR, Piepgras DG, Ivnik RJ: Dementia in bilateral carotid occlusive disease (abstract). Stroke 21(suppl 1):I99, 1990

Yao H, Sadoshima S, Kuwabara Y, et al: Cerebral blood flow and oxygen metabolism in patients with vascular dementia of the Binswanger type. Stroke 21:1694–1699, 1990

Yoshitake T, Kiyohara Y, Kato I, et al: Incidence and risk factors of vascular dementia and Alzheimer's disease in a defined elderly Japanese population: the Hisayama study. Neurology 45:1161–1168, 1995

CHAPTER

Dementia Pugilistica

Barry D. Jordan, M.D., M.P.H.

Introduction

Head trauma has a profound effect on memory function. Several clinical entities of memory dysfunction associated with head trauma have been described (Kapur 1988) (Table 9–1). However, ambiguity exists in the medical literature that delineates the clinical relationships between memory dysfunction and head trauma. Pretraumatic (retrograde) amnesia involves memory loss for recent events that preceded the head trauma and may represent a deficit in retrieval from labile short-term memory. In contrast, posttraumatic (anterograde) amnesia represents memory loss for events subsequent to head injury and probably reflects a deficit in learning, where there is a disruption of memory consolidation for ongoing events that may last for several months. Remote memory loss (retrograde memory deficit) can be defined as impaired memory for information acquired in a normal fashion beyond a period of 1 month. This remote memory loss probably represents a deficit in retrieval of information from the long-term memory storage. Posttraumatic dementia represents prolonged or persistent anterograde memory deficits status following head trauma and could be consid-

Table 9–1.   Clinical syndromes of memory dysfunction associated with
             head trauma

▌ Pretraumatic (retrograde) amnesia
▌ Remote memory loss (retrograde memory deficit)
▌ Posttraumatic (anterograde) amnesia
▌ Posttraumatic dementia (anterograde memory deficit)
▌ Dementia pugilistica (chronic traumatic encephalopathy)
▌ Head trauma–associated Alzheimer's disease

ered a clinical expression of unresolved posttraumatic amnesia. Head trauma has also been noted to be a risk factor or environmental trigger for AD (Van Duijn 1996). DP represents the long-term cumulative effects of repetitive head trauma. I describe the clinical aspects, pathology, pathophysiology and management of dementia pugilistica in this chapter.

Clinical Aspects

DP was first introduced into the clinical literature in the late 1920s by Martland (1928) when he described a 38-year-old retired boxer with parkinsonism. The full-blown clinical syndrome constitutes a variable presentation of dementia and/or personality changes, cerebellar dysfunction, extrapyramidal impairment, and pyramidal tract findings. This syndrome has been described primarily among retired boxers, but it may be anticipated in participants of other contact collision sports (e.g., American football, soccer, and ice hockey) where repetitive head trauma is typical.

Roberts (1969) randomly sampled 250 of 16,781 ex–professional boxers who were licensed by the British Board of Control for at least 3 years from 1929 through 1955. Among the 250 boxers, 224 were examined. Thirty-seven boxers, or 17%, had clinical evidence of central nervous system (CNS) lesions attributable to boxing. Clinically, these findings were relatively stereotypical, with predominantly cerebellar and extrapyramidal signs and less clearly defined impairment of intellectual function. Among the 37 subjects with traumatic encephalopathy, 16 showed some degree of impaired intellectual function or personality change. Two boxers demonstrated definite dementia that was complicated by paranoid illness. Nine boxers had severe memory impairment, and another five boxers displayed slow mentation and memory deficits suggestive of mild dementia. Roberts also demonstrated that the prevalence of DP varied according to age at examination. The percentage of boxers with DP aged 50 years and older at examination was 28%. The higher percentage of boxers aged 50 and older with DP may reflect the prolonged time period after the cessation of boxing required to develop neurological deterioration. Roberts (1969) also concluded that the frequency of DP increased according to other measures of occupational exposure that included the longer duration of career, later age at retirement, and higher number of total fights.

Critchley (1957), in his experience with 69 boxers suffering from chronic neurological disease, encountered various combinations of pyramidal, extrapyramidal, and cerebellar signs, with tremor and dysarthria representing the most common findings. His observations included the following:

1. Punch-drunkenness was more common among professionals than among amateurs.
2. These boxers are notorious for being able to take a punch.
3. They are usually sluggers and second- or third-rate boxers rather than intelligent, scientific boxers.
4. The syndrome is found in all weight divisions but is characteristic of smaller men who might fight heavier opponents.

Spillane (1962) reported on five former professional boxers, four of whom developed neurological abnormalities in later life, while the fifth experienced behavioral changes. Interestingly, four of the fighters had at least 300 fights, and all retired from the ring after the age of 32. Although this study only evaluated five boxers, it suggests that an extended career in boxing (i.e., large number of total fights or boxing beyond a certain age) increases the risk of neurological injury.

Johnson (1969) elaborated on the neuropsychiatric aspects of the punch-drunk syndrome in his evaluation of 17 former boxers. He described five overlapping organic psychosyndromes that he felt were attributable to boxing. They included chronic amnesia, dementia, morbid jealousy, rage reactions, and psychosis. Either a defect of memory affecting the retention and immediate recall of recent events or a progressive, irreversible disorganization of personality affecting cognitive function was noted in 14 of the 17 boxers. Usually the neurological manifestations preceded the psychiatric.

Mawdsley and Ferguson (1963) evaluated 10 former boxers, all of whom had neurological disease that was progressive and began when they were young, usually at the end of their boxing careers or shortly after retirement. Similar to the findings of Critchley (1957), predominant clinical features were dementia with extrapyramidal and/or cerebellar signs.

Table 9–2.   Clinical criteria of dementia pugilistica

	Definition	Clinical examples
Probable	Any neurologic process characterized by two or more of the following conditions: dementia, cerebellar dysfunction, pyramidal tract disease, or extrapyramidal disease; clinically distinguishable from any known disease process and consistent with the clinical description of DP	Dementia and extrapyramidal dysfunction suggestive of parkinsonism with associated cerebellar dysfunction that is inconsistent with parkinsonism
Possible	Any neurologic process that is consistent with the clinical description of DP but can be potentially explained by other known neurologic disease	Alzheimer's disease and other primary dementia, Parkinson's disease, primary cerebellar degeneration, and Wernicke-Korsakoff's
Improbable	Any neurologic process that is inconsistent with the clinical description of DP and can be explained by a pathophysiologic process unrelated to trauma	Cerebrovascular disease, multiple sclerosis, brain neoplasm, and inherited neurologic disorders

Since the clinical presentation of DP typically occurs after the cessation of a boxing career, the clinical diagnosis may be difficult to ascertain and must be distinguished from other neurological disorders. Table 9–2 provides a general outline for establishing the clinical criteria for probable, possible, and improbable DP.

Pathology

Among 15 former boxers, Corsellis (1978) and colleagues (1973) described four types of neuropathological changes categorized as septal and hypothalamic anomalies, cerebellar changes, degeneration of the substantia nigra, and regional occurrence of Alzheimer's neurofibrillary tangles (NFTs). Twelve subjects demonstrated a fenestrated septal cavum, and frequently the floor of the hypothalamus appeared stretched, while the fornix and mamillary bodies were atrophied. The cerebellum was notable for scarring of the folia in the region of the cerebellar tonsils, and there was a reduction of Purkinje cells on the inferior surface of the cerebellum. NFTs primarily involved parts of the hippocampus and the medial temporal gray matter. The substantia nigra tended to lack pigment, and nerve cells became glossed.

Roberts et al. (1990), utilizing immunocytochemical methods and an antibody raised to the beta-protein present in AD plaques, found that retired boxers with DP and substantial NFTs showed evidence of extensive beta-protein immunoreactive deposits (plaques). These diffuse plaques were not visible with Congo red or standard silver stains. Since the degree of beta-protein deposition was comparable to that seen in AD, it was postulated that in DP the pathogenic mechanism of tangle and plaque formation may be similar to that of AD. Support of this hypothesis was provided by Tokuda et al. (1991) when they demonstrated tau immunoreactive NFTs and beta-protein immunoreactive senile plaques in boxers exhibiting DP.

Another important neuropathological observation has been the presence of ubiquitin in the NFTs in the brains of boxers with DP and patients with AD (Dale et al. 1991). Ubiquitin, which has been identified as a component of NFTs in AD, is thought to be a protein involved in the ATP-dependent nonlysosomal degradation of abnormal proteins. It has been speculated that dementia may result from the dysfunction of cells bearing ubiquitin tangles. Among 16 boxers studied in this investigation, 11 exhibited dementia. Among the 11 boxers with dementia, 9 had evidence of ubiquitin immunoreactivity in the NFTs. None of the five boxers without dementia demonstrated staining of the NFTs with antiubiquitin.

Uhl et al. (1982) also presented evidence documenting similarities between DP and AD. These investigators conducted a pathological and neurochemical examination on the brain of a 52-year-old former boxer with well-documented DP. In addition to documenting NFTs in the cortex and the nucleus basalis of Meynert (nbM), they noted a significant reduction of choline acetyltransferase activity in the nbM and in several regions of the cerebral cortex. These findings are similar to those noted in AD.

Although, there are several similarities between AD and DP, Hof et al. (1992) reported that a more circumscribed population of cortical pyramidal neurons might be affected in DP than in AD. In DP the NFTs are concentrated primarily in the superficial layers (II and III) of the neocortex, whereas in AD the NFTs are distributed in the superficial and deep layers, with a predominance in the deeper layers. In the hippocampus, the distributions of NFTs in AD and DP are similar.

Pathophysiology

The pathophysiology of DP is unknown; however, one can develop hypotheses that might explain the pathological substrates for the clinical findings in boxers suffering from DP. The parkinsonian syndrome and ataxia or disequilibrium are related to changes in the substantia nigra and the cerebellum, respectively, whereas the cognitive and memory deficits could possibly be explained on the basis of the changes noted in the hippocampus, mamillary bodies, and fornix.

It has been hypothesized by Martland (1928) that this syndrome is secondary to single or repeated head blows resulting in multiple petechial hemorrhages in the deeper portions of the cerebrum that are later replaced by gliosis or a progressive degenerative lesion. Alternatively, it can be theorized that in order to develop clinical symptomatology of DP, a critical number or percentage of functional neurons must be damaged or experience cell death. Conceivably, a boxer who terminates a boxing career and has experienced some neuronal loss does not exhibit clinical symptoms consistent with DP because he has a critical number or percentage of functioning neurons. However, as he experiences a normal or accelerated neuronal dropout associated with aging, he may develop clinical signs of DP because he has less than the critical threshold level of functioning neurons. This theory would explain why DP appears to progress after the termination of a boxing career and the cessation of cerebral trauma.

Any account of the pathophysiology of DP would have to consider the pathologic role of abnormal amyloid deposition and central cholinergic systems. It has been speculated that potential blows to the head could conceivably produce local changes in the blood-brain barrier that may enable the deposition of beta-amyloid in the injured areas (Merz 1989). Alternatively, cerebral concussion may damage the blood-brain barrier, thus allowing the extravasation of serum proteins that may serve as antigenic initiators of a secondary immune response that attenuates normal CNS function (Mortimer et al. 1985). The role of the cholinergic system in the pathogenesis of DP is speculative. Animal studies indicate that concussive head injury has a profound effect on central cholinergic neurons (Saija et al. 1988). Furthermore, the cholinergic system has been implicated in the pathophysiology of AD (Smith and Swash 1978) and is probably involved in the physiological basis of learning and memory (Deutsch 1971). Accordingly, any theory on the pathogenesis of DP must delineate the interactions among head trauma, amyloid deposition, central cholinergic function, and cognitive impairment.

In addition to the previously mentioned factors, the potential role of apolipoprotein E (APOE) ε4 allele in the development of DP needs to be explored. Recent evidence suggests that the presence of the APOE ε4 allele may promote the deposition of cerebral amyloid in individuals experiencing traumatic brain injury (Nicoll et al. 1995). Mayeaux and colleagues (1995) noted a 10-fold increased risk of AD in those individuals with traumatic brain injury and the presence of APOE ε4. We have described a former world champion with progressive DP, extensive parenchymal cerebral amyloid deposition, and cerebral amyloid angiopathy that harbored an APOE ε4 allele (Jordan et al. 1995). Although only a case report, it raises the question of whether APOE ε4 is involved in the pathogenesis of DP. More recently, we demonstrated that the presence of APOE ε4 was associated with an increased severity of neurological impairment in a volunteer group of 30 boxers with high exposure to the sport (Jordan et al. 1997). Obviously, the investigation of the role of APOE ε4 in the development of DP would require a large population-based prospective study.

Neurodiagnostic Testing

Electroencephalogram.   Roberts (1969) performed 168 electroencephalograms (EEGs) on retired professional boxers and found no significant difference between subjects clinically diagnosed as suffering from the DP of boxing compared with normal former boxers. It was concluded that it was unwise to use a single EEG to support the diagnosis of boxers' encephalopathy. Similarly, Thomassen et al. (1979) compared the EEG patterns of 53 former amateur boxers with those of 53 former soccer players and noted no differences between the two groups.

Computed tomography.   Findings in retired boxers are usually nonspecific and may suggest brain atrophy and cavum septum pellucidum (CSP). Although the clinical significance of CSP on computed tomography (CT) scan in boxers is unknown, CSP may be a marker for brain atrophy (Jordan et al. 1992).

Magnetic resonance imaging.   The utilization of magnetic resonance imaging (MRI) scans in the evaluation of DP in boxing has been limited. The MRI scan can establish the antemortem diagnosis of diffuse axonal injury (DAI) in boxers. DAI, which is widespread damage to axons in the white matter of the brain, is a well-recognized consequence of nonmissile head injury (Adams et al. 1982) and has been noted in boxers (Jordan and Zimmerman 1990). According to Strich (1956), this diffuse degeneration of the cerebral white matter can be associated with dementia in patients following closed head injury. Levin et al. (1985), utilizing MRI scanning, demonstrated multifocal lesions in the white matter of the frontal, temporal, parietal, and occipital lobes in a young woman suffering from diffuse brain injury following a closed head injury. The relationship between white matter changes and the development of dementia needs to be established.

Cerebrospinal fluid.   Mawdsley and Ferguson (1963) noted that three of nine boxers had a slightly elevated cerebrospinal fluid (CSF) protein (50–70 mg/100 ml). The significance of this finding is unclear and probably nonspecific.

Treatment

The treatment of DP is largely supportive and remains to be established. Boxers exhibiting parkinsonian features that interfere with daily functioning should be empirically treated with levodopa or other antiparkinsonian medications. Friedman (1989) reported that treatment of progressive parkinsonism with levodopa produced no effect, while benztropine caused mild mental changes. However, Friedman also cites an unpublished case of parkinsonism in a retired boxer who was responsive to levodopa. The treatment of dementia is speculative. Goldberg et al. (1982) observed an improvement in verbal memory but not visual memory in a nonboxer, experiencing posttraumatic amnesia, who was treated with physostigmine and lecithin. Whether antidepressants or tranquilizers are effective in the treatment of psychiatric disorders associated with DP is unknown.

Discussion

In view of the similarities between AD and DP, the question of whether boxing is a risk factor for AD has been raised (Merz 1989). To further explore the association between AD and DP, Jordan et al. (1990) conducted a case-control study of patients with AD. This investigation failed to demonstrate an increased risk of AD associated with participation in boxing and other contact sports. However, the interpretation of these study results is limited by the small sample size.

Although a relationship between head trauma and dementia appears evident, clarification of terms of DP and posttraumatic dementia as distinct clinical entities with similar or dissimilar pathologic findings needs to be delineated. DP is applied to describe the long-term cumulative effects of repeated head trauma with probable complete cognitive recovery between episodes of recurrent mild cerebral trauma (e.g., concussion). In contrast, posttraumatic dementia implies that an individual has ongoing cognitive dysfunction and a progressive dementing illness after a single episode of more severe head trauma. Strich (1956) noted severe posttraumatic dementia following closed head injury that was pathologically associated with diffuse degeneration of the cerebral white matter. In contrast, Rudelli et al. (1982) reported neuropathological findings consistent with typical AD (i.e., NFTs and senile plaques) in a subject with posttraumatic dementia following a single episode of severe head trauma complicated by a skull fracture, subdural hematoma, intracerebral hematoma, and cerebral contusion. Rudelli et al. (1982) speculated that in posttraumatic dementia, trauma provided a provocative or permissive role in the development of the pathologic AD changes that may to some extent be cortical-subcortical demyelinating lesions indicative of axonal injury.

Conclusion

Head trauma exhibits a profound and detrimental effect on memory function and has been implicated in the etiology of traumatic dementias. The pathophysiology of this association is unknown and will be further elucidated upon continued delineation of the clinicopathologic relationship between DP, AD, and posttraumatic dementia.

References

Adams JH, Path FRC, Graham DL, et al: Diffuse axonal injury due to nonmissile head injury in humans: an analysis of 45 cases. Ann Neurol 12:557–563, 1982

Corsellis JAN: Alzheimer's disease: senile dementia and related disorders, in Posttraumatic Dementia. Edited by Katzman R, Terry RD, Bick KL. New York, Raven, 1978, pp 125–133

Corsellis JAN, Bruton CJ, Freeman-Browne D: The aftermath of boxing. Psychol Med 3:270–303, 1973

Critchley M: Medical aspects of boxing, particularly from neurological standpoint. Br Med J 1:357–362, 1957

Dale GE, Leigh PN, Luthert P, et al: Neurofibrillary tangles in dementia pugilistica are ubiquinated. J Neurol Neurosurg Psychiatry 54:116–118, 1991

Deutsch JA: The cholinergic synapse and the site of memory. Science 174: 788–794, 1971

Friedman JH: Progressive parkinsonism in boxers. South Med J 82:543–546, 1989

Goldberg E, Gerstman LJ, Mattis S, et al: Effect of cholinergic treatment on posttraumatic anterograde amnesia. Arch Neurol 39:581, 1982

Hof PR, Bouras C, Buee L, et al: Differential distribution of neurofibrillary tangles in the cerebral cortex of dementia pugilistica and Alzheimer's disease cases. Acta Neuropathol 85:23–30, 1992

Johnson J: Organic psychosyndromes due to boxing. Br J Psychiatry 115: 45–53, 1969

Jordan BD, Zimmerman RD: Computed tomography and magnetic resonance imaging comparison in boxers. JAMA 263:1670–1674, 1990

Jordan BD, Baker FM, Barclay L, et al: Head trauma and participation in contact sports as risk factors for Alzheimer's disease (abstract). Neurology 40(suppl 1):S347, 1990

Jordan BD, Jahre C, Hauser WA, et al: CT of 338 active professional boxers. Radiology 185:509–512, 1992

Jordan BD, Kanick AB, Horwich MS, et al: Apolipoprotein E ε4 and fatal cerebral amyloid angiopathy associated with dementia pugilistica. Ann Neurol 38:698–699, 1995

Jordan BD, Relkin NR, Ravdin LD, et al: Apolipoprotein E ε4 associated with chronic traumatic brain injury in boxing. JAMA 278:136–140, 1997

Kapur N: Memory Disorders in Clinical Practice. London, Butterworth, 1988

Levin HS, Handel SF, Goldman AM, et al: Magnetic resonance imaging after "diffuse" nonmissile head injury: a neurobehavioral study. Arch Neurol 42:963–968, 1985

Martland HS: Punch drunk. JAMA 91:1103–1107, 1928

Mawdsley C, Ferguson FR: Neurological disease in boxers. Lancet 2:795–801, 1963

Mayeaux R, Ottoman R, Maestre G, et al: Synergistic effects of traumatic head injury and apolipoprotein ε4 in patients with Alzheimer's disease. Neurology 45:555–557, 1995

Merz B: Is boxing a risk factor for Alzheimer's? JAMA 261:2597–2598, 1989

Mortimer JA, French LR, Hutton JT, Schuman LM: Head injury as a risk factor for Alzheimer's disease. Neurology 35:264–267, 1985

Nicoll JAR, Roberts GW, Graham DI: Apolipoprotein E ε4 allele is associated with deposition of amyloid beta protein following head injury. Nat Med 1:135–137, 1995

Roberts AH: Brain Damage in Boxers. London, Pitman, 1969

Roberts GW, Allsop D, Bruton C: The occult aftermath of boxing. J Neurol Neurosurg Psychiatry 53:373–378, 1990

Ross RJ, Cole M, Thompson JS, Kim KH: Boxers: computed tomography, EEG, and neurosurgical evaluation. JAMA 249:211–213, 1983

Rudelli R, Strom JO, Welch PT, et al: Posttraumatic premature Alzheimer's disease: neuropathologic findings and pathogenetic considerations. Arch Neurol 39:570–575, 1982

Saija A, Hayes RL, Lyeth BG, et al: The effects of concussive head injury on central cholinergic neurons. Brain Res 452:303–311, 1988

Smith CM, Swash M: Possible biochemical basis of memory disorder in Alzheimer's disease. Neurology 3:471–473, 1978

Spillane JD: Five boxers. Br Med J 12:1205–1210, 1962

Strich AJ: Diffuse degeneration of the cerebral white matter in severe dementia following head injury. J Neurol Neurosurg Psychiatry 19:163–185, 1956

Thomassen A, Juul-Jensen P, Olivarius B, et al: Neurological electroencephalographic and neuropsychological examination of 53 former amateur boxers. Acta Neurol Scand 60:352–362, 1979

Tokuda T, Ikeda S, Yanagisawa N, et al: Re-examination of ex-boxers' brain using immunohistochemistry with antibodies to amyloid beta protein and tau protein. Acta Neuropathol 82:280–285, 1991

Uhl GR, McKinney M, Hedreen JC, et al: Dementia pugilistica: loss of basal forebrain cholinergic neurons and cortical cholinergic markers (abstract). Ann Neurol 12:99, 1982

Van Duijn CM: Epidemiology of the dementias: recent developments and new approaches. J Neurol Neurosurg Psychiatry 60:478–488, 1996

CHAPTER

10

Head Trauma as a Risk Factor for Alzheimer's Disease

Albert Heyman, M.D.

Although patients with severe head trauma have occasionally been reported to develop Alzheimer's disease (AD) within a few years after their injuries, few if any prospective follow-up studies have been undertaken to determine whether head trauma is indeed a risk factor for this form of dementia. Several case-control studies have addressed this issue. A few of them concluded that severe head injury was indeed a significant risk factor for AD. Other case-control studies, however, failed to confirm this finding. Since many of the early studies comprised relatively small numbers of subjects and various types and degrees of severity of head injury, reanalyses were made by pooling information from several European and U.S. case-control studies. The pooled data strongly supported an association between head injury and subsequent AD. There were few plausible explanations for this relationship until recently. Neuropathologic studies in Britain have now shown a significantly increased deposition of β amyloid protein in the brains of patients with severe head injury, as compared to the brains of age-matched control subjects without head trauma.

The purpose of this chapter is to summarize these investigations and to discuss possible mechanisms for the relationship between severe head injury and the development of AD.

Case Reports

Table 10–1 lists the few published case reports in which autopsy-confirmed AD followed a severe head injury. The most recent case report appeared in 1982 (Rudelli et al. 1982) and described the clinical course of a 22-year-old man who had a very severe head injury caused by an automobile accident. The injury was associated with loss of consciousness, skull fracture, and small acute subdural hemorrhages. After discharge from the hospital a month after the accident, the patient was able to return to work. Eight years later, he was observed to have severe behavioral changes, marked language deficits, cognitive impairment, and myoclonic jerking of the trunk and limbs. He died at age 38, 16 years after his injury. Neuropathological study of the brain at autopsy showed the typical findings of severe AD, with the presence of neurofibrillary tangles,

Table 10–1. Alzheimer's disease following head trauma

Source and year	Age at trauma	Age at onset of dementia	Age at death	Neuritic plaques	Fibrillary tangles
Rudelli et al. 1982	22	30	37	+	+
Claude et al. 1939	50	51	57	+	+
Corsellis et al. 1959	50	51	55	+	+
Hollander et al. 1970	69	69	72	+	+
Khaime et al. 1976	62	64	66	+	+
Khaime et al. 1976	57	58	64	+	+
Khaime et al. 1976	58	69	69	+	+

Source.   Adapted from Rudelli R, Strom JO, Welch PT, et al: Posttraumatic premature Alzheimer's disease: neuropathologic findings and pathogenetic considerations. Arch Neurol 39:570–575, 1982. Used with permission. Copyright 1982, American Medical Association.

neuritic plaques, and other characteristic histological evidence of this disorder. A review of the literature revealed six other subjects who also developed AD following head injury (Claude and Cuel 1939; Corsellis and Brierley 1959; Hollander and Strich 1970; Khaime 1976). The ages at death of these patients ranged from 55 to 72 years, and thus the possibility of a coincidental senile dementia could not be entirely excluded.

Case-Control Studies

An early case-control study of risk factors associated with AD was conducted at Duke University Medical Center and published in 1984 (Heyman et al. 1984). It was designed to determine the possible roles of various environmental factors, prior illnesses, use of medications, and personal habits in the development of AD. Information was collected from 40 patients, almost all of whom had presenile onset of dementia (i.e., before age 65), and from 80 matched community control subjects. No significant differences were found between patients and controls in their exposures to toxic or environmental hazards, animal contacts, smoking, drinking, or unusual dietary habits. As shown in Table 10–2, a history of head injury was seen significantly more often among the patients with AD than among the controls (15.0% versus 3.8%). The head injuries in this study were usually caused by automobile accidents several decades before the onset of dementia. In most, but not all, instances, the head trauma was quite severe, with loss of consciousness, retrograde amnesia, and multiple fractures of the limbs and trunk.

Table 10–2 also shows a significantly greater frequency of thyroid disease in the patients with AD than in the control subjects (18.0% versus 6.3%). Aside from these differences, there were no major premorbid demographic or clinical factors associated with the subsequent development of AD. There was, however, evidence of a genetic factor, which was manifested by a higher frequency of dementia and mental retardation (including Down's syndrome) in

Table 10–2.   Frequency of selected illnesses and accidents
                  in a case-control study of Alzheimer's disease

| Prior illness and accidents | Frequency (%) | | Odds ratio |
	Patients	Controls	
Head injury	15.0	3.8	5.31*
Thyroid disease	18.0	6.3	3.50*
Diabetes	7.5	8.8	0.84
Stomach ulcer	7.5	10.3	0.71
Migraine	20.5	35.1	0.49
Hypertension	15.0	36.7	0.26*
Influenza (WWI)	7.9	1.4	3.65
Arthritis	41.0	36.7	1.19

*$P < .05$. With educational and residential variables as covariates, the odds ratios
for head injury, thyroid disease, and hypertension were 11.52, 6.87, and 0.19, respectively, each with $P < .05$.
Source.   Adapted from Heyman et al. 1984.

the families of patients with AD than in the families of controls.
Two other case-control studies (Graves et al. 1990; Mortimer et al.
1985) also found a positive association between head trauma and
AD. Such an association, however, was not confirmed statistically
in six other studies conducted in recent years. In three of them
(Amaducci et al. 1986; Broe et al. 1990; Shalat et al. 1987), head
trauma was noted more frequently in subjects than in controls, but
the difference was not statistically significant. In the remaining
three cases (Chandra et al. 1989; Ferini-Strambi et al. 1990; Soininen and Heinonen 1982), no association between head injury and
AD was noted.

The data from 11 case-control studies in the United States and
Europe were reanalyzed by the EURODEM Risk Factors Research
Group (Breteler et al. 1992; van Duijn et al. 1992). As seen in Table
10–3, the pooled relative risk of head injury with unconsciousness
was found to be 1.8, with a 95% confidence interval of 1.3–2.7. This
reanalysis also confirmed the original Duke study (Heyman et al.
1984), in which the likelihood of dementia or mental retardation
(including Down's syndrome) was found to be greater in relatives
of subjects with AD than in those of the controls. It also confirmed
the finding in the Duke study that thyroid disease (hypothyroidism) may be a risk factor in the development of AD.

Table 10–3.   Risk factors for Alzheimer's disease: results from the
EURODEM reanalysis of case-control studies

Risk factor defined	Relative risk	95% confidence interval	Exposure frequency	
			Cases	Controls
Head trauma with unconsciousness	1.8	1.3–2.7	87/1,059	50/1,059
Dementia in first-degree relatives	3.5	2.6–4.6	305/814	140/894
Down's syndrome or mental retardation in first-degree relatives	2.7	1.2–5.7	20/588	7/615
History of hypothyroidism	2.3	1.0–5.4	17/655	8/732

Source.   Adapted from Breteler et al. 1992.

One of the major problems in case-control studies of this type is the possibility of biased recall; that is, the patients' families or informants may be eager to find an explanation for the dementia and thus may overreport an exposure, such as head trauma, that they believe to be a causative factor (van Duijn et al. 1992). For this reason, the case-control studies listed in Table 10–3 restricted analysis to subjects with head injury with loss of consciousness, since it seems unlikely that relatives of patients would report such a serious event if it had not occurred.

The design of one case-control study (Chandra et al. 1989) attempted to minimize the possibility of biased recall by reviewing the history of patients and controls in the medical record linkage system at Mayo Clinic. This study failed to find any significant differences in the frequency of head injury between patients with AD and controls enrolled in that institution.

Possible Explanations for the Association of Head Injury and AD

It has been suggested (Mortimer et al. 1991; van Duijn et al. 1992) that head injury may be associated with subsequent AD because of possible damage to the blood-brain barrier caused by severe brain trauma. Such damage may permit entry of toxic products or make the brain more susceptible to the effects of aging, resulting in pathological findings of AD. It has also been suggested that head injury may significantly decrease the brain's functional reserves and thus shorten the time for developing clinically diagnosable dementia. This hypothesis is supported by studies (Gedye et al. 1989; Sullivan et al. 1987) that show that patients with a history of head injury have earlier onset of dementia.

Recent studies from Britain (Gentleman et al. 1993; Roberts et al. 1994) may provide a linkage between head injury and AD. These studies have shown that the brains of patients with severe head injury have a greater deposition of beta amyloid protein (βAP) in one or more areas of the cortex than do those of age-matched control subjects without a history of head trauma. The frequency and extent of βAP deposits increased with age, particularly in patients over 60 years old. A small group of subjects with head injury were examined for evidence of beta amyloid precursor protein (βAPP) activity; the subjects showed a generalized increase in βAPP immunoactivity in the perikarya of neurons in the vicinity of βAP deposits. Although the precise relationship of these newly observed neuropathologic findings to the development of AD following trauma remains to be determined, these findings may provide a useful model for further studies and a better understanding of the neuropathologic changes in AD.

References

Amaducci LA, Fratiglioni L, Rocca WA, et al: Risk factors for clinically diagnosed Alzheimer's disease: a case-control study of an Italian population. Neurology 36:922–931, 1986

Breteler MMB, Claus JJ, van Duijn CM, et al: Epidemiology of Alzheimer's disease. Epidemiol Rev 14:59–82, 1992

Broe GA, Henderson AS, Creasey H, et al: A case-control study of Alzheimer's disease in Australia. Neurology 40:1698–1707, 1990

Chandra V, Kokmen E, Schoenberg BS, Beard CM: Head trauma with loss of consciousness as a risk factor for Alzheimer's disease. Neurology 39:1576–1578, 1989

Claude H, Cuel J: Demence pre-senile post-traumatique apres fracture du crane: considerations medico-legales. Annales de Medecine Legale, Criminologie, Police, Scientifique, et Toxologie 19:173–184, 1939

Corsellis JAN, Brierley JB: Observations on the pathology of insidious dementia following head injury. Journal of Mental Science 105:714–720, 1959

Ferini-Strambi L, Smirne S, Garancini P, et al: Clinical and epidemiological aspects of Alzheimer's disease with presenile onset: a case-control study. Neuroepidemiology 9:39–49, 1990

Gedye A, Bettie BL, Tuokko H, et al: Severe head injury hastens age of onset of Alzheimer's disease. J Am Geriatr Soc 37:970–973, 1989

Gentleman SM, Graham DI, Roberts GW: Molecular pathology of head trauma: altered BAPP metabolism and the aetiology of Alzheimer's disease, in Progress in Brain Research. Edited by Kogure K, Hossmann A, Siesjo BK. Amsterdam, Elsevier, 1993, pp 96, 237–246

Graves AB, White E, Koepsell TD, et al: The association between head trauma and Alzheimer's disease. Am J Epidemiol 131:491–501, 1990

Heyman A, Wilkinson WE, Stafford JA, et al: Alzheimer's disease: a study of epidemiological aspects. Ann Neurol 15:335–341, 1984

Hollander D, Strich S: Atypical Alzheimer's disease with congophilic angiopathy presenting with dementia of acute onset, in Alzheimer's Disease and Related Conditions. Edited by Wolstenholme GEW, O'Connor M. New York, Churchill Livingstone, 1970, pp 105–135

Khaime TSB: Role of craniocerebral trauma in the development of Alzheimer's disease. Zh Nevropatol Psikhiatr Im S S Korsakova 76:1028–1032, 1976

Mortimer JA, French LR, Hutton JT, Schuman LM: Head injury as a risk factor for Alzheimer's disease. Neurology 35:264–267, 1985

Mortimer JA, van Duijn CM, Chandra V, et al: Head trauma as a risk factor for Alzheimer's disease: a collaborative re-analysis of case-control studies. Int J Epidemiol 20:S28–S35, 1991

Roberts GW, Gentleman SM, Lynch A, et al: β amyloid protein deposition in the brain after severe head injury: implications for the pathogenesis of Alzheimer's disease. J Neurol Neurosurg Psychiatry 57:419–425, 1994

Rudelli R, Strom JO, Welch PT, Ambler MW: Posttraumatic premature

Alzheimer's disease: neuropathologic findings and pathogenetic considerations. Arch Neurol 39:570–575, 1982

Shalat SL, Seltzer B, Pidcock C, Baker EI: Risk factors for Alzheimer's disease: a case-control study. Neurology 37:1630–1633, 1987

Soininen H, Heinonen OP: Clinical and etiological aspects of senile dementia. Eur Neurol 21:401–410, 1982

Sullivan P, Petitti D, Barbaccia J: Head trauma and age of onset of dementia of the Alzheimer type (letter). JAMA 257:2289–2290, 1987

van Duijn CM, Tanja TA, Haaxma R, et al: Head trauma and the risk of Alzheimer's disease, in Risk Factors for Alzheimer's Disease: A Genetic-Epidemiologic Study. Am J Epidemiol 135:775–782, 1992

11

Implications of the AIDS Dementia Complex Viewed as an Acquired Genetic Neurodegenerative Disease

Richard W. Price, M.D.

The acquired immunodeficiency syndrome (AIDS) epidemic has provoked one of the most intensive biomedical research and treatment efforts ever undertaken. Naturally, this effort initially borrowed its models of disease pathogenesis and therapy from other disciplines. However, because of its medical and sociopolitical impact, and likely also because it attracted some of the best and brightest investigators and received priority from the National Institutes of Health (NIH) and other funding agencies, the AIDS re-

---

My studies of the AIDS dementia complex are supported by USPHS Grant NS-25701. I would like to thank Dr. John J. Sidtis for his valuable comments and for his help in conceptualizing and constructing Figure 11–1.

search effort has moved from this position of borrower to that of innovator and, in some areas, to that of leadership, particularly in application of newer technologies. AIDS research has thus begun to provide lessons for other research disciplines. In this chapter, I explore how this process of initial borrowing from and then returning to other disciplines applies to work on human immunodeficiency virus type 1 (HIV-1) infection and its effect on the brain. My starting point is the simple conceit that the AIDS dementia complex (ADC) can be viewed as an *acquired genetic neurodegenerative disease*. This view serves to highlight certain similarities between ADC and other neurodegenerative diseases and, in turn, to stimulate interchange of information pertaining to disease mechanisms and sharing of approaches to their treatment. (For the sake of brevity, references to general concepts of HIV-1 disease in this text are to review articles and thus do not pretend to be either comprehensive or inclusive of the original work.)

Definition and Classification of ADC Among the Dementias

The term *AIDS dementia complex* was proposed because it combined three important aspects of a clinical syndrome recognized in HIV-1–infected patients (Navia et al. 1986b). *AIDS* was included not only to highlight the relation to HIV-1 infection but also in recognition of the morbidity of this neurological disorder, which is comparable to other clinical AIDS-defining complications (Neaton et al. 1994). The term *dementia* was added because cognitive dysfunction underlies its most common symptoms and signs and is its most important cause of disability. Although ADC may not fit easily into the contours of dementia defined by DSM IV (American Psychiatric Association 1994), largely because the latter is narrowly based on the model of Alzheimer's disease, it conforms to a broader lay definition that emphasizes "deterioration of intellectual faculties, such as memory, concentration and judgment, resulting from an organic disease or a disorder of the brain" (American Heritage

Dictionary 1992, p. 496). It is an acquired, progressive brain disorder that prominently compromises cognition. The third component of ADC, *complex,* was included because of additional features of the syndrome, including particularly the motor abnormalities that are invariably present.

The combined presence of 1) motor abnormalities notable for early slowing and imprecision of rapid extremity and eye movements, and later by frank spastic ataxia or weakness in some patients, and 2) cognitive difficulty characterized by slowing and problems with attention and concentration provide the justification for classifying ADC among the *subcortical dementias* (Benson 1987). Although this is largely a clinical designation, it may have a biological basis given the prominence of pathology in the diencephalon and deep white matter (Brew et al. 1995; Kure et al. 1990). The slowness of both movement and thought parallels aspects of the other dementias in this class, including Parkinson's disease and hydrocephalus. A simple, but very useful, ADC staging scheme, ranging from stage 0 (normal) to stage 4 (end stage), has been devised to categorize the functional severity of the syndrome (Price and Brew 1988; Price and Sidtis 1990).

HIV-1 Infection and ADC as an Acquired Genetic Neurodegenerative Disease

All viral diseases can, in fact, be considered *acquired* genetic diseases since they are caused by a transmitted, exogenous viral genome. However, this designation is particularly apt in the case of HIV-1 infection because of its protracted course involving long-term persistence and expression of the integrated proviral DNA. As in many true inherited genetic disorders, the effects of this chronic gene expression increase over time, although in the case of HIV-1 infection this relates to progressive amplification of the genome by its replication as well as to the cumulative sequelae of its expression. Eventually HIV-1 replication in combination with gene expression results in a lethal disease, AIDS, characterized by

destruction of selected targets in the immune system and consequent vulnerability to opportunistic infections and other secondary
diseases. AIDS also differs from hereditary genetic diseases, including those causing late-life neurodegeneration, in resulting not
from expression (or loss of expression) of a single altered gene but
rather from the action of a complex viral genome containing structural, replicative, and regulatory genes that together confer its capacity to both persist in the host genome, thereby avoiding its removal, and also to replicate and package itself for transmission to
the next host. These processes exploit the normal host cell ma-
chinery, including particularly that of the immune system and its
regulatory signals (Nabel 1993).

HIV-1 Infection of the Brain

In addition to its critical effect on the immune system, HIV-1 also
invades the brain and causes a primary degenerative disease, although the mechanisms linking infection and brain injury remain
enigmatic in many of their details. Exposure of the brain, or at least
the leptomeninges, early in infection has been well documented by
a number of studies of cerebrospinal fluid (CSF) obtained from
asymptomatic HIV-1–infected subjects (Appleman et al. 1988; Elovaara et al. 1987; Resnick et al. 1988). However, at this early time,
CNS invasion is usually innocent and unaccompanied by clinically
evident brain dysfunction. Indeed, it is likely that the persistent
and continued very active lymphatic infection that is now understood to occur in the period of clinical latency results in repeated
exposure of the brain to virus. Yet it is only late in the course of
infection that florid parenchymal brain infection, true HIV-1 encephalitis accompanied often by distinct multinucleated-cell histopathology, develops in some patients (Budka et al. 1991; Navia
et al. 1986a; Price et al. 1988; Rosenblum 1990). In this setting,
HIV-1 replicates principally, if not exclusively, in macrophages and
microglial cells originating in the bone marrow rather in neuroec-
trodermally derived neurons or macroglia that perform the major
specialized work of the CNS (Dickson et al. 1994). However, astro-

cytes may support limited expression of regulatory viral genes, including *nef* (Saito et al. 1994; Tornatore et al. 1994). Moreover, recent studies using the technique of combined in situ hybridization with polymerase chain reaction (PCR) amplification may indicate that infection is more promiscuous, involving not only astrocytes and vascular endothelial cells but also neurons (Nuovo et al. 1994). Understanding the pathogenetic significance of infection detected by this technique requires further study.

An important additional aspect of late HIV-1 brain infection relates to the role of genetic variants of HIV-1 that are isolated from the brain (O'Brien 1994). These variants are generally characterized by their capacity to replicate well in macrophages and related cells, including microglia, but poorly in lymphocyte-derived cell lines, a property referred to as *macrophage tropism*. Each AIDS patient is populated by a viral swarm or quasispecies derived from the original inoculum that changes over time. An evolving genetic profile results from rapid viral turnover, a high mutation rate conferred by the poor fidelity of the viral RNA-DNA polymerase or reverse transcriptase (RT), and immune selection by the host. Macrophage-tropic variants infect and replicate in the brain during the late stage of disease and are identified in cases of multinucleated-cell encephalitis. However, while this cell tropism is important, it is clearly not the sole determinant of late brain infection, since macrophage-tropic variants are usually present during the early phase of infection without causing brain disease. Therefore, either other changes in the virus confer true brain tropism or neuropathogenicity (i.e., special predilection to replicate in microglia and brain macrophages and to subsequently cause disease) (Power et al. 1994) or infection by such strains must be combined with immunosuppression or other unknown cofactors to permit late, productive HIV-1 encephalitis (Price 1995).

Brain Injury in ADC

Perhaps the most intriguing questions regarding ADC pathogenesis center on how the brain is injured and how this injury relates to

HIV-1 infection (Price 1994; Price et al. 1988). In more severely infected patients, brain atrophy is nearly universal, although often better appreciated by neuroimaging during life than at autopsy (Gelman and Guinto 1992). Diffuse pallor of the white matter is very common and may correlate with the degree of clinical impairment (Navia et al. 1986a; Power et al. 1993), but gray matter changes with neuronal loss are now very well documented (Everall et al. 1993; Masliah et al. 1996). Cortical and diencephalic neurons are reduced in number, and reactive astroglioses and microglioses are prominent. These changes are not homogeneously distributed in the brain (Brew et al. 1995), and Kure and colleagues (1990) and others have pointed out a topological predilection for the pathology resembling that found in multisystem atrophy. In addition to simple neuronal loss, neuronal dendrites are altered, with simplification of their processes, and synapses are also reduced (Masliah et al. 1996). Vacuolar changes may be prominent in the spinal cord and also in the brain in some cases (Petito et al. 1985). Thus, there are several types of pathologies justifying the inclusion of ADC among neurodegenerative conditions, although both gray and white matter are affected.

HIV-1 Infection and the Immune System

In considering how HIV-1 infects and damages the brain, it is necessary to take into account the interactions of the virus with the immune system. Indeed, one can view ADC as an epiphenomenon of the more central interactions between the invading virus and the cells of the immune system. The roles played by the immune system in AIDS and ADC can be divided into three types. First, certain cells of the immune system cells are the principal points of viral attack. CD4$^+$ T lymphocytes and cells of the monocyte-macrophage lineage are the direct targets of HIV-1 and are capable of supporting a variable degree of viral gene expression and replication (Pantaleo et al. 1993). Depending on both the cell type and cell state, the profile of infection may be latent, chronically productive, or lytically productive. Eventually this infection results in selective damage of cell-mediated immune defenses.

Second, the immune system also acts as the principal defensive arm of the host against HIV-1. Immune defenses eliminate some infected cells and reduce extracellular virus by a variety of mechanisms, including particularly cytotoxic T cells (Schooley 1995); they also modify viral gene expression and replication through elaboration of cytokines that can either promote or suppress HIV-1 (Pantaleo et al. 1994). The complex interplay of the virus and the immune system, with the latter serving as both target and defender, evolves over time. After an initial stage of major viremia, active infection is suppressed and confined principally to lymph nodes for a period of years (Embretson et al. 1993; Pantaleo et al. 1993). However, there is gradual attrition of antiviral immune defenses until the late phase when they eventually fail and, once again, high-titer viremia and extranodal infection reappear.

Third, the immune system is a source of immunopathology that may be particularly important in damaging the nervous system. In considering this third aspect of immune reactions, it is important to emphasize that the effect of the virus on the immune system is not simply one of causing loss of function, but rather it entails induction of a more general state of immune dysregulation. As part of this dysregulation, certain immune reactions are, in fact, *increased.* The latter includes increased production of certain cytokines (Pantaleo et al. 1994). Increased concentration of some cytokines and some markers of cytokine activity in body fluids have been well documented for some time and have been shown to be indicators of prognosis. For example, elevated blood concentrations of β_2-microglobulin (β_2M) and neopterin, both markers of macrophage activation, indicate poor prognosis (Fahey et al. 1990). As discussed later in this chapter, these cytokine reactions are likely involved in the brain injury and dysfunction of ADC, and these same markers are elevated in the CSF of ADC patients (Brew et al. 1990, 1992).

Models of HIV-1 Pathogenesis

From the considerations outlined previously, three basic elements can be isolated to begin formulations of ADC pathogenesis: 1) *HIV-1 infection,* the prime mover in initiating and sustaining disease; 2) the *immune system,* with its tripartite role of viral target, defender, and origin of immunopathological reactions; and 3) the *CNS,* with its degenerative pathology (Price 1994; Spencer and Price 1992). Although each of these elements appears to be important, a number of observations raise questions regarding the details of how they interact and how infection eventuates in brain injury. As discussed earlier, HIV-1 and the immune system have a reciprocal interaction that evolves with time from early immunodominance (after the initial viremia) with suppression of infection to late viral dominance in the face of severely crippled defense against the virus. In this late phase, CNS injury may result from effects of the virus or from immunopathological reactions.

Considerable evidence has accumulated supporting the general hypothesis that HIV-1, itself, rather than some other opportunistic infection, causes ADC. However, this evidence also suggests that the virus causes injury by *indirect* mechanisms rather than by simple lytic infection of neurons as in, for example, poliovirus infection. Some of the principal observations leading to these conclusions are summarized in Table 11–1 and have been discussed elsewhere (Epstein and Gendelman 1993; Price 1994; Tyor et al. 1995). A model of ADC viral pathogenesis that takes these findings into account and transforms the three interacting elements into cellular terms is diagrammed in Figure 11–1. This model divides ADC pathogenesis into two principal components: a *primary* component encompassing HIV-1 infection and immune defenses and a *secondary* component dealing with neuropathic processes. This bipartite division is important to considerations of the relation of ADC to other neurodegenerative conditions and to the approaches to therapy to be discussed later (Price 1995, 1996).

Primary Processes: Infection and Defense

The primary processes depicted in Figure 11–1 relate to HIV-1 infection and include entry of virus into the CNS, local infection and replication of virus in an initiator cell within the brain, and a de-

Table 11–1.　　Pathogenetic basis of ADC therapy: hypothesis of HIV-1 causation

Evidence favoring HIV-1 as the *cause* of ADC:
1. ADC is unique to HIV-1 infection.
2. There is precedent in animal lentivirus CNS infection and diseases.
3. HIV-1 infects the brain.
   a. The CNS exposed early, and perhaps continuously to HIV-1.
   b. Productive brain infection can correlate with severe clinical ADC.
   c. Infection has a predilection for subcortical structures.
   d. It involves neuropathic, macrophage-tropic strains.
4. No alternative etiology has been identified.
5. Cell culture and animal models have shown neurotoxic effect of viral gene products.
6. Treatment with antiretroviral drugs may prevent and reverse ADC.

Evidence suggesting that HIV-1 causes ADC by *"indirect"* mechanisms:
1. Productive HIV-1 infection is confined largely and perhaps exclusively to macrophage/microglia.
2. Neuroectodermal cells are largely spared.
3. The extent of productive brain HIV-1 infection is sometimes "less than anticipated."
   a. Infection may be minimal or undetectable in mild cases.
4. Immune activation of cytokine pathways correlates with disease severity.
5. Some HIV-1–associated neurotoxicity noted in cell culture requires the presence of noninfected intermediary cells.

Note.　　For review of these observations and literature references see Price 1995.

fender cell representing the immune responses that down-regulate HIV-1 infection in the brain. A number of questions related to each of these steps remain unanswered. Thus, the form in which the virus enters the brain is uncertain, although most evidence favors entry within trafficking cells (the Trojan horse) rather than as a cell-free virion (Haase 1986). The factors enhancing infection likely involve lymphocyte and monocyte activation that allow their promiscuous entry into the brain, along with alterations of vascular endothelium and their surface receptors (Williams and Hickey 1996). The brain sites of entry at different stages of infection are likewise uncertain. Early appearance in the CSF, along with more direct observations in human and animal models, suggests that the choroid plexus serves as the major portal (Petito 1996). This find-

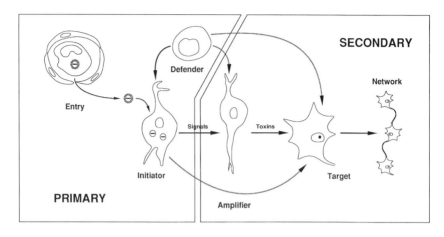

Figure 11-1. Cell model of ADC viral pathogenesis. Model of ADC pathogenesis involving six functional cell types (or organelles) that form a basis for classifying therapeutic strategies. It also divides these processes into two broad groups or compartments. *Primary* processes involve entry of the virus into the central nervous system (CNS), initiator cells that express viral genes, and defender cells that eliminate and reduce infection. These primary reactions are part of the fundamental viral disease process and involve mechanisms parallel to those of the evolving systemic HIV-1 infection but metastatic to the CNS. *Secondary* processes are initiated by products of the virus-infected initiator cell but involve an unspecific host neurotoxic pathway. The functional cell components include amplifier cells that transduce and amplify signals from the infected cell, the primary target cells that react to and are altered by toxic signals from the amplifier, and the downstream neural networks that are physiologically perturbed as a result of changes in the primary target and account for the clinical disease phenotype.

Source.   Adapted from Price 1996.

ing may also partially explain the predilection for viral replication and pathological changes in the deep gray and white matter, if the incoming infected cells then migrate centrifugally from the lateral ventricles into the adjacent brain parenchyma. In late disease, foci of macrophage infection cluster around small blood vessels; this might be due either to local entry of these infected cells or to migration of susceptible monocyte macrophages into sites of already established infection and subsequent secondary local propagation.

The principal initiator cells are the macrophage and microgliocyte, related cell types derived from bone marrow rather than neuroectodermal lineage but migrating to the brain at different times in ontogeny (Dickson and Lee 1996). As noted previously, productive brain HIV-1 infection involves viral variants adapted to these cells. Not only might these cells produce progeny virus, thereby sustaining and augmenting local infection, but they serve as sources of important signals that act on other cells. The genetic origin of these signals may be the viral genome or cell genes that are up-regulated by infection. Whatever the coding source, the model emphasizes the role of HIV-1 gene expression as the force that drives the entire pathogenetic process. Among the viral gene products that have been proposed as putative neurotoxic signals, the viral external glycoprotein, gp120, has received the most attention. This glycoprotein is secreted by productively infected cells and clearly can produce neuronal toxicity both in cell culture and animal models, including transgenic mice (Brenneman et al. 1988; Lipton et al. 1994; Toggas et al. 1994). Other potential neurotoxins include the products of two regulatory viral genes, *tat* and *nef* (Sabatier et al. 1991; Werner et al. 1991).

As cited earlier, other cells, including neuroectodermally derived macroglia and neurons and vascular endothelial cells may also be infected by HIV-1 (Nuovo et al. 1994). However, such infection likely occurs at a very low level or is characterized by an incomplete replication cycle without production of viral progeny. Nonetheless, it is possible that this type of infection could alter important cell functions. If so, cell types other than macrophage-microglia could act as pathogenic initiators, and some of the paths depicted in the model could be short-circuited by more direct effects of the viral genome on functional neuroectodermal cells, including neurons.

While the immune system has several roles, the defender cell in Figure 11–1 emphasizes the protective role in down-regulating infection in the brain. Whether by eliminating infected cells or secreting products such as the interferons that suppress replication in neighboring cells, this system modifies infection and likely prevents its development in the brain until late in the course of systemic infection. It is only when these defenses collapse near the end of the patient's course that productive HIV-1 encephalitis can flourish. Factors, whether endogenous or therapeutic, that augment this defensive activity will reduce infection and brain injury.

The primary processes in Figure 11–1 are depicted as occurring within the brain. However, they also mirror processes that occur outside of the brain. Indeed, brain infection can be considered to be a *metastatic process* involving extralymphatic infection that spreads to the CNS; both the virus and the defensive cells that suppress infection are derived from the systemic circulation. It is additionally possible that these same processes outside of the brain also cause CNS injury. If extracerebral infection produces signals that traverse the blood-brain barrier, particularly if the integrity of the latter is compromised, then the neurotoxic pathway to be discussed in a subsequent section may be activated. This toxic effect is likely to be less potent than that produced within the brain but still might account for the characteristic diffuse white matter pallor and glioses that can occur in the absence of detectable productive brain within the brain. Foci of metastatic brain infection would then superimpose more severe injury because of a higher local concentration of signals and toxins.

Secondary Processes: The Neurotoxic Pathway

The secondary pathway includes a number of hypothetical steps, some likely involving complex cellular circuits, that connect the infection (at the input end) with the disturbed brain function that manifests as the ADC syndrome (at the output end). For modeling purposes, this pathway is divided into several representative cells or steps in Figure 11–1. The first of these is designated the *amplifier* cell, which represents the major link between infection and the downstream neurotoxic processes and serves to both transduce and increase signals. It receives signals from the initiator cell and converts them into additional signals that have neurotoxic properties, either directly or through further amplifying circuits. It also activates a wider range and number of cells, thereby increasing the effects of the signals from the initiator. Its insertion in the model is justified by the paucity of active infection found in some brains at autopsy despite functionally important antemortem ADC (Brew et al. 1995; Glass et al. 1993) and by observations indicating that some of the neurotoxic effects of gp120, for example, require participation of intermediary uninfected cells (Genis et al. 1992; Lipton et al. 1994).

Both macrophage microglia and astrocytes are major cell type candidates for this amplification role. Studies of nitric oxide (NO) neurotoxicity even suggest that NO-producing neurons may serve as neurotoxicity amplifiers (Dawson et al. 1993). Endothelial cells can also be viewed as amplifier cells since their alteration in the course of infection might enhance not only viral entry but also the penetration of toxic molecules from the bloodstream as their blood-brain barrier role is compromised (Moses et al. 1996). Based on identification of their expression in brain or CSF and on cell culture and animal experiments, a number of signals have been identified that might serve as important intermediary signals or neurotoxins, including quinolinic acid and other unidentified NMDA receptor agonists; TNF-α; eicosinoids; NO; pteridines; and interferons and other interleukins (Price 1995). There are thus now more than enough candidate molecules for this hypothesized role in indirect brain injury and others likely will be added to the list. Future work will need to determine which of these are more or less important in patients. A common theme in considering these putative toxins is that most are intermediaries or products of cytokine pathways that involve redundant intermediaries, many of which have pleiotropic effects. These reactions are likely important in causing brain dysfunction in many infections and other neurological conditions that involve immune reactions in the brain, but their effect is particularly enhanced in late HIV-1 infection in which their activation is chronic rather than phasic. In the broad sense, these reactions can be considered to be immunopathological, since they involve mechanisms that are usually part of the host's defense but become

harmful to the delicate CNS when present in unusually high concentration for long time periods.

These neurotoxic mechanisms converge on the primary *target*
cells, which in the case of ADC include populations of neurons as
already discussed and likely also oligodendrocytes. These functional elements that mediate reception, modulation, and generation of signals and assure their rapid conduction are thus altered
as a result of infection and its consequent effects on neighboring
cells that support and sustain the local internal milieu. The phenotype of clinical disease then depends on the particular effects of
these target-cell alterations on neural networks, including on their
character, location, and time course.

Therapeutic Lessons for ADC and Other Neurodegenerative Diseases From the ADC Model

Although the primary processes initiating ADC differ in a number
of respects from those of the traditional neurodegenerative diseases, examination of the retroviral disease may still illuminate
aspects of the latter. Whereas ADC is driven by the complex lentivirus genome, its principal neurotoxic determinant may be the
product of only one of the component viral genes, thus resembling
the mechanism of a one-gene hereditary disorder. The other viral
genes can then be viewed as involved in supporting and modulating
the expression of this neuropathic gene. In fact, these viral genes
likely originate in cellular genes. One avenue of potential therapeutic attack being explored in HIV-1 infection involves attempts
to influence various regulatory genes and their products to reduce
viral replication. This approach might also hold lessons for modi-
fying expression of inherited disease genes.

In considering treatment of ADC itself, the model emphasizes
the principal importance of the acquired genetic material in pathogenesis. Since active virus replication and gene expression drives
pathogenesis, likely the most effective approach to treatment should
be directed at this process, which in fact is being done. Current

therapy for HIV-1 and AIDS involves antiretroviral therapy that inhibits viral RT and protease genes (Concorde Coordinating Committee 1994; Fischl 1995; Winslow and Otto 1995). As with systemic infection, this is also the most promising approach to ADC, with at least one of these drugs, zidovudine, having shown efficacy in reversing and perhaps also preventing this neurological disease (Gray et al. 1994; Pizzo et al. 1988; Schmitt et al. 1988; Sidtis et al. 1993). More innovative approaches are also being pursued, including attempts to interfere with other steps in the virus life cycle, including gene transcription. As these approaches are developed and tested, thought should be given to whether similar strategies can be applied to mutant neurodegenerative disease genes. Ultimately, the goal should be to inactivate, replace, or eliminate the proviral genome or these mutant genes.

As emphasized earlier, the integrity of antiviral immune defenses are likely important in protecting against HIV-1 encephalitis and ADC. A number of strategies are being explored to augment these defenses therapeutically, including cytokine infusion and cell transplantation. Although general damage to the immune system is clearly not a feature of most neurodegenerative disorders, the model encourages examination of whether enhancing targeted immune surveillance might have some place in therapy, for example, by eliminating cells expressing dominantly inherited disease genes. This approach might be feasible if the cells elaborating high levels of mutant gene products could be eliminated safely. Additionally, other surveillance mechanisms acting within cells may have analogous functions to the immune system in protecting cells against expression of harmful gene products. If so, a search for strategies analogous to immune enhancement may be worthwhile.

More clearly shared between ADC and neurodegenerative diseases are components of the secondary neurotoxic pathway. Many seem to be participants in a range of brain diseases, including immune-mediated, vascular, and degenerative disorders. Recognition of this potential commonality is, of course, evidenced by some of the work on neurotoxicity in ADC already discussed involving NMDA agonists, NO, and other mechanisms. These investigations have been guided by observations first made in pursuing the causes of other diseases. In the case of ADC, these neurotoxic mechanisms are linked to immune reactions and, more particularly, to cytokine pathways. While the severe immunosuppression of AIDS results in sustained and generalized up-regulation of certain cytokine pathways, other neurological diseases might activate some of these pathways in a more circumscribed manner. These diseases may vary from conditions that are more closely related and clearly involve immunopathology, such as multiple sclerosis, to more traditional degenerative diseases in which less-prominent inflammatory reactions are likely to serve as secondary, supplementary pathogenic forces rather than the principal cause of nervous system injury. Nonetheless, even in the latter conditions, suppression of secondary inflammatory reactions may have a place in easing morbidity or slowing the pace of disease progression.

Beyond the inflammatory component represented by the initiator-amplifier connection, the mechanisms of neuronal injury and secondary effects on neural networks are clearly shared between ADC and neurodegenerative diseases. They form a final common pathway to cell dysfunction, cell death, and neurological impairment. Efforts at more general neuroprotection and at compensating for cell dysfunction are strategies with potential widespread application and are now being pursued in relation to a number of disorders. Observations related to ADC should be applied to other disorders when possible, and, vice versa, those related to experimental and naturally occurring neurodegenerative diseases should continue to be tested for their value in relation to ADC.

In the case of ADC, therapeutic protocols based on this general neurotoxicity hypothesis have been proposed, and a few have been initiated. They include the use of nimodipine to block pathological activation of Ca^{2+} channels, memantine and dextramethorphan on the basis of their NMDA receptor antagonism, and peptide-T rationalized by its VIP-like neuroprotective effect (Dreyer et al. 1990; Glowa et al. 1992; Lipton 1994). Similarly, more proximally in the pathway, efforts to block cytokine pathways with pentoxiphylline or thalidomide have been suggested. None of these has yet been shown to be effective, but this effort is in its very earliest phase.

On the other hand, a view of this model emphasizes the importance of the primary disease process in pathogenesis and thus as a therapeutic target. While common and therefore potentially serving as therapeutic targets in a variety of conditions, the steps in the neuropathic pathway are nonetheless truly secondary and likely involve physiological processes that are difficult to selectively inhibit. The cytokine pathways also tend to be highly redundant, so that elimination of one intermediary might not have a great effect on eventual neurotoxin production. This is not to say that efforts to target these and the reactions further downstream pharmacologically are not worthwhile but only that their ultimate effect on chronic disease may be limited. The lesson in relation to ADC is that the most important strategy for therapy is likely the one currently being pursued most vigorously, antiviral therapy. If the virus can be inhibited, then the stimulus to the neurotoxic pathway will be reduced. This belief is suggested by the observations that treatment of ADC with zidovudine results in reduction of elevated CSF concentrations of β_2M, neopterin, and quinolinic acid (Brew 1990, 1992; Heyes et al. 1991).

Conclusion

Although there are major differences in the mechanisms underlying ADC and those of the genetic and sporadic neurodegenerative disorders, there are enough shared or parallel processes to allow each to hold important lessons for the other. Work on AIDS and ADC has provided insight into mechanisms that link immune reactions to neurodegeneration. Both the traditional and more innovative approaches that are being developed for HIV-1 should also provide new information relevant to the pathogenesis and therapy of neurodegenerative diseases. It therefore behooves the neuroscientist interested in disease pathogenesis and therapy to monitor the advances in AIDS research and consider how they might apply to their own work.

References

American Heritage Dictionary of the English Language, 3rd Edition. Boston, Houghton Mifflin, 1992, p 496

American Psychiatric Association: Diagnostic and Statistical Manual of Mental Disorders, 4th Edition. Washington, DC, American Psychiatric Press, 1994

Appleman M, Marshall D, Brey R, et al: Cerebrospinal fluid abnormalities in patients without AIDS who are seropositive for the human immunodeficiency virus. J Infect Dis 158:193–199, 1988

Benson D: The spectrum of dementia: a comparison of the clinical features of AIDS dementia and dementia of the Alzheimer's type. Alzheimer Dis Assoc Disord 14:217–220, 1987

Brenneman D, Westbrook G, Fitzgerald S, et al: Neuronal cell killing by the envelope glycoprotein of HIV and its prevention by vasoactive intestinal peptide. Nature 335:639–642, 1988

Brew B, Bhalla R, Paul M, et al: Cerebrospinal fluid neopterin in human immunodeficiency virus type 1 infection. Ann Neurol 28:556–560, 1990

Brew BJ, Bhalla RB, Paul M, et al: Cerebrospinal fluid beta 2-microglobulin in patients with AIDS dementia: an expanded series including response to zidovudine treatment. AIDS 6:461–465, 1992

Brew BJ, Rosenblum M, Cronin K, Price RW: AIDS dementia complex (ADC) and human immunodeficiency virus type 1 (HIV-1) brain infection: clinical-virological correlations. Ann Neurol 38:563–570, 1995

Budka H, Wiley C, Kleihues P, et al: HIV-associated disease of the nervous system: review of nomenclature and proposal for neuropathology-based terminology. Brain Pathol 1:143–152, 1991

Concorde Coordinating Committee: Concorde: MRC/ANRS randomized double-blind controlled trial of immediate and deferred zidovudine in symptom-free infection. Lancet 343:871–881, 1994

Dawson V, Dawson T, Uhl G, Snyder S: Human immunodeficiency virus type 1 coat protein neurotoxicity mediated by nitric oxide in primary cortical cultures. Proc Natl Acad Sci U S A 90:3256–3259, 1993

Dickson D, Lee S: Microglia and HIV-related CNS neuropathology: an update. Journal of Neuro-AIDS 1:57–83, 1996

Dickson D, Lee S, Hatch W, et al: Macrophages and microglia in HIV-related neuropathology, in HIV, AIDS, and the Brain. Edited by Price RW, Perry S. New York, Raven, 1994, pp 99–118

Dreyer E, Kaiser P, Offermann J, Lipton S: HIV-1 coat protein neurotoxicity prevented by calcium channel antagonists. Science 248:364–367, 1990

Elovaara I, Iivanainen M, Valle S, et al: CSF protein and cellular profiles in various stages of HIV infection related to neurological manifestations. J Neurol Sci 78:331–342, 1987

Embretson J, Zupancic M, Ribas J, et al: Massive covert infection of helper T lymphocytes and macrophages by HIV during the incubation period of AIDS. Nature 362:359–362, 1993

Epstein L, Gendelman H: Human immunodeficiency virus type 1 infection of the nervous system: pathogenetic mechanisms. Ann Neurol 33:429–436, 1993

Everall I, Luthert P, Lantos P: A review of neuronal damage in human immunodeficiency virus infection: its assessment, possible mechanism and relationship to dementia. J Neuropath Exp Neurol 52:561–566, 1993

Fahey J, Taylor J, Detels R, et al: The prognostic value of cellular and serologic markers in infection with human immunodeficiency virus type 1. N Engl J Med 322:166–172, 1990

Fischl M: Treatment of HIV infection, in The Medical Management of AIDS. Edited by Sande M, Volberding P. Philadelphia, WB Saunders, 1995, pp 141–160

Gelman B, Guinto FJ: Morphometry, histopathology, and tomography of cerebral atrophy in the acquired immunodeficiency syndrome. Ann Neurol 31:32–40, 1992

Genis P, Jett M, Bernton EW, et al: Cytokines and arachidonic metabolites produced during human immunodeficiency virus (HIV)-infected macrophage-astroglia interactions: implications for the neuropathogenesis of HIV disease. J Exp Med 176: 1703–1718, 1992

Glass J D, Wesselingh SL, Selnes OA, McArthur JC: Clinical-neuropathologic correlation in HIV-associated dementia. Neurology 43:2230–2237, 1993

Glowa J, Panlilio L, Brenneman D, et al: Learning impairment following intracerebral administration of the HIV envelope protein gp120 or a VIP antagonist. Brain Res 570:49–53, 1992

Gray F, Belec L, Keohane C, et al: Zidovudine therapy and HIV encephalitis: a 10-year neuropathological survey. AIDS 8:489–493, 1994

Haase A: Pathogenesis of lentivirus infections. Nature 322:130–136, 1986

Heyes M, Brew B, Martin A, et al: Increased cerebrospinal fluid concentrations of the excitotoxin quinolinic acid in HIV infection and AIDS dementia complex. Ann Neurol 29:202–209, 1991

Kure K, Weidenhiem K, Lyman W, Dickson D: Morphology and distribution of HIV-1 gp41-positive microglia in subacute AIDS encephalitis. Acta Neuropathologica (Berl) 80:393–400, 1990

Lipton SA: HIV-related neuronal injury-potential therapeutic intervention with calcium channel antagonists and NMDA antagonist. Mol Neurobiol 8:181–196, 1994

Lipton S, Yeh M, Dreyer E: Update on current models of HIV-related neuronal injury: platelet-activating factor, arachidonic acid and nitric acid. Advances in Neuroimmunology 4:181–188, 1994

Masliah E, Ge N, Achim C, et al: Patterns of neurodegeneration in HIV encephalitis. Journal of Neuro-AIDS 1:161–173, 1996

Moses A, Stenglein S, Nelson J: HIV infection of the brain microvasculature and its contribution to the AIDS dementia complex. Journal of Neuro-AIDS 1:85–99, 1996

Nabel G: The role of cellular transcription factors in the regulation of human immunodeficiency virus gene expression, in Human Retroviruses. Edited by Cullen BF. New York, Oxford University Press, 1993, pp 49–73

Navia B, Cho EW, Petito C, Price RW: The AIDS dementia complex, II: neuropathology. Ann Neurol 19:525–535, 1986a

Navia B, Jordan B, Price RW: The AIDS dementia complex, I: clinical features. Ann Neurol 19:517–524, 1986b

Neaton J, Wentworth D, Rhame F, et al: Methods of studying interventions: considerations in choice of a clinical endpoint for AIDS clinical trials. Stat Med 13:2107–2125, 1994

Nuovo G, Gallery F, MacConnel P, Braun A: In situ detection of polymerase chain reaction-amplified HIV-1 nucleic acids and tumor necrosis factor-a RNA in the central nervous system. Am J Pathol 144:659–666, 1994

O'Brien W: Genetic and biologic basis of HIV-1 neurotropism, in HIV, AIDS, and the Brain. Edited by Price RW, Perry S. New York, Raven, 1994, pp 47–70

Pantaleo G, Graziosi C, Demarest J, et al: HIV infection is active and progressive in lymphoid tissue during clinically latent stages of the disease. Nature 362:355–358, 1993

Pantaleo G, Graziosi C, Demarest J, et al: Role of lymphoid organs in the pathogenesis of human immunodeficiency virus (HIV) infection. Immunol Rev 140:105–130, 1994

Petito C: Ependyma and choroid plexus. Journal of Neuro-AIDS 1:101–110, 1996

Petito C, Navia B, Cho E, et al: Vacuolar myelopathy pathologically resembling subacute combined degeneration in patients with acquired immunodeficiency syndrome (AIDS). N Engl J Med 312:874–879, 1985

Pizzo P, Eddy J, Fallon J, et al: Effect of continuous intravenous infusion of zidovudine (AZT) in children with symptomatic HIV infection. N Engl J Med 319:889–896, 1988

Power C, Kong P, Crawford T, et al: Cerebral white matter changes in acquired immunodeficiency syndrome dementia: alterations of the blood-brain barrier. Ann Neurol 34:339–350, 1993

Power C, McArthur JC, Johnson RT, et al: Demented and nondemented patients with AIDS differ in brain-derived human immunodeficiency virus type 1 envelope sequences. J Virol 68:4643–4649, 1994

Price R: Understanding the AIDS dementia complex (ADC): the challenge of HIV and its effects on the central nervous system, in HIV, AIDS, and the Brain. Edited by Price RW, Perry S. New York, Raven, 1994, pp 1–45

Price R: Management of AIDS dementia complex and HIV-1 infection of the nervous system. AIDS 9(suppl A):S221–S236, 1995

Price R: The cellular basis of central nervous system HIV-1 infection and the AIDS dementia complex: introduction. Journal of Neuro-AIDS 1:128, 1996

Price RW, Brew BJ: The AIDS dementia complex. J Infect Dis 158:1079–1083, 1988

Price R, Sidtis JJ: Early HIV infection and the AIDS dementia complex. Neurology 40:323–326, 1990

Price R, Brew B, Sidtis J, et al: The brain in AIDS: central nervous system HIV-1 infection and AIDS dementia complex. Science 239:586–592, 1988

Resnick L, Berger J, Shapshak P, Tourtellotte W: Early penetration of the blood-brain barrier by HIV. Neurology 38:9–14, 1988

Rosenblum M: Infection of the central nervous system by the human immunodeficiency virus type 1: morphology and relation to syndromes of progressive encephalopathy and myelopathy in patients with AIDS. Pathology Annual 25:117–169, 1990

Sabatier JM, Vives E, Marbrouk K, et al: Evidence for neurotoxic activity of tat from human immunodeficiency virus type 1. J Virol 65:961–967, 1991

Saito Y, Sharer L, Epstein L, et al: Overexpression of nef as a marker for restricted HIV-1 infection of astrocytes in postmortem pediatric central nervous system tissues. Neurology 44:474–481, 1994

Schmitt F, Bigleg J, McKinnis R, et al: Neuropsychological outcome of azidothymidine (AZT) in the treatment of AIDS and AIDS-related complex: a double blind, placebo-controlled trial. N Engl J Med 319: 1573–1578, 1988

Schooley R: HIV-1-specific cytotoxic T-cell responses. AIDS 9(suppl A): S113–S116, 1995

Sidtis JJ, Gatsonis C, Price RW, et al: Zidovudine treatment of the AIDS dementia complex: results of a placebo-controlled trial. Ann Neurol 33:343–349, 1993

Spencer DC, Price RW: Human immunodeficiency virus and the central nervous system. Annu Rev Microbiol 46:655–693, 1992

Toggas S, Masliah E, Rockenstein E, et al: Central nervous system damage produced by expression of the HIV-1 coat protein gp120 in transgenic mice. Nature 367:188–193, 1994

Tornatore C, Chandra R, Berger J, Major E: HIV-1 infection of subcortical astrocytes in the pediatric central nervous system. Neurology 44:481–487, 1994

Tyor W, Wesselingh S, Griffin J, et al: Unifying hypothesis for the pathogenesis of HIV-associated dementia complex, vacuolar myelopathy, and sensory neuropathy. J Acquir Immune Defic Syndr Hum Retrovirol 9:379–388, 1995

Werner T, Ferroni S, Saermark T, et al: HIV-1 nef protein exhibits structural and functional similarity to scorpion peptides interacting with K+ channels. AIDS 5:1301–1308, 1991

Williams K, Hickey W: Traffic of lymphocytes into the CNS during inflammation and HIV infection. Journal of Neuro-AIDS 1:31–55, 1996

Winslow D, Otto M: HIV protease inhibitors. AIDS 9(suppl A):S183–S192, 1995

12

Brain Imaging in Alzheimer's Disease

Stanley I. Rapoport, M.D.

Introduction

Before the introduction of in vivo brain imaging, information was limited about the metabolic and anatomic brain abnormalities that underlie the signs and symptoms of Alzheimer's disease (AD) in a given individual, and diagnostic accuracy of AD and other dementias was limited. Indeed, structural imaging in the form of computed tomography (CT), introduced some 20 years ago (Hounsfield 1973), contributed to an increase in diagnostic accuracy for AD from 43% to more than 70% (Boller et al. 1989).

With regard to functional imaging, a low-resolution ^{133}Xe clearance technique provided initial evidence for a relation between reduced regional cerebral blood flow (rCBF) and dementia severity in AD (Hagberg and Ingvar 1976). This technique was replaced in the early 1980s by the more quantitative and higher resolution positron-emission tomography (PET), which provided values for rCBF, regional cerebral metabolic rates for glucose (rCMR$_{glc}$) and for O$_2$ (rCMRO$_2$), and regional oxygen extraction fractions (rOER) in AD (Duara et al. 1986; Frackowiak et al. 1981; Malison et al. 1994). Furthermore, PET has elucidated blood-brain barrier integrity, dopamine metabolism, and receptor density in brains of AD patients (Mueller-Gaertner et al. 1991; Nordberg et al. 1992; Schlageter et al. 1987; Tyrrell et al. 1990). More recently, single photon emission computed tomography (SPECT) has been introduced as a less expensive and more available imaging tool than PET (Holman et al. 1991; Malison et al. 1994).

In this chapter, we consider how each of these in vivo imaging techniques has helped to elucidate the nature and diagnosis of AD. Imaging has been especially informative when related to the cognitive profile of the individual patient. Imaging with PET, for example, has demonstrated that resting-state metabolic reductions in specific neocortical areas predict and reflect alterations in neuropsychological abilities that are subserved by these areas (see later section) (Haxby et al. 1985, 1988, 1990). Individual profiles should be taken into account because AD is a heterogeneous disease with regard to severity and the pattern of neuropsychological deficits (Haxby et al. 1992; Mayeux et al. 1985). Dementia severity can be defined by scores on the Mini-Mental State Examination (MMSE): mild, 22–30; moderate, 11–21; and severe, 0–10 (Folstein et al. 1975). Mean cognitive profiles based on severity are illustrated in Table 12–1 (Haxby et al. 1990). Patients with moderate dementia had significantly reduced mean scores on each neuropsychological test that was administered, whereas patients with mild dementia had reduced mean scores only on measures of memory, attention, and planning.

Computed Tomography and Magnetic Resonance Imaging

Quantitative Volumetric Imaging

Computed Tomography

Computed tomography (CT) cannot reliably distinguish AD patients with mild or moderate dementia from healthy age-matched

Table 12–1. Cognitive profiles for Alzheimer's patients with mild or moderate dementia

Neuropsychological test	Controls (N = 21–29)	Mild AD (N = 11)	Moderate AD (N = 13)
Omnibus tests			
Wechsler Intelligence Scale			
Full-scale IQ	126 ± 10	117 ± 8	92 ± 17**
Deviation quotients			
Verbal comprehension	129 ± 10	123 ± 9	102 ± 17**
Memory and distractibility	116 ± 13	113 ± 8	90 ± 15**
Perceptual organization	119 ± 13	109 ± 13	84 ± 26**
Memory			
Wechsler Memory Scale			
Immediate story recall	22 ± 15	11 ± 5**	5 ± 3**
Immediate figure recall	10 ± 3	7 ± 4*	1 ± 2**
Delayed story recall	17 ± 5	2 ± 4**	1 ± 1**
Delayed figure recall	7 ± 3	1 ± 1**	0 ± 1**
Attention, planning, and abstract reasoning			
Trailmaking (trail A), s	40 ± 17	54 ± 30	153 ± 98**
Trailmaking (trail B), s	82 ± 40	192 ± 155*	428 ± 139**
Stroop color-word interference, no/45s	37 ± 8	24 ± 8*	12 ± 8**
Porteus mazes, age in years	15.4 ± 1.6	12.8 ± 3.9	7.7 ± 3.8**
Language			
Syntax comprehension	24 ± 2	23 ± 2	17 ± 5**
Controlled word association	42 ± 2	34 ± 13	25 ± 12**
Boston naming	37 ± 4	35 ± 7	25 ± 8**
Visuospatial function			
Extended range drawing	21 ± 2	19 ± 4	13 ± 5**
Hiskey-Nebraska block patterns	15 ± 4	11 ± 5	4 ± 3**
Benton facial recognition	44 ± 4	42 ± 5	9 ± 5*

Note. Neuropsychological tests classified by cognitive sphere that they are considered to evaluate.

Mean ± SD differs from control mean; $*P < .05$, $**P < .001$.

Source. Haxby et al. 1990.

controls when causes of dementia other than AD are excluded (DeCarli et al. 1990; Luxenberg et al. 1986). This lack of sensitivity is due largely to a marked overlap in brain atrophy between AD patients and healthy elderly (Creasey et al. 1986; Drayer 1988; Kaye et al. 1992). Nevertheless, cross-sectional CT has demonstrated statistically significant reductions in mean gray matter volume and in the mean gray/white matter volume ratio, and increases in lateral ventricular volume in relation to dementia severity (Creasey et al. 1986).

In one longitudinal study, the mean rate of enlargement of lateral ventricle volume on CT (cm^3/year) completely separated a group of 12 male AD patients, (including 8 with mild dementia) examined during a mean interval of 1.4 years, from controls who were examined during a mean interval of 3.3 years (Luxenberg et al. 1987). Rates of enlargement in individual patients were correlated significantly with rates of decline on a composite neuropsychological test battery. In a follow-up study (DeCarli et al. 1992b), the rate of lateral ventricle enlargement (cm^3/year) differed significantly between patients and controls, with a 94% specificity (the ability to make a correct positive diagnosis) and a 90% sensitivity (the ability to correctly exclude AD). However, the diagnostic power of volumetric measurements from two CT scans taken 1 year apart was only 0.33 in patients with mild dementia (DeCarli et al. 1992b).

Magnetic Resonance Imaging

Limitations of CT include its low spatial resolution, low tissue contrast differences, and an artifactual elevation of brain CT density adjacent to the skull ("bone hardening artifact") that renders CT unreliable for measuring subarachnoid cerebral spinal fluid (CSF) volume and cortical atrophy. MRI can overcome some of these limitations, because it requires no ionizing radiation, repeated measures are without known risk, and images are free of a bone-hardening artifact (although MRI scans contain spectral inhomogeneities) (Drayer 1988; Murphy et al. 1993b). A thorough description of MRI methodology and its limitations and advantages is presented elsewhere (Lim et al. 1994). MRI but not CT can be used to quantitate lobar and cortical atrophy as well as volumes of subarachnoid cerebrospinal fluid. MRI is more costly than CT and should be used clinically when CT is considered inadequate for diagnosis.

Whereas a cross-sectional volumetric CT study of the brain demonstrated no significant difference between AD patients with mild dementia and controls (Creasey et al. 1986), a comparable cross-sectional MRI study showed that AD patients with mild dementia had smaller mean cerebral brain matter and temporal lobe volumes and larger volumes of the lateral ventricles and of temporal lobe CSF than did controls (Murphy et al. 1993b), suggesting that MRI is more sensitive than CT for early diagnosis.

Discriminant analysis is a statistical procedure that constructs a linear combination of observed variables that best describes group differences and can classify group membership of any individual. When applied to MRI volumetric data, a discriminant analysis distinguished each of 31 AD patients with mild dementia from gender- and age-matched controls (DeCarli et al. 1995). Age and brain volume were more significant discriminators for men, whereas temporal lobe and CSF volumes were more significant for women. Because 10 of the patients had a diagnosis of possible AD, with impaired memory as the only apparent cognitive deficit, a discriminant analysis using volumetric MRI variables can add diagnostic certainty in possible AD patients with mild dementia using National Institute of Communicative Disorders and Stroke–Alzheimer's Disease and Related Disorders Association (NINCDS-ADRDA) criteria (McKhann et al. 1984).

CT and MRI Densities to Distinguish AD From Vascular Dementia

Of 2,143 patients with dementia reported as of 1988 with a diagnosis of AD and/or vascular dementia with 15% pathological confirmation, 51% had a diagnosis of AD alone, 23% of vascular dementia alone, and 15% of AD plus cerebrovascular disease (Boller et al. 1989). Thus, vascular disease contributes to about 38% of reported dementias, and its distinction from AD is a diagnostic problem. Causes of vascular dementia include arteriosclerotic encephalopathy (lacunar state, multiple small infarcts, large cerebral infarcts), hypertensive arteriosclerosis (including mixed cortical and subcortical leukoencephalopathy of Binswanger), and congophilic angiopathy (Chui et al. 1992; Jellinger 1976). In subcortical disease (leukoencephalopathy), CT and T_2-weighted MRI images demonstrate periventricular and deep white matter changes, referred to as *leukoaraiosis*. Although imaging criteria to distinguish vascular dementia from AD have not formally been incorporated into neuroimaging, published data demonstrate these criteria can be very helpful (Chui et al. 1992; McKhann et al. 1984; Rosen et al. 1980).

The relation between white matter hyperintensities on CT or MRI and cognitive and metabolic function is not clear. Studies indicate that 30%–80% of elderly individuals without neurologic signs have focal density abnormalities in cerebral white matter and that the frequency of these abnormalities increases with hypertension (Chui et al. 1992). Abnormalities, which can be small focal or confluent areas of increased signal intensity on T_2-weighted MRI, are found more frequently than on CT (Drayer 1988). However, cognitive testing has failed to demonstrate differences between healthy aged adults with and without white matter hyperintensities (Almkvist et al. 1992).

Normotensive AD patients do not demonstrate a higher frequency of grade 2–3 white matter abnormalities (17%) than do elderly nonhypertensive healthy controls (27%) (Kozachuk et al. 1990). On autopsy, each of three normotensive AD patients with leukoencephalopathy in life demonstrated the senile plaques and tangles of AD, as well as extensive myelin pallor in white matter in the area of distribution of the white matter hyperintensities (DeCarli et al. 1996). In each brain, Congo red staining revealed striking amyloid deposition (amyloid angiopathy) in meningeal and cerebral perforating arteries but normal-appearing arteries in white matter and in the lenticulostriate vasculature. There was no evidence of hypertensive lipohyalinosis or atherosclerosis in these vessels.

Grading of white matter lesions on MRI to distinguish AD from vascular dementia has been of limited success. In one study, the grade of periventricular lesions could not distinguish the two groups; scores of subcortical lesions, although somewhat better, showed too much overlap to be useful (Bowen et al. 1990). Forty percent of the AD patients did not have subcortical white matter changes, whereas such changes were present in all the vascular dementia patients. In another study, vascular dementia patients compared with AD patients had significantly more infarcts and lacunae, and more focal signal hyperintensities in the basal ganglia and thalamus (Lechner and Bertha 1991).

Magnetic Resonance Spectroscopy

In vivo magnetic resonance spectroscopy (MRS) produces spectra of relatively weak magnetic signals from nuclei of phosphorus, carbon, or nonwater hydrogen (the signals are weak because of the small concentrations of these nuclei). These spectra can provide information about chemical compounds and the energy state within localized brain regions (Shulman et al. 1993).

Phosphomonoesters (e.g., phosphoethanolamine and phosphocholine) are considered anabolic precursors of membrane phospholipids, whereas phosphodiesters (e.g., glycerol-3-phosphoethanolamine and glycerol-3-phosphocholine) are thought to represent catabolic products from the breakdown of phospholipids (Pettegrew et al. 1988). Using in vivo ^{31}P MRS, AD patients were reported to have a larger-than-normal concentration of phosphomonoesters in the temporoparietal cortex (Brown et al. 1989). This observation, as well as evidence that phosphomonoesters and phosphodiesters are abnormal in the postmortem AD brain (Pettegrew et al. 1988; Smith et al. 1993), suggested that regenerative processes involving phospholipids occur early in AD, whereas degenerative processes occur later on. The phosphocreatine-to-inorganic phosphorus ratio with ^{31}P MRS was reported to distinguish AD from vascular dementia patients (Brown et al. 1989).

Disturbed phospholipid metabolism also is suggested by ^{1}H MRS evidence of a 50% increased concentration of myoinositol in the parietal and occipital cortices of AD patients compared with controls, related to an 11% decreased concentration of the neuronal marker N-acetylaspartate (Moats et al. 1994). Because myoinositol is part of the phosphatidylinositol molecule and participates in the phosphatidylinositide cycle (Berridge and Irvine 1984), its increased brain concentration in AD could reflect accelerated breakdown of phosphatidylinositol.

Despite reported abnormal findings with ^{13}P MRS, a study that used ^{1}H MRS to localize and calculate dimensions of a brain volume of interest and ^{31}P MRS to quantitate phosphorus metabolites in this volume of interest when employing internal standards found no significant difference between AD patients and controls in absolute concentrations of adenosine triphosphate, phosphocreatine, inorganic phosphate, phosphomonoesters, or phosphodiesters (Murphy et al. 1993a). Nor was any absolute concentration or concentration ratio in AD related to dementia severity, or to rCMR$_{glc}$ as measured with PET, in the volume of interest. It was concluded that reduced rCMR$_{glc}$ in AD (see later section) is not due to rate-limited delivery of glucose or oxygen to brain and that normal levels of high-energy phosphorus metabolites are maintained even with severe dementia. A quantitative MRS study of association cortex in patients with severe dementia is needed to confirm these conclusions.

Functional Imaging: PET

PET Methods

With PET, a positron-emitting compound administered intravenously is taken up by brain in relation to functional activity or receptor density, where it releases positrons (positively charged electrons). These positrons collide with electrons and are annihilated to release two gamma rays at 180° to each other. Radiation detectors surrounding the head identify by coincidence, counting the quantities and locations of radioactivity within the brain. ^{18}F-2-fluoro-2-deoxy-D-glucose (^{18}F-FDG, radioactive half-life of ^{18}F is 110 minutes) and ^{11}C-DG (radioactive half-life of ^{11}C is 20 minutes) have been used to measure rCMR$_{glc}$ with PET, whereas H$_2$^{15}0 and ^{15}O$_2$ or ^{15}O-CO$_2$ (radioactive half-life of ^{15}0 is 2.03 minutes) have been used to generate rCMRO$_2$ and rCBF images, respectively.

In the absence of acute functional activation or an acute pathological condition, rCBF is proportional (coupled) to both rCMR$_{glc}$ and rCMRO$_2$ (Raichle et al. 1976). During focal stimulation, however, coupling is maintained between rCBF and rCMR$_{glc}$ but appears to be disrupted between each of these measures and rCMRO$_2$ (Fox et al. 1988), implying glycolytic metabolism at the expense of oxidative metabolism. Thus, rCBF or rCMR$_{glc}$, but not rCMRO$_2$, can be employed to quantify focal activation.

Resting Cerebral Metabolism in AD

Data from more than 20 cross-sectional PET studies have demonstrated reductions in resting-state metabolism or rCBF throughout the neocortex in AD patients, more so in association than in primary areas (Rapoport 1991). Reductions were more severe in relation to dementia severity, ranging from −17% in the prefrontal association cortex of patients with mild dementia to −54% in the parietal association cortex of patients with severe dementia. Reductions in frontal association cortex correlated with atrophy of the anterior corpus callosum on MRI, whereas those in the parietal-occipital association cortex correlated with atrophy of the posterior corpus callosum (Yamauchi et al. 1993).

Representative rCMR$_{glc}$ data from the most complete study with a high-resolution multislice PET scanner (Kumar et al. 1991) on 47 carefully screened AD patients of differing dementia severity and 30 controls are illustrated in Table 12–2. With the exception

Table 12-2. Glucose metabolism in Alzheimer's patients of different dementia severity, in relation to metabolism in age-matched healthy controls

Region	Controls (N = 30)	Mild AD (N = 17)	Moderate AD (N = 19)	Severe AD (N = 11)
		$rCMR_{glc}$(mg/100 g/min)		
Association neocortex				
Prefrontal	7.96 ± 1.09	6.59 ± 1.34(83)[a],*	6.22 ± 1.40(78)*	4.69 ± 1.64(59)*
Premotor	8.69 ± 1.16	6.90 ± 1.46(79)*	6.26 ± 1.43(72)*	4.70 ± 1.74(54)*
Parietal	8.27 ± 1.13	6.09 ± 1.37(74)*	5.36 ± 1.28(65)*	3.83 ± 1.46(46)*
Temporal	7.53 ± 0.79	5.98 ± 0.91(79)*	5.63 ± 1.23(75)*	3.97 ± 1.28(52)*
Occipital	7.72 ± 0.94	6.65 ± 1.28(86)*	6.13 ± 1.23(79)*	5.00 ± 1.83(65)*
Allocortex				
Ant cingulate	7.72 ± 1.24	6.71 ± 1.15(87)	6.53 ± 1.41(85)*	5.38 ± 1.72(80)*
Primary neocortex				
Sensorimotor	8.31 ± 1.00	7.27 ± 1.03(87)*	6.75 ± 1.14(82)*	5.61 ± 1.71(68)*
Calcarine	8.06 ± 1.12	7.02 ± 1.09(87)*	7.09 ± 1.12(88)*	6.52 ± 1.89(81)*
Subcortical nuclei				
Caudate	9.24 ± 1.64	8.35 ± 1.26(90)	7.72 ± 1.87(84)*	6.45 ± 1.21(70)*
Lenticular	9.41 ± 1.37	8.76 ± 1.45(93)*	8.71 ± 1.85(93)*	6.87 ± 1.48(73)*
Thalamus	8.99 ± 1.37	8.27 ± 1.46(92)*	8.15 ± 0.94(91)*	6.42 ± 2.05(71)*

[a]Mean ± SD (percentage of control mean).
*Differs significantly from control mean ($P < .05$), corrected for six comparisons.
Source.   Kumar et al. 1991.

of the caudate nucleus, mean metabolic rates even in AD patients with mild dementia were significantly less than in controls. Involvement of the posterior but not anterior cingulate cortex early in disease likely represents limbic dysfunction (Minoshima et al. 1994). At each level of dementia severity, rCMR$_{glc}$ was lower in association than primary neocortices or subcortical nuclei, consistent with reported gradients in neuropathology (Lewis et al. 1987; DeCarli et al. 1992a). Figure 12–1 illustrates that association neocortex is metabolically worse relative to primary neocortex and subcortical

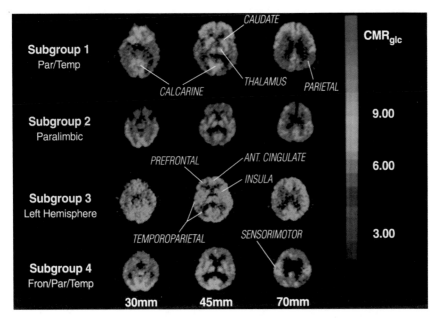

Figure 12–1. PET scan images from 36 AD patients that best characterize four independent subgroups of metabolic patterns. Three planes are shown for each subject: *left,* at level of orbitofrontal cortex 30 mm above inferior orbitomeatal (IOM) line; *middle,* at level of basal ganglia 45 mm above IOM line; *right,* at level of centrum ovale 70 mm above IOM line. rCMR$_{glc}$ scale in mg/100 g/minute.

Source. Reprinted from Grady CL, Haxby JV, Schapiro MB, et al: Subgroups in dementia of the Alzheimer type identified using positron emission tomography. J Neuropsychiatry Clin Neurosci 2:373–384, 1990. Used with permission.

basal ganglia and thalamic regions, regardless of the pattern of metabolic deficits in AD.

In dementia patients with autopsy-confirmed AD, neurofibrillary tangle densities were common in cortical association areas that had the most reductions in $rCMR_{glc}$ before death but were much less common in primary cortical areas (DeCarli et al. 1992a). This correlation is consistent with other reports on gradients of tangle distribution and atrophy associated with loss of layer III and layer V pyramidal neurons in the neocortex in AD (Lewis 1987). Because focal atrophy in AD may artificially reduce PET metabolic values due to partial voluming, anatomic registration will be needed in future PET studies to obtain true estimates of metabolism or flow per gram tissue (Lim et al. 1994; Malison et al. 1994).

Can PET Distinguish AD From Vascular Dementia?

Independently of clinical history and evaluation and of CT or MRI scans, PET (like SPECT, see later section) cannot easily distinguish AD from vascular dementia. Both syndromes demonstrate global reductions in brain metabolism and flow in relation to dementia severity (Frackowiak et al. 1981), as well as heterogeneous cognitive and local metabolic deficits. Asymmetric metabolic or flow reductions that correspond to CT or MRI abnormalities, or reductions in the basal ganglia or thalamus, suggest vascular dementia, whereas sparing of primary compared with association cortical areas suggests AD (Benson et al. 1983). Neither AD nor vascular dementia is accompanied by an elevated rOER (Frackowiak et al. 1981; Fukuyama et al. 1994). However, before the appearance of dementia in some subjects with leukoaraiosis and hypertension (a major risk factor for vascular dementia), rOER can be elevated (Yao et al. 1992), suggesting that vascular dementia can be preceded by hypoperfusion (O'Brien and Mallett 1970). The rCBF response to hypercapnia is normal in AD but defective in vascular dementia of the Binswanger type (Kuwabara et al. 1992).

Metabolic and Cognitive-Behavioral Correlations in AD

Group Patterns

As illustrated in Figure 12–1, four statistically significant patterns have been identified by a principal-components analysis of high-resolution $rCMR_{glc}$ data from 16 regions of 36 AD patients with mild to severe dementia (Grady et al. 1990). The most common pattern (Group 1, 17 patients) had $rCMR_{glc}$ reduced in superior and inferior parietal lobules and posterior medial temporal lobe. Group 2 (paralimbic) patients (8 of 36) had reduced metabolism in orbitofrontal and anterior cingulate gyri, whereas parietal regions were relatively spared. Group 3 (5 of 36) patients showed reduced left-hemisphere metabolism, whereas Group 4 (6 of 36) patients had reductions in frontal, parietal, and temporal cortices. In each group, association neocortex was metabolically spared compared with primary neocortex, thalamus, and caudate nucleus.

Each patient group demonstrated a characteristic neuropsychological-behavioral profile, consistent with the principle that a profile in an individual patient is related to his or her pattern of brain metabolic deficits (Table 12–3). Group 2 patients had poorer verbal performance and fluency than Group 1 (parietal/temporal) patients but better visuospatial performance and spatial memory. Group 3 patients (left hemisphere) had worse verbal memory, verbal fluency, and calculating ability than Group 1 patients but better visuoperceptual performance and drawing. Group 1 patients were likely to be depressed, whereas Group 4 patients tended to show inappropriate behavior and psychotic symptoms. Group 2 patients demonstrated agitation, inappropriate behavior, and personality change, whereas those in Group 3 frequently had depressive symptoms (Grady et al. 1990). PET metabolic patterns are not related to etiology early- or late-onset (Grady et al. 1988), or familial or sporadic forms of AD (Hoffman et al. 1989). Although the biparie-

Table 12–3. Percentage of Alzheimer's patients in each subgroup (see Figure 12–1) showing behavioral disturbances; subgroup is defined by predominant pattern of metabolic deficits

	Subgroup			
Symptom	1 (Parietotemporal) (N = 13)[a]	2 (Paralimbic) (N = 8)	3 (Left hemisphere) (N = 5)	4 (Frontal parietotemporal) (N = 5)
	Percentage of subgroup			
Anxiety/agitation	13	25	20	20
Inappropriate behavior	7	25	0	40
Personality change	13	25	0	20
Depression	33	0	60	20
Psychosis	20	0	0	40
At least one symptom	67	50	60	100

[a]Number of subjects in parentheses (total N = 31).
Source. Grady et al. 1990.

totemporal hypometabolism in the appropriate clinical setting indicates a high likelihood of AD, it is not necessarily specific for AD. Biparietotemporal hypometabolism has been reported in a patient with clinical signs of slowly progressive dementia and Parkinson's disease, who on autopsy had pathological findings only of Parkinson's disease (Schapiro et al. 1993).

Metabolic-Cognitive Correlations in Individual Patients

Based on evidence that extended range drawing and visual recall tests reflect right neocortical function and that syntax comprehension and verbal recall tests reflect left neocortical function, AD patients and controls were ranked separately on these test scores and differences between ranks were quantified as a "drawing/comprehension discrepancy" or a "visual recall/verbal recall discrepancy" to calculate hemispheric functional asymmetry (Haxby et al. 1990). These discrepancies then were correlated with a metabolic asymmetry index, where $rCMR_{glc,right}$ is the metabolic rate in a right-hemisphere region and $rCMR_{glc,left}$ the rate in the homologous left-hemisphere region:

$$\text{Metabolic asymmetry index (\%)} = \frac{rCMR_{glc,right} - rCMR_{glc,left}}{(rCMR_{glc,right} + rCMR_{glc,left})/2} \times 100 \qquad (1)$$

Metabolic asymmetry indices for four association and two primary cortical areas are illustrated in Figure 12–2 for AD patients with mild to severe dementia and for controls. As shown by asterisks, patients had significantly greater variances (SD^2) than controls in association but not in primary cortices. Distinct metabolic asymmetries were visually evident in PET scans of individual patients (Figure 12–2, Group 3). Abnormal variances of metabolic asymmetry were found at each dementia severity (Table 12–4), but the asymmetry was correlated significantly and in the expected directions, with a cognitive discrepancy in patients with moderate

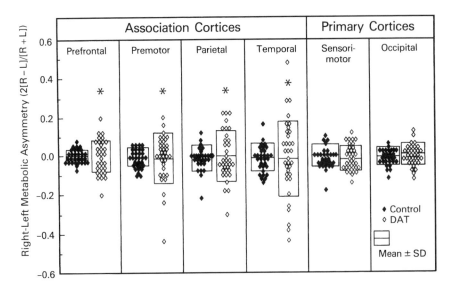

Figure 12–2. Right-left metabolic asymmetry indexes (Eq. 1) in association and primary cortical regions in AD patients with mild to severe dementia and in control subjects. R, $rCMR_{glc, right}$; L, $rCMR_{glc, left}$; *, coefficient of variation differs from control value ($P < .05$). High-resolution Scanditronix PC 1024–7B data from Haxby et al. (1990).

but not mild dementia (Table 12–5). In the patients with moderate dementia, a lower right-sided metabolism corresponded to worse drawing and visual recall test scores, compared with syntax comprehension and verbal recall test scores, respectively. The opposite was true for patients with left-sided hypometabolism (Haxby et al. 1990).

PET scans of AD patients frequently display gradients in metabolism between the parietal and frontal lobes (Figure 12–1, Groups 1 and 3). Accordingly, cognitive tests of parietal lobe function—arithmetic subtest of the Wechsler Adult Intelligence Scale (WAIS), syntax comprehension test, extended range drawing test, and block tapping span test—were compared in terms of rank ordering and cognitive discrepancies (see earlier section) with tests of prefrontal integrity—Controlled Word Association (FAS) and Trailmaking (Trail A) tests. As noted in Table 12–6, statistically significant correlations in the expected directions were evident be-

Table 12–4. Right-left metabolic asymmetries (Equation 1) in control subjects and in Alzheimer's patients of differing dementia severity

Brain regions	Controls (31)	Right-left metabolic asymmetries		
		Mild AD (11)	Moderate AD (13)	Severe AD (8)
Association cortex				
Prefrontal	0.01 ± 0.03	−0.01 ± 0.07*	−0.01 ± 0.08***	0.05 ± 0.10***
Premotor	0.01 ± 0.05	−0.01 ± 0.10**	−0.02 ± 0.16***	0.05 ± 0.11**
Orbitofrontal	−0.01 ± 0.06	−0.03 ± 0.08	−0.03 ± 0.11**	0.00 ± 0.11*
Parietal	−0.01 ± 0.06	−0.01 ± 0.11*	−0.03 ± 0.13**	0.08 ± 0.13*
Lateral temporal	−0.01 ± 0.07	−0.05 ± 0.17***	−0.03 ± 0.18***	0.08 ± 0.23***
Primary cortex				
Sensorimotor	−0.02 ± 0.05	−0.01 ± 0.07	0.00 ± 0.06	0.01 ± 0.06
Occipital[a]	−0.01 ± 0.04	0.00 ± 0.05	−0.01 ± 0.03	0.03 ± 0.08*

Note. Values are means ± SD (number of subjects).
[a]Primary and unimodal association cortex.
Variance greater than in controls: *$P < .05$; **$P < .01$; ***$P < .001$.
Source. Scanditronix PC 1024-7B data from Haxby et al. 1990.

Table 12–5.   Spearman rank-sum correlations between right-left
                 metabolic asymmetries (Equation 1) and drawing/syntax
                 comprehension or visual recall/verbal recall discrepancies
                 in Alzheimer's patients of varying dementia severity

Neuropsychological discrepancy	Right-left metabolic asymmetry			
	Prefrontal	Premotor	Parietal	Lateral temporal
	Correlation coefficient			
Controls (N = 15–16)				
Drawing versus comprehension	−0.10	−0.33	0.00	0.12
Visual versus verbal recall	−0.30	−0.39	−0.40	−0.17
AD with mild dementia (N = 10)				
Drawing versus comprehension	0.04	−0.15	0.04	−0.24
Visual versus verbal recall	−0.22	−0.21	−0.16	−0.18
AD with moderate dementia (N = 13)				
Drawing versus comprehension	0.76**	0.76**	0.79**	0.53
Visual versus verbal recall	0.49	0.55*	0.69**	0.48

Note.   Positive correlation indicates that better drawing capacity or better visual
recall is associated with relatively higher right-sided metabolism.
Spearman rank-sum correlation differs from zero: *$P < .05$; **$P < .01$.
Source.   Scanditronix PC 1024-7B data from Haxby et al. 1990.

tween cognitive discrepancies and the parietal/prefrontal metabolic ratios in patients with moderate but not mild dementia
(Haxby et al. 1988).

Furthermore, longitudinal PET studies of 11 AD patients demonstrated retention of the initial direction of right/left metabolic
asymmetry and parietal/frontal metabolic ratios for up to 4 years
(Figure 12–3) (Grady et al. 1988). Likewise, Spearman correlations
between initial and follow-up metabolic ratios at least 1.5 years
later ranged from 0.67 to 0.86 ($P < .01$) (Haxby et al. 1988).

This consistency explains why metabolic asymmetries in AD
patients with initial mild dementia were significant predictors of

Table 12–6. Spearman correlations between parietal/prefrontal rCMR$_{glc}$ ratios and parietal/prefrontal neuropsychological test score discrepancies in Alzheimer's patients

Neuropsychological discrepancy	Parietal/prefrontal metabolic ratio					
	Controls (14–17)[a]		Mild AD (10)		Moderate AD (14)	
	Right	Left	Right	Left	Right	Left
	Correlation coefficient					
Arithmetic versus						
Verbal fluency	−0.02	0.00	−0.14	−0.04	0.63*	0.57*
Attention (trail A)	−0.34	−0.08	−0.02	−0.21	0.43	0.46
Verbal comprehension versus						
Verbal fluency	0.00	0.03	−0.30	−0.06	0.66*	0.67*
Attention (trail A)	−0.12	0.11	0.04	−0.01	0.51	0.56*
Drawing versus						
Verbal fluency	−0.02	0.11	−0.02	0.22	0.66*	0.57
Attention (trail A)	−0.21	0.20	0.42	0.32	0.44	0.43
Immediate memory span for visuospatial location (block tapping) versus						
Verbal fluency	0.16	0.05	−0.25	−0.11	0.62*	0.54
Attention (trail A)	0.14	0.32	0.26	0.11	0.73**	0.72**

Note. Neuropsychological discrepancy equals rank on a test of arithmetic, syntax comprehension score, extended range drawing, or minus rank on controlled word association or attentional trailmaking (Trail A) test score.
[a]Number of subjects in parentheses.
Spearman correlation coefficient in AD differs from control: *$P < .05$; **$P < .01$.
Source. Scanditronix PC 1024-7B data from Haxby et al. 1988a.

expected cognitive discrepancies that appeared 1 to 3 years later (language worse with initial left-sided hypometabolism, visuospatial function worse with initial right-sided hypometabolism), and why lower parietal as compared with frontal metabolism in patients with mild dementia accurately predicted worse scores on cognitive tests of parietal than of frontal integrity (Grady et al. 1988; Haxby et al. 1990). Thus, in AD patients with initially mild dementia in whom the direction of metabolic asymmetry was maintained (Figure 12–3), Spearman rank-sum correlations between asymmetries and appropriate neuropsychological discrepancies were significant

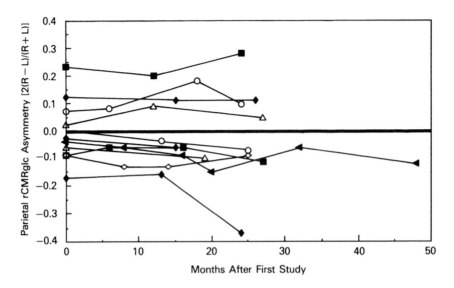

Figure 12–3.   Stability over time of right-left metabolic asymmetries in parietal association cortex of 11 AD patients with initially mild dementia. *Source.*   Reprinted from Haxby JV, Grady CL, Koss E, et al: Longitudinal study of cerebral metabolic assymetries and associated neuropsychological patterns in early dementia of the Alzheimer type. Arch Neurol 47:753–760, 1990. Used with permission. Copyright 1990 American Medical Association.

at the last but not at the first evaluation (Table 12–5) (Haxby et al. 1990).

PET Identification of AD in Possible AD Patients and Subjects at Risk for AD

A patient who presents with a history of memory decline and a singular memory disorder would be diagnosed as having possible AD according to NINCDS-ADRDA criteria (McKhann et al. 1984). However, if this patient also has an abnormal metabolic asymmetry (2 SD from mean as noted in Figure 12–2) or an abnormal parietal or frontal metabolic gradient, each shown to predict patterns of later cognitive dysfunction that would lead to a probable diagnosis, the early metabolic abnormalities could convert the "possible" to a "probable" diagnosis of AD.

Another way to statistically identify an abnormal metabolic PET pattern in an individual with only a memory deficit, and to reliably make an early probable diagnosis of AD, is by using a discriminant function involving $rCMR_{glc}$ in frontal and parietal association areas (Azari et al. 1993). Such a function could correctly identify 87% of AD patients with mild to moderate dementia and controls and convert possible to probable AD diagnoses in patients with mild dementia (Azari et al. 1993).

This same function later identified as having AD an at-risk individual with an isolated memory impairment and a family history for autosomal dominant AD; whose PET scan showed normal absolute and ratio values of $rCMR_{glc}$. The patient subsequently developed severe dementia and parietal hypometabolism (Pietrini et al. 1993). Further, a comparable discriminant function identified individual at-risk older Down's syndrome subjects without dementia as having AD (Azari et al. 1994b). Thus, discriminant analysis should be of use for deciding if and when to initiate pharmacotherapy in at-risk subjects or subjects with an isolated memory deficit (Azari et al. 1993, 1994b).

More recently, group mean abnormalities in resting $rCMR_{glc}$ have been demonstrated in at-risk subjects. In one study, subjects with a family history of probable AD, and in many cases with memory impairment, were divided according to their apolipoprotein ε4 allele status: ε4 heterozygotes and noncarriers of this allele (Reiman et al. 1996). Compared with the noncarriers, the heterozygotes had abnormally low and asymmetric mean $rCMR_{glc}$ in a preselected parietal region. In another study, middle-aged cognitively normal subjects homozygous for the ε4 allele were shown to have an AD-like PET pattern on metabolic projection maps of $rCMR_{glc}$ (Small et al. 1995). A third study reported that subjects at risk for familial AD, due to chromosome 14 linkage, known APP mutations, or other genetic factors, had reduced mean global and parietotemporal metabolism compared with age-matched controls but less so than in subjects with diagnosed AD (Kennedy et al.

1995). Follow-up will be necessary to establish whether there is a relation between individual metabolic rates in at-risk subjects and later development of AD.

Brain Activation in AD

Synaptic markers are reduced in the postmortem AD brain in relation to dementia severity in life (Terry et al. 1991). In biopsy tissue representing middle-stage disease, presynaptic elements have been reported to be reduced in number, with remaining elements hypertrophied so as to maintain a normal area of apposition with postsynaptic elements (DeKosky and Scheff 1990). These and other data suggested to us that metabolic reductions early in AD reflect reduced efficacy of synaptic transmission, which might be overcome by appropriate cognitive stimulation or by medication that modulates synaptic transmission (Rapoport and Grady 1993). Consistent with this hypothesis is in vitro evidence that $rCMR_{glc}$ represents functional activity of terminal synapses and their postsynaptic dendritic connections (Malison et al. 1994) and that AD patients compared with controls have fewer significant positive correlations between pairs of PET-derived $rCMR_{glc}$ values (Horwitz et al. 1987).

We used $H_2^{15}O$ and PET to examine rCBF in occipitotemporal visual association regions that subserve object recognition, while AD patients or healthy subjects performed a control or face-matching task (Figure 12–4) (Grady et al. 1993; Rapoport and Grady 1993; J. VanMeter, S. I. Rapoport, and C. Grady, unpublished results, 1994). rCBF during the control task (a button was pressed alternately with right and left thumbs in response to a neutral visual stimulus) was subtracted from rCBF during the face-matching task (the button was pressed with the appropriate thumb after deciding whether the right or left face was to be matched) to produce a "difference" image (Figure 12–5). AD patients with mild to moderate dementia were capable of performing the face-matching task

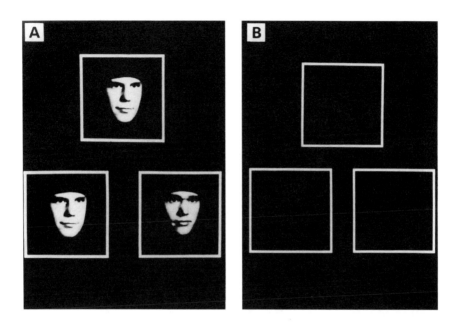

Figure 12–4. Sample items from face-matching *(A)* and control tasks *(B)*. Responses during face matching were with the right or left thumb depending on which of the two choice items seen below (right or left) was a correct match to the top face. Right and left button presses were alternated during the control task.

Source. Reprinted with permission from Neurobiology of Aging, Vol. 14, Grady CL, Haxby JV, Horwitz B, et al., Activation of cerebral blood flow during a visuoperceptual task in patients with Alzheimer-type dementia, pp. 35–44, 1993. Elsevier Science Inc.

as accurately (85% ± 8% [SD] correct choices) as controls (92% ± 5%), although reaction times during the task were more variable than in the controls, 3.34 ± 1.46 (SD) seconds compared with 2.07 ± 0.54 seconds.

As illustrated in Table 12–7, in the control task, rCBF was lower in occipitotemporal regions (Brodmann areas 17, 19, and 37) in AD than in control subjects, consistent with functional activity in these areas. Nevertheless, during face matching, the mean increment ΔrCBF (ml/100 g/minute) did not differ significantly or differed only minimally between patients and controls. Thus, the affected AD

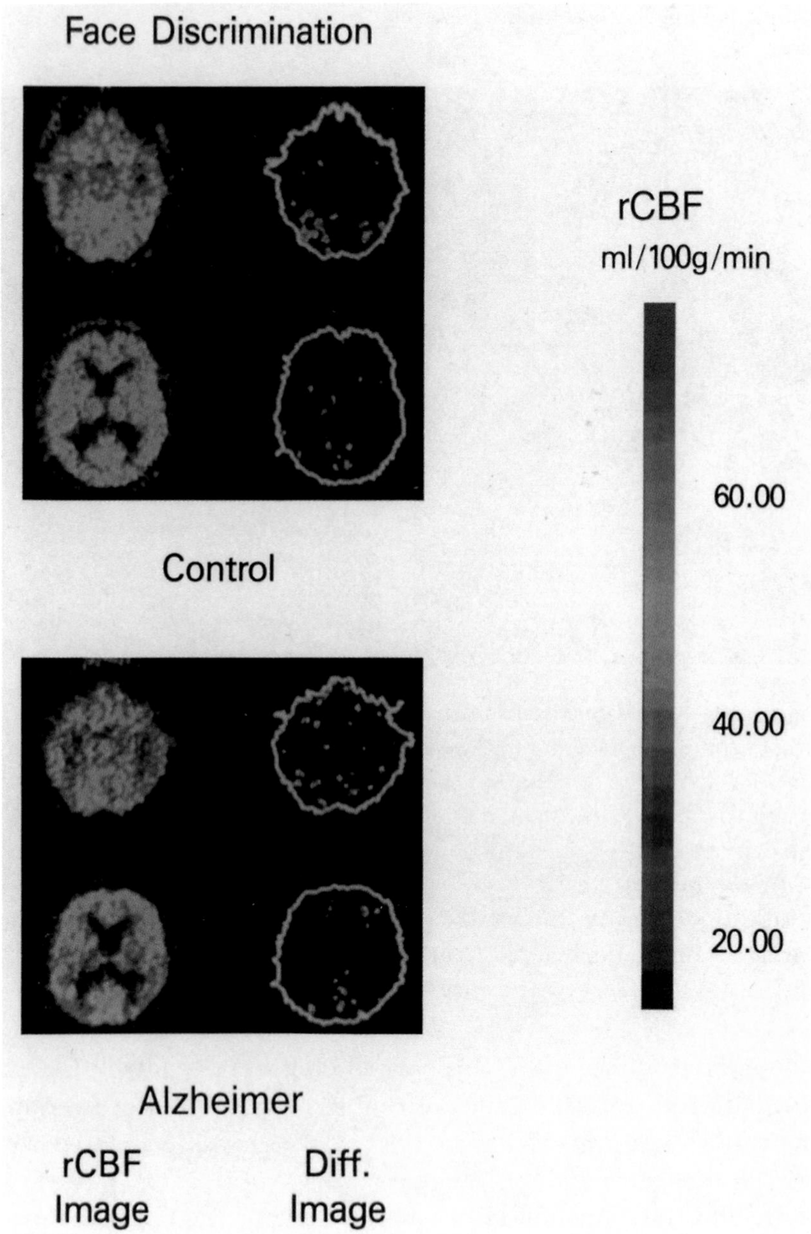

Face Discrimination

Control

Alzheimer

rCBF
Image

Diff.
Image

rCBF
ml/100g/min

60.00

40.00

20.00

Figure 12–5. rCBF and ΔrCBF (difference between face discrimination and control rCBF) images in control and AD subjects. Parietotemporal rCBF was reduced in lower rCBF image from AD subject. Difference image identifies pixels in which flow was increased by more than 30% above baseline. rCBF in units of ml/100 g/minute.
Source. Grady et al., unpublished 1993.

Table 12–7. rCBF in occipitotemporal visual association areas in Alzheimer's patients and control subjects performing control or face-matching tasks

Parameter	Controls (N = 13)	Alzheimer (N = 11)
	rCBF (ml/100 g/min)	
Baseline control task	48.4 ± 0.9	40.1 ± 1.1*
Face-matching task	53.1 ± 0.9	44.1 ± 1.2*
Difference Δ rCBF, face matching–control task	4.7 ± 0.2	4.0 ± 0.4

[a]rCBF measured in occipitotemporal visual association areas (Brodmann 19 and part of 37).
*Mean ± SE differs significantly from control mean, $P < .001$.
Source. Van Meter et al., unpublished results, 1994, and Rapoport and Grady 1993.

areas were capable of being fully activated during the task, suggesting a degree of reversibility of functional failure (Rapoport and Grady 1993).

Stimulation-response relations in hippocampal slices in vitro suggest that a wide range of measurable (parameterized) stimulus intensities would be required to determine the extent and reversibility of synaptic failure due to changes in synaptic efficacy in an AD patient (Pellmar 1986), just as a range of medication doses would be needed to examine differences in the K_D and maximum effect of a drug (Benet et al. 1990). Over a certain stimulus range, rCBF (a measure of firing) of a homogeneous population of synapses might be expected to be a monotonic function (F) of test difficulty and subject effort. This is represented in the left side of Figure 12–6 as a sigmoidal curve in normal subjects (Rapoport and Grady 1993). In early AD in which failure of synaptic efficacy could be overcome, the curve would be shifted to the right without a reduction in the maximum response. For the middle activation in the figure, the increment ΔrCBF would be equal in the control and the AD subject (e.g., Table 12–7), whereas to the left of that activation, ΔrCBF would be less in AD patients than in controls and to the right of that activation the reverse would occur. Only at extreme levels of F might total flow be equal between AD and controls.

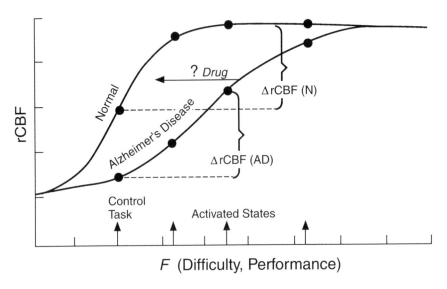

Figure 12–6. Hypothetical relations between function F of task difficulty or task performance on the one hand, and rCBF on the other, in normal subject and in an AD patient with mild dementia. The normal curve is shifted to the right in AD, but rCBF nevertheless can be maximally activated at high values of F. A control task and three activated states are illustrated by upward arrows. The middle activated state results in an increment ΔrCBF, which is the same in the AD patient and control subject. ΔrCBF in the left activated state is less in the patient than in the control subject, whereas it is higher in the patient than control subject in the right activated state. Horizontal arrow suggests that a drug that can increase synaptic efficacy would tend to return the AD curve toward the normal curve.
Source. Modified from Rapoport et al. 1993.

Figure 12–6 also suggests that mediations that enhance synaptic efficacy might normalize an AD curve that is shifted to the right.

Pharmacology

Limited data are available on drug effects measured with PET in AD. In one study, patients who were scanned before and during physostigmine infusion demonstrated increments as well as decrements of normalized (related to global) rCMR$_{glc}$ (Tune et al. 1991). In another study of six AD patients, acutely administered physostigmine (5 µg/kg/hour) reduced rCMR$_{glc}$ below its already reduced value in the neocortex (Blin et al. 1994). With regard to cholinergic therapy, AD patients with mild to moderate dementia, treated orally with the cholinesterase inhibitor tetrahydroaminoacridine for several months, were shown to have improved neuropsychological performance and increased rCMR$_{glc}$ but unchanged rCBF by PET. There was increased uptake of $(+)$-^{11}C-nicotine in frontal and temporal cortices, suggesting partial restoration of nicotinic cholinergic receptors (Nordberg 1993). In another study, phosphatidylserine administered to 18 AD patients over a 6-month period did not affect rCMR$_{glc}$, at rest or during visual stimulation, or cognitive performance (Heiss et al. 1994).

Positron-emitting ligands for receptors have been developed for PET, but few have as yet been applied to AD. ^{11}C-carfentanil has been used to demonstrate early loss of mµ opiate receptors in the amygdaloid complex of AD patients (Mueller-Gaertner et al. 1991). Binding of ^{18}F-setoperone, a 5-HT$_2$ antagonist, was reduced by 31%–46% in association cortical areas of nine patients with AD (Blin et al. 1993).

SPECT in AD: Comparison With PET and Utility for Clinical Diagnosis

SPECT has been introduced into clinical settings to estimate rCBF and receptor densities because it is less expensive than PET and requires less personnel and technical support. High-sensitivity gamma cameras can be used with ^{133}Xe gas to image single slices during 4 to 7.5 minutes with a resolution approaching 8 mm (Malison et al. 1994). Alternatively, low-sensitivity rotating gamma cameras can provide volumetric information, using commercially available long-lived ^{123}I- or ^{99m}Tc-labeled radiopharmaceuticals (Holman et al. 1991, 1992). The use of long-lived isotopes with a need for long signal acquisition times extends scanning time to 30 to 60 minutes and allows only one scan per day. However, SPECT is not truly quantitative because photon scatter and attenuation compensation have not been adequately addressed in its reconstruction paradigms. Ratios of radioactivity between one brain region and another usually are determined, and arterial input functions for absolute flow calculations generally are not obtained.

Whereas four statistically distinct PET patterns of $rCMR_{glc}$ have been reported in AD (see earlier section) (Grady et al. 1990), seven qualitative rCBF patterns have been identified using ^{99m}Tc–hexamethyl-propyleneamine oxime (HMPAO) SPECT from a prospective study of 132 consecutive patients of varying dementia severity (Holman et al. 1992). Probability of AD was 82% for bilateral temporoparietal defects, 72% for bilateral temporoparietal plus additional defects, 57% for unilateral temporoparietal defects, 43% for frontal defects, 18% for large focal defects, and 0% for multiple small cortical defects. Because a normal SPECT pattern has been reported in 45% of patients with mild dementia (Reed et al. 1989), ^{99m}Tc-HMPAO SPECT has minimal diagnostic utility in AD patients with mild dementia except when there is considerable diagnostic doubt (Claus et al. 1993).

A temporoparietal reduction in SPECT rCBF is more likely with AD, whereas a patchy whole brain reduction involving the motor cortex and thalamus is more likely with vascular dementia (Lechner and Bertha 1991; Kawabata et al. 1993). But normal SPECT images occur in mildly demented AD patients and vascular dementia patients, and an asymmetric presentation in an AD patient may be indistinguishable from a pattern of cerebral infarction in another patient (Holman et al. 1991). In AD and vascular dementia patients matched for dementia severity, ^{99m}Tc-HMPAO ratios of temporoparietal cortex, parietal cortex, or frontal cortex to cerebellar radioactivity did not distinguish between the two groups (Weinstein et al. 1991). On the other hand, a discriminant analysis of ^{99m}Tc-HMPAO-derived flows correctly identified 100% of controls and 87% of AD patients with mild dementia (O'Mahony et al. 1994).

The muscarinic M_2 presynaptic receptor subtype is selectively lost in AD, leaving the M_1 postsynaptic subtype in place (Mash et al. 1985). Intravenous physostigmine, 0.5 mg, was shown by SPECT to increase rCBF in the left posterior parietotemporal region of AD patients whose baseline rCBF was reduced, but not of normals, suggesting up-regulation of postsynaptic cholinergic sensitivity (Geaney et al. 1990). The radioligand ^{123}I-3-quinuclidinyl-4-iodobenzilate (QNB) has different binding to M_1 compared with M_2 receptors, which may allow SPECT with this tracer to quantitate loss of the M_2 subtype AD. This is unlikely in the parietal cortex, however, where $M_1 = 88$ nM and $M_2 = 12$ nM in normal brain (Zeeberg et al. 1992). Focal reductions of ^{123}I-QNB binding by SPECT, in the thalamus and frontal cortex of AD patients, suggest selective loss of M_2 receptors in these regions (Weinberger et al. 1992).

References

Almkvist O, Wahlund L-O, Andersson-Lundman G, et al: White-matter hyperintensity and neuropsychological functions in dementia and healthy aging. Arch Neurol 49:626–632, 1992

Azari NP, Pettigrew KD, Schapiro MB, et al: Early detection of Alzheimer's disease: a statistical approach using positron emission tomographic data. J Cereb Blood Flow Metab 13:438–447, 1993

Azari NP, Horwitz B, Pettigrew KD, et al: Abnormal pattern of cerebral glucose metabolic rates involving language areas in young adults with Down syndrome. Brain Lang 46:1–20, 1994a

Azari NP, Pettigrew KD, Horwitz B, et al: Detection of an Alzheimer disease pattern of cerebral metabolism in Down syndrome. Dementia 5:69–78, 1994b

Benet LZ, Mitchell JR, Sheiner LB: Pharmacokinetics: the dynamics of drug absorption, distribution, and elimination, in Goodman and Gilman's The Pharmacological Basis of Therapeutics, 8th Edition. Edited by Gilman AG, Rall TW, Nies AS, Taylor P. New York, McGraw-Hill, 1990, pp 1–32

Benson DF, Kuhl DE, Hawkins RA, et al: The fluorodeoxyglucose ^{18}F scan in Alzheimer's disease and multi-infarct dementia. Arch Neurol 40: 711–714, 1983

Berridge MJ, Irvine RF: Inositol triphosphate, a novel second messenger in cellular signal transduction. Nature 312:315–321, 1984

Blin J, Baron JC, Dubois B, et al: Loss of brain 5-HT$_2$ receptors in Alzheimer's disease. Brain 116:497–510, 1993

Blin J, Piercey MF, Giuffra MA, et al: Metabolic effects of scopolamine and physostigmine in human brain measured by positron emission tomography. J Neurol Sci 123:44–51, 1994

Boller F, Lopez OL, Moossy J: Diagnosis of dementia: clinicopathologic correlations. Neurology 39:76–79, 1989

Bowen BC, Barker WW, Loewenstein DA, et al: MR signal abnormalities in memory disorder and dementia. AJR Am J Roentgenol 154:1285–1292, 1990

Brown GG, Levine SR, Gorell JM, et al: *In vivo* ^{31}P NMR profiles of Alzheimer's disease and multiple subcortical infarct dementia. Neurology 39:1423–1427, 1989

Chui HC, Victoroff JI, Margolin D, et al: Criteria for the diagnosis of ischemic vascular dementia proposed by the state of California Alzheimer's disease diagnostic and treatment centers. Neurology 42:473–480, 1992

Claus JJ, Hasan D, van Harskamp FH, et al: SPECT with ^{99m}Tc-HMPAO is of limited diagnostic value in mild Alzheimer's disease: a population-based study (abstract). Neurology 43(suppl 2):A406, 1993

Creasey H, Schwartz M, Frederickson H, et al: Quantitative computed tomography in dementia of the Alzheimer type. Neurology 36:1563–1568, 1986

DeCarli C, Kaye JA, Horwitz B, et al: Critical analysis of the use of computer-assisted transverse axial tomography to study human brain in aging and dementia of the Alzheimer type. Neurology 40:872–883, 1990

DeCarli CS, Atack JR, Ball MJ, et al: Post-mortem regional neurofibrillary tangle densities but not senile plaque densities are related to regional cerebral metabolic rates for glucose during life in Alzheimer's disease patients. Neurodegeneration 1:113–121, 1992a

DeCarli C, Haxby JV, Gillette JA, et al: Longitudinal changes in lateral ventricular volume in patients with dementia of the Alzheimer type. Neurology 42:2029–2036, 1992b

DeCarli C, Murphy DGM, McIntosh AR, et al: Discriminant analysis of MRI measures determines the presence of dementia of the Alzheimer type in males and females. Psychiatry Res 57:119–130, 1995

DeCarli C, Grady CL, Clark CM, et al: Comparison of positron emission tomography, cognition, and brain volume in Alzheimer disease with and without severe abnormalities of white matter. J Neurol Neurosurg Psychiatry 60:158–167, 1996

DeKosky ST, Scheff SW: Synapse loss in frontal cortex biopsies in Alzheimer's disease: correlation with cognitive severity. Ann Neurol 27:457–464, 1990

Drayer BP: Imaging of the aging brain, II: pathologic conditions. Radiology 166:797–806, 1988

Duara R, Grady C, Haxby J, et al: Positron emission tomography in Alzheimer's disease. Neurology 36:879–887, 1986

Folstein MF, Folstein SE, McHugh PR: Mini Mental State: a practical method for grading the cognitive state of patients for the clinician. J Psychiatr Res 12:189–198, 1975

Fox PT, Raichle ME, Mintun MA, et al: Nonoxidative glucose consumption during focal physiologic neural activity. Science 241:462–464, 1988

Frackowiak RSJ, Pozzilli C, Legg NJ, et al: Regional cerebral oxygen supply and utilization in dementia: a clinical and physiological study with oxygen-15 and positron tomography. Brain 104:753–778, 1981

Fukuyama H, Ogawa M, Yamauchi H, et al: Altered cerebral energy metabolism in Alzheimer's disease: a PET study. J Nucl Med 35:1–6, 1994

Geaney DP, Soper N, Shepstone BJ, et al: Effect of central cholinergic stimulation on regional cerebral blood flow in Alzheimer's disease. Lancet 335:1484–1487, 1990

Grady CL, Haxby JV, Horwitz B, et al: Longitudinal study of the early neuropsychological and cerebral metabolic changes in dementia of the Alzheimer type. J Clin Exp Neuropsychol 10:576–596, 1988

Grady CL, Haxby JV, Schapiro MB, et al: Subgroups in dementia of the Alzheimer type identified using positron emission tomography. J Neuropsychiatry Clin Neurosci 2:373–384, 1990

Grady CL, Haxby JV, Horwitz B, et al: Activation of cerebral blood flow during a visuoperceptual task in patients with Alzheimer-type dementia. Neurobiol Aging 14:35–44, 1993

Hagberg BO, Ingvar DH: Cognitive reduction in presenile dementia related to regional abnormalities of the cerebral blood flow. Br J Psychiatry 128:209–222, 1976

Haxby JV, Duara R, Grady CL, et al: Relations between neuropsychological and cerebral metabolic asymmetries in early Alzheimer's disease. J Cereb Blood Flow Metab 5:193–200, 1985

Haxby JV, Grady CL, Koss E, et al: Heterogeneous anterior-posterior metabolic patterns in dementia of the Alzheimer type. Neurology 38:1853–1863, 1988

Haxby JV, Grady CL, Koss E, et al: Longitudinal study of cerebral metabolic asymmetries and associated neuropsychological patterns in early dementia of the Alzheimer type. Arch Neurol 47:753–760, 1990

Haxby JV, Raffaele K, Gillette J, et al: Individual trajectories of cognitive decline in patients with dementia of the Alzheimer type. J Clin Exp Neuropsychol 14:575–592, 1992

Heiss W-D, Kessler J, Mielke R, et al: Long-term effects of phosphatidylserine, pyritinol, and cognitive training in Alzheimer's disease. Dementia 5:88–98, 1994

Hoffman JM, Guze BH, Baxter L, et al: Metabolic homogeneity in familial and sporadic Alzheimer's disease: an FDG-PET study (abstract). Neurology 39(suppl 1):S167, 1989

Holman BL, Nagel JS, Johnson KA, et al: Imaging dementia with SPECT. Ann N Y Acad Sci 620:165–174, 1991

Holman BL, Johnson KA, Gerada B, et al: The scintigraphic appearance of Alzheimer's disease: a prospective study using technetium-99m-HMPAO SPECT. J Nucl Med 33:181–185, 1992

Horwitz B, Grady CL, Schlageter NL, et al: Intercorrelations of regional cerebral glucose metabolic rates in Alzheimer's disease. Brain Res 407:294–306, 1987

Hounsfield GN: Computerized transverse axial scanning (tomography), I: description of system. Br J Radiol 46:1016–1022, 1973

Jellinger K: Neuropathological aspects of dementias resulting from abnormal blood and cerebrospinal fluid dynamics. Acta Neurol Belg 76:83–102, 1976

Kawabata K, Tachibana H, Sugita M, et al: A comparative I-123 IMP SPECT study in Binswanger's disease and Alzheimer's disease. Clin Nucl Med 18:329–336, 1993

Kaye JA, DeCarli C, Luxenberg JS, et al: The significance of age-related enlargement of the cerebral ventricles in healthy men and women measured by quantitative computed X-ray tomography. J Am Geriatr Soc 40:225–231, 1992

Kennedy AM, Frackowia RSJ, Newman SK, et al: Deficits in cerebral glucose metabolism demonstrated by positron emission tomography in individuals at risk of familial Alzheimer's disease. Neurosci Lett 186:17–20, 1995

Kozachuk WE, DeCarli C, Schapiro MB, et al: White matter hyperintensities in dementia of Alzheimer's type and in healthy subjects without cerebrovascular risk factors: a magnetic resonance imaging study. Arch Neurol 47:1306–1310, 1990

Kumar A, Schapiro MB, Grady C, et al: High-resolution PET studies in Alzheimer's disease. Neuropsychopharmacology 4:35–46, 1991

Kuwabara Y, Ichiya Y, Otsuka M, et al: Cerebrovascular responsiveness to hypercapnia in Alzheimer's dementia and vascular dementia of the Binswanger type. Stroke 23:594–598, 1992

Lechner H, Bertha G: Multiinfarct dementia. J Neural Transm Suppl 33: 49–52, 1991

Lewis DA, Campbell MJ, Terry RD, et al: Laminar and regional distributions of neurofibrillary tangles and neuritic plaques in Alzheimer's disease: a quantitative study of visual and auditory cortices. J Neurosci 7:1799–1808, 1987

Lim KO, Rosenbloom M, Pfefferbaum A: In vivo structural brain assessment, in Psychopharmacology: The Fourth Generation of Progress. Edited by Bloom FE, Kupfer DJ. New York, Raven, 1994, pp 881–894

Luxenberg JS, Friedland RP, Rapoport SI: Quantitative X-ray computed tomography (CT) in dementia of the Alzheimer type (DAT). Can J Neurol Sci 13:570–572, 1986

Luxenberg JS, Haxby JV, Creasey H, et al: Rate of ventricular enlargement in dementia of the Alzheimer type correlates with rate of neuropsychological deterioration. Neurology 37:1135–1140, 1987

Malison RT, Laruelle M, Innis RB: Positron and single photon emission tomography: principles and applications in psychopharmacology, in Psychopharmacology: The Fourth Generation of Progress. Edited by Bloom FE, Kupfer DJ. New York, Raven, 1994, pp 865–880

Mash DC, Flynn DD, Potter LT: Loss of M_2 muscarine receptors in the cerebral cortex in Alzheimer's disease and experimental cholinergic denervation. Science 228:1115–1117, 1985

Mayeux R, Stern Y, Spanton S: Heterogeneity in dementia of the Alzheimer type: evidence of subgroups. Neurology 35:453–461, 1985

McKhann G, Drachman D, Folstein M, et al: Clinical diagnosis of Alzheimer's disease: report of the NINCDS-ADRDA work group under the auspices of Department of Health and Human Services task force on Alzheimer's disease. Neurology 34:939–944, 1984

Minoshima S, Foster NL, Kuhl DE: Posterior cingulate cortex in Alzheimer's disease. Lancet 344:895, 1994

Moats RA, Ernst T, Shonk TK, et al: Abnormal cerebral metabolite concentrations in patient with probable Alzheimer disease. Magn Reson Med 32:110–115, 1994

Mueller-Gaertner HW, Mayberg HS, Tune L, et al: Mu opiate receptor binding in amygdala in Alzheimer's disease: in vivo quantification by 11C carfentanil and PET (abstract). J Cereb Blood Flow Metab 11(suppl 2):S20, 1991

Murphy DGM, Bottomley PA, Salerno JA, et al: An in vivo study of phosphorus and glucose metabolism in Alzheimer's disease using magnetic resonance spectroscopy and PET. Arch Gen Psychiatry 50:341–349, 1993a

Murphy DGM, DeCarli CD, Daly E, et al: Volumetric magnetic resonance imaging in men with dementia of the Alzheimer type: correlations with disease severity. Biol Psychiatry 34:612–621, 1993b

Nordberg A: Effect of long-term treatment with tacrine (THA) in Alzheimer's disease as visualized by PET. Acta Neurol Scand 149(suppl):62–65, 1993

Nordberg A, Lilja A, Lundqvist H, et al: Tacrine restores cholinergic nicotinic receptors and glucose metabolism in Alzheimer patients as visualized by positron emission tomography. Neurobiol Aging 13:747–758, 1992

O'Brien MD, Mallett BL: Cerebral cortex perfusion rates in dementia. J Neurol Neurosurg Psychiatry 33:497–500, 1970

O'Mahony D, Coffey J, Murphy J, et al: The discriminant value of semiquantitative SPECT data in mild Alzheimer's disease. J Nucl Med 35:1450–1455, 1994

Pellmar T: Electrophysiological correlates of peroxide damage in guinea pig hippocampus in vitro. Brain Res 364:377–381, 1986

Pettegrew JW, Moossy J, Withers G, et al: ^{31}P nuclear magnetic resonance study of the brain in Alzheimer's disease. J Neuropathol Exp Neurol 47:235–248, 1988

Pietrini P, Azari NP, Grady CL, et al: Pattern of cerebral metabolic interactions in a subject with isolated amnesia at risk for Alzheimer's disease: a longitudinal evaluation. Dementia 4:94–101, 1993

Raichle ME, Grubb RL Jr, Gado MH, et al: Correlation between regional cerebral blood flow and oxidative metabolism. Arch Neurol 33:523–526, 1976

Rapoport SI: Brain evolution and Alzheimer's disease. Rev Neurol (Paris) 144:79–90, 1988

Rapoport SI: Positron emission tomography in Alzheimer's disease in relation to disease pathogenesis: a critical review. Cerebrovascular Brain Metabolism Reviews 3:297–335, 1991

Rapoport SI, Grady CL: Parametric in vivo brain imaging during activation to examine pathological mechanisms of functional failure in Alzheimer disease. Int J Neurosci 70:39–56, 1993

Reed BR, Jagust WJ, Seab JP, et al: Memory and regional cerebral blood flow in mildly symptomatic Alzheimer's disease. Neurology 39:1537–1539, 1989

Reiman EM, Caselli RJ, Yun LS, et al: Preclinical evidence of Alzheimer's disease in persons homozygous for the ε4 allele for apolipoprotein E. N Engl J Med 334:752–758, 1996

Rosen WG, Terry RD, Fuld PA, et al: Pathological verification of ischemic score in differentiation of dementias. Ann Neurol 7:486–488, 1980

Schapiro MB, Pietrini P, Grady CL, et al: Reductions in parietal and temporal cerebral metabolic rates for glucose are not specific for Alzheimer's disease. J Neurol Neurosurg Psychiatry 56:859–864, 1993

Schlageter NL, Carson RE, Rapoport SI: Examination of blood-brain barrier permeability in dementia of the Alzheimer type with [68-Ga]EDTA and positron emission tomography. J Cereb Blood Flow Metab 77:1–8, 1987

Shulman RG, Blamire AM, Rothman DL, et al: Nuclear magnetic resonance imaging and spectroscopy of human brain function. Proc Natl Acad Sci U S A 90:3127–3133, 1993

Small GW, Mazziotta JC, Collins MT, et al: Apolipoprotein E type 4 allele and cerebral glucose metabolism in relatives at risk for familial Alzheimer disease. JAMA 273:942–947, 1995

Smith CD, Gallenstein LG, Layton WJ, et al: ^{31}P magnetic resonance spectroscopy in Alzheimer's and Pick's disease. Neurobiol Aging 14:85–92, 1993

Terry RD, Masliah E, Salmon DP, et al: Physical basis of cognitive alterations in Alzheimer's disease: synapse loss is the major correlate of cognitive impairment. Ann Neurol 30:572–580, 1991

Tune L, Brandt J, Frost JJ, et al: Physostigmine in Alzheimer's disease: effects on cognitive functioning, cerebral glucose metabolism analyzed by positron emission tomography and cerebral blood flow analyzed by single photon emission tomography. Acta Psychiatr Scand Suppl 366:61–65, 1991

Tyrrell PJ, Sawle GV, Ibanez V, et al: Clinical and positron emission tomography studies in the "extrapyramidal syndrome" of dementia of the Alzheimer type. Arch Neurol 47:1318–1323, 1990

Weinberger DR, Jones D, Reba RC, et al: A comparison of FDG PET and IQNB SPECT in normal subjects and in patients with dementia. J Neuropsychiatry Clin Neurosci 4:239–248, 1992

Weinstein HC, Haan J, van Royen EO, et al: SPECT in the diagnosis of Alzheimer's disease and multi-infarct-dementia. Clin Neurol Neurosurg 93:39–43, 1991

Yamauchi H, Fukuyama H, Harada K, et al: Callosal atrophy parallels decreased cortical oxygen metabolism and neuropsychological impairment in Alzheimer's disease. Arch Neurol 50:1070–1074, 1993

Yao H, Sadoshima S, Ibayashi S, et al: Leukoaraiosis and dementia in hypertensive patients. Stroke 23:1673–1677, 1992

Zeeberg BR, Kim H-J, Reba RC: Pharmacokinetic simulations of SPECT quantitation of the M_2 muscarinic neuroreceptor subtype in disease states using radioiodinated (R,R)-4IQNB. Life Sci 51:661–670, 1992

13

Diagnostic Markers for Alzheimer's Disease

Norman Relkin, M.D., Ph.D.

One of the long-standing goals of Alzheimer's disease (AD) research has been the development of an objective and accurate antemortem diagnostic test. Despite considerable progress in the discovery of AD biological markers, this goal has not been accomplished. The clinical diagnosis of AD is only 75%–85% accurate in routine practice and depends primarily on the exclusion of other causes of dementia rather than the positive identification of AD. The unrivaled gold standard for confirming the diagnosis of AD continues to be autopsy examination to establish the presence of excessive quan-

I express my appreciation to Dr. Sam Gandy and Dr. Fred Plum for their many helpful discussions and to Ms. Younga Kwon and Julia Tsai for their assistance in the preparation of this manuscript. I would also like to thank Dr. Michael Boss for the literature he provided concerning the CSF tau assay and the Athena ADMark battery.

This work was supported in part by a grant from the C.V. Starr Foundation (The Starr Program for Neurogeriatric Studies).

tities of neuritic plaques (NPs) and neurofibrillary tangles (NFTs) in the brain of a patient who had dementia during life (Khachaturian 1985). In this chapter, I review the major strategies now being employed in the search for a more accurate means of diagnosing AD antemortem.

Arguably, the greatest impediment to the development of an accurate laboratory test for AD has been the lack of a confirmed causal explanation for the disease. As in the parable of the blind men and the elephant, current theories tend to explain isolated aspects of AD's pathogenesis without capturing the essential nature of the beast. Consequently, most of the proposed laboratory tests for AD have been based on *surrogate markers,* that is, those whose appearance or level of expression parallels the occurrence of the disease without necessarily occupying a position on its causal pathway (Schatzkin et al. 1993). Although many such markers have been identified in recent years (see reviews by Percy 1993; Pirozzolo 1988; Thal and Davies 1987; Van Gool and Bolhius 1991), none have led to the development of an effective antemortem diagnostic test for AD. The sensitivity and specificity of surrogate markers may be limited by the heterogeneity of AD's presentation and course, as well as by the clinical and neuropathologic similarities that exist between AD, "normal" aging, and other forms of dementia.

The use of multiple biological markers may be an inherent part of the AD diagnostic process. For example, documentation of excessive NPs and NFTs in the brain at autopsy in itself involves multiple markers and must be supplemented by additional information confirming the presence of dementia during life. Can a single antemortem laboratory test carried out in isolation be expected to accomplish the same? To do so would require the identification of a biological marker that is an obligate cause of AD and is expressed specifically and exclusively when AD becomes clinically manifest. Since AD appears to be a multifactorial illness fostered by the complex interaction of inborn susceptibilities, age-related processes, and lifelong exposures to provocative factors, there is reason to doubt that such a marker can be found.

Genetic Tests

At least one group of biological markers that appear to be causally related to AD have been identified. Three gene mutations that lead to the development of early-onset familial forms of AD have been found on chromosomes 21, 14, and 1. The gene products associated with these mutations have also been identified (Goate et al. 1991; Levy-Lahad 1995; Sherrington et al. 1995). These mutations are inherited in an autosomal dominant fashion and are expressed with almost complete penetrance before age 60. The chromosome 21 APP-V717F mutation has been shown to induce many of the neuropathologic features of AD in transgenic mice (Games et al. 1995). Studies are under way to determine whether these mice are cognitively impaired, which would provide further evidence of a causal link between AD and the APP-V717F gene.

A relatively small fraction of the total population of AD patients (an estimated 2%) possess early onset genes, limiting their potential diagnostic use. Technically speaking, an assay for an early onset AD gene does not constitute a true diagnostic test because genes are *trait markers,* that is, they indicate the carrier's predisposition to AD, not whether an individual is actually affected. Confirmation of diagnosis in a carrier requires measurement of *state markers,* that is, indicators of the onset or progression of disease. Despite the evident predictive value of trait markers, it has been proposed recently that a genetic trait marker for late-onset AD known as apolipoprotein E (APOE) be used as an adjunctive diagnostic test and not for predictive purposes (Roses 1995).

APOE genotyping. APOE is the first identified genetic susceptibility locus for late-onset familial and sporadic forms of AD (Strittmatter et al. 1993). The ApoE lipoprotein is produced in brain and liver and is encoded by a gene (*APOE*) on chromosome 19. ApoE has long been known to play a role in cholesterol transport and is now thought to influence such diverse processes as cerebral amyloid deposition, cytoskeletal integrity, neuronal plasticity, cholinergic activity, and other processes that may be related to AD's pathophysiology. There are three common allelic forms of APOE, designated ε2, ε3, and ε4. Everyone inherits a single APOE allele from each parent and therefore possesses one of six possible genotypes (ε2/ε2, ε2/ε3, ε2/ε4, ε3/ε3, ε3/ε4, ε4/ε4). An individual's genotype can be determined by relatively inexpensive and widely available polymerase chain reaction (PCR)-based assays performed on DNA extracted from leukocytes. Approximately one-fifth of the general population possesses the APOE ε3/ε4 genotype and is at moderately increased relative risk of developing AD as a consequence. The 2% of the population who are homozygotes for ε4 (APOE ε4/ε4) are at relatively high risk for AD as well as moderately increased risk of heart disease. APOE appears to modulate the average age at onset of AD symptoms, with ε4 carriers being affected the earliest. APOE ε2 may exert a protective effect against AD.

The role of APOE genotyping in the diagnosis and prediction of AD is a continuing matter of controversy. Although APOE is a trait marker, genotyping of asymptomatic individuals to predict future risk of AD is not recommended currently except in the context of clinical research protocols (Relkin et al. 1996). Before predictive use can be recommended, additional prospective studies are needed to evaluate the influence of age, gender, ethnicity, and other factors on APOE-related AD risk. APOE genotyping lacks the sensitivity and specificity to be used in isolation as a diagnostic test (van Gool and Hijdra 1994). However, APOE ε4 is clearly overrepresented among AD patients relative to patients with other forms of dementia and normals, which has led to the suggestion that it might be useful as an adjunct to current clinical diagnostic procedures (Roses 1995). According to analyses based on Bayesian theory, the 75%–85% accuracy of diagnosis currently achieved when a patient meets clinical criteria for AD may be increased to 90%–95% or more if subjects are found to possess one or more APOE ε4 alleles (van Gool and Hijdra 1994). The actual positive predictive value of APOE for AD is unknown, and several factors may confound its use in standard clinical practice. There may be an age window in which APOE genotyping is most useful, perhaps in the range of 60–75 years. At more advanced ages, APOE ε4's representation in the AD population decreases.

Roses (1995) have suggested that adjunct use of APOE genotyping could prove cost-effective in the diagnostic evaluation of AD if it reduces reliance on more expensive ancillary tests, such as brain imaging. This proposal has been questioned on the grounds that the possession of APOE ε4 does not preclude the presence of other potentially treatable causes of cognitive decline, such as cerebrovascular disease, communicating hydrocephalus, and space-occupying lesions (Bird 1995). Although APOE genotyping would not eliminate the need for such studies, it is conceivable that clinicians might refrain from ordering magnetic resonance imaging (MRI) scans in uncomplicated cases of subjects found to possess two copies of APOE ε4. The American College of Medical Genetics has issued a statement against all clinical use of APOE genotyping in relation to AD (Farrer 1995). However, a working group of the National Institute on Aging and the Alzheimer's Association has acknowledged a possible clinical role and recommended that physicians consider the use of APOE genotyping as an adjunct to current diagnostic procedures at their own discretion (Relkin 1996). Most experts agree that further prospective studies with autopsy correlation are required before APOE genotyping can be recommended for routine use in the clinical evaluation of dementia.

Plaque- and Tangle-Based Tests

Excessive quantities of intracerebral plaques and tangles are a defining feature of AD neuropathology. In the absence of a direct means of visualizing these changes in the brain of living patients, many researchers have focused on the assayable components of NPs and NFTs in blood, cerebrospinal fluid (CSF), skin, and other tissues. Several factors may undermine the success of this approach, however. Plaques, tangles, and most of their known macromolecular constituents are not entirely specific to AD. Plaque-

and tangle-related biological markers can vary widely in their level of expression across patients, particularly at different stages of the disease, and levels in peripheral tissues and fluids do not necessarily correlate with the extent of brain pathology. Nevertheless, a test battery intended for AD incorporating assays for CSF tau protein and Aβ42 has been developed and marketed in the United States under the trade name ADmark (Athena Diagnostics, Massachusetts).

Tau protein.　Neurofibrillary tangles in AD are composed of paired helical filaments, the principal component of which is a highly phosphorylated form of the microtubule-associated protein, tau. Tau plays a physiological role in the formation and stabilization of microtubules, and it has been proposed as a candidate biological marker for AD (Trojanowski et al. 1993). Levels of tau have been shown to be increased in brain tissue of AD patients relative to controls (Khatoon et al. 1992), and elevations of tau proteins have been documented by immunoassay in the CSF of AD patients (Motter et al. 1995; Vandermeeren et al. 1993; Vigo-Pelfrey et al. 1995).

From a diagnostic standpoint, the first encouraging implementation of a tau-based assay employed a commercially available (Innogenetics, Belgium) double-sandwich enzyme-linked immunosorbent assay (ELISA) that nonspecifically detects both phosphorylated and unphosphorylated forms of tau (Jensen et al. 1995). Elevations of total tau were found in the CSF of patients with familial as well as sporadic forms of AD. Within the familial cohort tested, asymptomatic carriers of the $APP_{670/671}$ mutation had higher CSF tau concentrations than normal controls, suggesting that total tau in CSF could prove to be an early marker of AD pathology. However, significant elevations of immunoreactivity were also detected in association with other neurological disorders, making this particular tau-based assay sensitive but not specific for AD. High sensitivity but low specificity was also reported in a larger study using monoclonal antibodies against recombinant human tau as the basis of an ELISA on CSF (Vigo-Pelfrey et al. 1995).

In theory, assays targeting AD-associated isoforms of tau could convey greater specificity to this test, but this idea has not been proven in practice so far. The A68 protein (PHF-tau) is an antigenic target of the Alz-50 antibody and appears to be a highly phosphorylated form of tau occurring with high specificity in AD brain. The Alz-50 antigen was once identified as a promising AD biomarker (Thal and Davies 1987) and was detected in low concentrations in the CSF of AD patients (Wolozin et al. 1986), but it has not proven useful as a clinical diagnostic test. A more recent study employing AT8, another monoclonal antibody that reacts with A68, failed to detect significant levels of the protein in the CSF of AD patients (Vandermeeren et al. 1993). It appears at this time that measurement of specific phosphorylation states of tau does not add significantly to the clinical value of tau-based assays.

Elevated CSF tau levels have now been documented in about 50%–60% of AD patients in subsequent studies collectively involving several hundred AD patients (Arai 1995; Monroe 1995; Mori 1995; Tato 1995). Although the low sensitivity effectively disqualifies measurement of CSF tau from consideration as a sole diagnostic test for AD, the reported greater-than-90% specificity of this test makes it appealing as an adjunct diagnostic measure. CSF tau levels do not show a significant correlation with severity of disease (Arai 1995; Motter et al. 1995), creating the potential for use throughout the course of the illness.

Amyloid precursor, amyloid peptide, and β-amyloid.   The amyloid core of NPs in the brains of AD patients is composed largely of aggregated and nonaggregated insoluble forms of beta amyloid (Aβ), a group of 4-kD peptide fragments of a large transmembrane amyloid precursor protein (APP). Soluble forms of Aβ (sAβ) and soluble derivatives of APP (sAPP or sβPP) derived from posttranslational processing of the amyloid precursor are present in CSF and have been studied as putative AD biomarkers.

No consistent relationship has been found between the amount of sAβ in the CSF and amyloid turnover as measured directly in brain tissue of AD patients and controls (Tabaton et al. 1994). Clinical studies have further established that there is considerable overlap between CSF sAβ levels in AD patients and normal controls and controls with dementia (Nitsch et al 1995; Pirttila et al. 1994; Van

Gool et al. 1995). Therefore, CSF sAβ does not appear to be the basis of a clinically useful diagnostic test for AD.

sβPP has been found to be reduced in the CSF of clinically diagnosed sporadic and familial AD patients relative to normals, based on results of a monoclonal antibody-based immunoassay (Hendricksson et al. 1991). sβPP is also lowered in cases of hereditary cerebral hemorrhage with amyloidosis (Dutch type) and the spongiform disorder Gerstmann-Sträussler-Scheinker syndrome (Van Nostrand et al. 1992). Since the overall prevalence of the latter two disorders is low compared to AD, it is still conceivable that sβPP could prove useful as a diagnostic marker in clinical practice. Prospective testing with autopsy correlation does not appear to support the use of the CSF sβPP assay alone as a diagnostic test for AD.

Aβ peptides terminating at the 42nd amino acid (Aβ42) have been postulated to be more relevant to the pathophysiology of AD than the more prevalent 40 amino acid peptides (Aβ40) because of the increased propensity of Aβ42 to aggregate and precipitate in vitro. Aβ42 is reportedly decreased in the CSF of AD patients relative to normals and neurologically diseased controls (Motter et al. 1995). Levels do not correlate with severity or duration of dementia, age, or possession of the APOE ε4 allele. Although the assay for Aβ42 has been marketed as part of the ADmark battery, the studies supporting its combined use with tau as a surrogate marker have not been widely replicated and its predictive value as an AD diagnostic test has not been conclusively established. Caution is therefore advised in interpreting this test until further studies are completed.

Other plaque-associated markers.   Other components of the NPs, such as the endosomal-lysosomal proteinase cathepsin D (cat D), have come under investigation as possible AD surrogate markers. Dysregulation of the lysosomal system has been cited as a possible mechanism for accelerated production of Aβ in AD (Nixon et al. 1992). Cat D levels averaged four-fold higher in the ventricular CSF of AD patients compared to normal controls, but the range of values among patients and controls shows considerable overlap (Schwagerl et al. 1995). This finding makes it unlikely that cat D levels will prove diagnostically useful in isolation.

Acute phase reactants have also been detected in the amyloid deposits, CSF, and serum of AD patients. Inflammatory markers have therefore continued to receive scrutiny as possible diagnostic markers for AD. Increased serum alpha-1-antichymotrypsin and interleukin-6 are among the markers showing significant but non-specific associations with AD. A diagnostic role for these markers in relation to AD diagnosis is unlikely, although it is conceivable that they could assist treatment trials involving anti-inflammatory medications.

Structural and Functional Brain Imaging

Assays of CSF or other peripheral markers provide little or no information about the neuroanatomic distribution of Alzheimer-related pathology in the brain. The latter is of considerable importance to the diagnosis of AD, as evidenced by the fact that brain biopsies confined to a small region of the cerebral cortex are significantly less conclusive than autopsy examinations of brain that permit examination of multiple brain regions to detect characteristic neuropathological changes. Currently available whole brain imaging methods reveal structural as well as functional correlates of Alzheimer-related neuropathology but do not permit the direct visualization of NPs or NFTs in a living person.

Magnetic resonance imaging volumetry.   The advent of computed tomography (CT) and magnetic resonance imaging (MRI) improved the differential diagnosis of dementia but has not had a comparable impact on the inclusionary diagnosis of AD. The information derived from visual inspection of structural brain images can be augmented by computer-assisted quantification of regional brain volumes. There has been some suggestion that volumetric techniques may prove useful as adjunct diagnostic measures for AD. Generalized cerebral atrophy is concomitant with normal aging, but selective reductions in the volume of various temporal lobe subregions have been reported to be specific to AD (Jack et al. 1992; Killiany et al. 1993). Age and gender appear to be important variables in the process of dissociating AD-related changes in brain volumes from those occurring in the course of normal aging (DeCarli et al. 1994). Confining measurements to the hippocampus may be undesirable in light of the variability in hippocampal volume among normals. The protocol for obtaining optimal diagnostic discrimination has yet to be determined, and most studies to date have examined normal and AD brains to the exclusion of non-AD dementias. Currently, MRI volumetry is a research tool that will require further development before its value as a diagnostic test for AD can be assessed objectively.

Magnetic resonance spectroscopy. Magnetic resonance spectroscopy (MRS) permits measurement of the concentration and chemical properties of metabolites containing certain atomic species in tissue volumes on the order of 1 to 3 cm^3. Although preliminary work with phosphorous MRS failed to provide sensitive or specific AD markers (Pettigrew et al. 1988), proton MRS has demonstrated reduced levels of the neuronal marker N-acetylaspartate (NAA) and increased concentrations of myoinositol (MI) in the brains of AD patients. NAA reduction is hypothesized to reflect loss of neurons in affected brain regions (Parnetti et al. 1995; Urenjak et al. 1993), while the pathological significance of increased MI levels in AD is uncertain. Shonk and co-workers (1995) found 83% sensitivity, 95% specificity, and a positive predictive value of 98% in distinguishing AD patients from normals using MRS measurement to measure the ratio of MI to NAA. However, when distinguishing AD from other dementias, specificity fell to 64%. MI alone (referenced to creatinine levels) provided a sensitivity of 82%, a negative predictive value of 80%, and a positive predictive value of 74% in distinguishing AD from other dementias. Owing to technical considerations, these measurements were carried out on the occipital lobe, which has a paucity of AD-related neuropathology relative to areas such as the medial temporal lobe. Nevertheless, temporoparietal regions are accessible to this technique, and the respectable predictive values in these preliminary studies suggest that proton MRS could play a role in the clinical diagnosis of AD if additional prospective large-scale studies and postmortem correlations can be carried out.

Single photon emission computed tomography and positron-emission tomography. Alterations in cerebral perfusion and metabolism as measured by single photon emission computed tomography (SPECT) and positron-emission tomography (PET) correlate with the distribution of NFTs and other aspects of Alzheimer neuropathology in the temporal and parietal cortices of mildly affected AD patients. Decreases in resting cerebral metabolism and blood flow can predate the development of cognitive deficits and can be detected by PET (Small et al. 1995). This theory was convincingly demonstrated in a recent PET study by Reiman and co-workers (1996) in which cognitively normal late-middle-aged APOE ε4 homozygotes with a family history of AD were found to have the same pattern of decreased regional glucose utilization as symptomatic patients with probable AD. This study involved analysis of group data and does not establish the technique's utility for predicting the development of AD in individual cases. This study nevertheless demonstrates the power of combining a trait marker such as APOE with a state marker such as PET.

Although PET can be used to determine both cerebral metabolic and perfusion alterations in association with AD, SPECT perfusion studies are more widely available and less costly, which may make them better suited for clinical diagnostic purposes. Hanyu and colleagues (1993) investigated the accuracy of SPECT in the diagnosis of AD in 219 neurological patients and normals, including 56 with probable AD. The presence of resting temporoparietal hypoperfusion, as judged by the qualitative interpretation of SPECT scans obtained using the perfusion tracer N-isopropyl-p-[^{123}I] (IMP), correlated with a diagnosis of AD with an overall sensitivity of 82% and specificity of 89%. The sensitivity of the test was least in the mildest cases (69%), and false positives occurred in 2 of 25 normals and 1 of 3 patients with Parkinson's disease with dementia. In another study, the accuracy of diagnosis of AD by SPECT alone (blinded to the clinical history) was compared to the strict application of National Institute of Communicative Disorders and Stroke–Alzheimer's Disease and Related Disorders Association (NINCDS-ADRDA) diagnostic criteria using autopsy correlation. Clinical criteria were found to be only slightly more sensitive than interpretation of SPECT in the absence of additional clinical data.

SPECT can be a valuable adjunctive tool in the differential diagnosis of AD and vascular dementia. In the study by Hanyu et al. (1993), only 10% of vascular dementia cases studied showed temporoparietal hypoperfusion. The presence of three or more zones of pronounced cortical hypoperfusion in association with dementia is highly suggestive of a cerebrovascular etiology. Most SPECT perfusion studies are currently performed in a nonquantitative fashion, and, as such, diagnostic accuracy is dependent on the skills of the interpreter. Quantitation of cerebral perfusion can be achieved with dynamic SPECT or PET but at considerably greater expense and effort. The cost and limited availability of PET, SPECT, and MRS have to a great extent limited the clinical application of these methods. Alternate means of obtaining cerebral perfusion measurements, including functional MRI techniques, are currently being evaluated and could eclipse SPECT's clinical role in the future.

Lessons From a Cholinergic Marker

Although cholinergic deficiency is no longer considered to be the primary cause of AD, early and accentuated loss of cholinergic projections to the cerebral cortex are among the best-documented neurochemical abnormalities in AD. Some evidence for an association between cholinergic abnormalities and classical AD neuropathology has emerged, including demonstration of acetylcholinesterase and butylcholinesterase activity in association with the NPs and alteration of amyloid precursor metabolism in vitro by cholinergic agonists. A variety of autonomic abnormalities attributable to cholinergic abnormalities have also been described in AD patients (Vitiello et al. 1993).

Past reports of an exaggerated response to mydriatics in patients with Down's syndrome, a group at risk for AD, inspired Scinto and colleagues (1994) to examine whether the cholinergic antagonist tropicamide would induce distinctive pupillary responses in AD patients. They placed a highly dilute solution of tropicamide, a synthetic analogue of atropine, in one eye of 14 AD patients, 32 cognitively normal elderly controls, and 12 patients with various other kinds of memory impairments. A saline solution was placed in the other eye for control purposes. An automated pupillometer was then employed to accurately measure the changes in pupil size over the course of 1 hour following introduction of the tropicamide drops. The relative magnitude of pupillary dilation 29 minutes after tropicamide administration was said to distinguish 95% of AD patients from 94% of controls, which led the investigators to suggest that tropicamide could provide a "possible neurobiological test for Alzheimer's disease" (Scinto et al. 1994, p. 1051). These statistics are by no means equivalent to prospectively measured clinical sensitivity and specificity. This study was not carried out in a blinded fashion or in a population with equivalent disease prevalence to that encountered clinically, as would be necessary to determine its true predictive power. Subjects with potentially confounding conditions such as primary autonomic or ophthalmologic disorders were excluded from the study, and results were analyzed using a retrospectively defined time point and cutoff that was chosen to minimize the overlap between AD and control groups. Even under these biased conditions, one out of four of the non-Alzheimer's dementia patients tested had a larger mydriatic response to tropicamide than the majority of AD patients in the study, and only 1%–2% changes in pupillary size separated the least dramatic responders among the AD patients from normal controls.

These considerations reduce the likelihood that this test would prove useful in the clinical diagnosis of AD, and the test's lack of diagnostic utility has now been suggested by other studies. The tropicamide test could still prove useful as a noninvasive, inexpensive screening test or alternate end point, particularly if it proves sensitive to AD pathology before the onset of clinical symptoms. One initially normal elderly control subject in the study by Scinto and colleagues (1994) showed the same degree of pupillary hyperresponsivity to tropicamide as AD patients and developed cognitive symptoms consistent with AD 9 months later. The likelihood that tropicamide sensitivity represents a true early marker of AD with long-term predictive value seems small, although the test could very well be sensitive to physiologic changes beginning a few months before the onset of cognitive symptoms becomes apparent.

Conclusions

In the foreseeable future, antemortem AD diagnosis is likely to involve the combination of trait markers, such as deterministic and susceptibility genes, with clinical and laboratory tests based on state markers. This approach should improve the accuracy of antemortem diagnosis and could also prove useful for identifying high-risk, asymptomatic individuals who are the best candidates for future preventative therapies.

The biological markers discussed in this chapter represent only a small fraction of those currently under study. In recent years, several markers that lack sufficient sensitivity or specificity to be used for direct diagnosis have been proposed for clinical use as adjunctive diagnostic tests. This trend may be dangerous. The inherent complexities of diagnosis based on multiple markers make exaggerated claims about the utility of individual tests more difficult to discern. It is useful to distinguish among tests that are based on robust biological markers (such as APOE genotyping) and those involving surrogate markers with only tenuous links to AD or its known neuropathology. Although the latter are potentially interesting and useful in other contexts, most have failed to provide significant improvements in the diagnostic accuracy for AD when applied clinically.

While APOE genotyping should not be used as the sole diagnostic test for AD, the strength of its association with AD provides a rationale for considering its adjunct diagnostic use. As yet, there have not been adequate clinical trials with autopsy correlation to permit recommendation of the combined use of APOE with other positive AD markers in routine clinical practice. The Bayesian approach to AD diagnosis awaits further prospective studies to assess validity of the method and the interactions between markers, as well as to establish the best means of applying various combinations of tests in a real-world setting. The combination of trait markers such as APOE genotyping with state markers such as functional brain imaging would appear to be a particularly promising inroad to pursue. Whether this approach will prove cost-effective and provide clinically meaningful improvement in AD diagnostic accuracy remains to be determined.

References

Arai H, Terajima M, Miura M, et al: Tau in cerebrospinal fluid: a potential diagnostic marker in Alzheimer's disease. Ann Neurol 38:649–652, 1995

Bird TD: Apolipoprotein E genotyping in the diagnosis of AD: a cautionary view. Ann Neurol 38:2–4, 1995

DeCarli C, Murphy DGM, McIntosh AR, et al: Descriminant analysis of Alzheimer's disease. Arch Neurol 51:1088–1089, 1994

Farrer LA: Statement on the use of apolipoprotein E testing for Alzheimer's disease. JAMA 274:1627–1629, 1995

Games D, Adams D, Alessandrini R, et al: Alzheimer-type neuropathology in transgenic mice overexpressing V717F beta-amyloid precursor protein. Nature 373:523–527, 1995

Goate A, Chartier-Harlin M, Mullan M, et al: Segregation of a missense mutation in the amyloid precursor protein gene with familial Alzheimer's disease. Nature 349:704–706, 1991

Hanyu H, Abe S, Arai H, et al: Diagnostic accuracy of single photon emission computed tomography in Alzheimer's disease. Gerontology 39: 260–266, 1993

Hendricksson T, Barbour RM, Braa S, et al: Analysis and quantitation of the β-amyloid precursor protein in the cerebrospinal fluid of Alzheimer's disease patients with a monoclonal antibody based immunoassay. J Neurochem 56:1037–1042, 1991

Jack CR Jr, Petersen RC, O'Brien PC, et al: MR-based hippocampal volumetry in the diagnosis of Alzheimer's disease. Neurology 42:183–188, 1992

Jensen M, Basun H, Lannfelt L: Increased cerebrospinal fluid tau in patients with Alzheimer's disease. Neurosci Lett 186:189–191, 1995

Khachaturian ZS: Diagnosis of Alzheimer's disease. Arch Neurol 42:1097–1106, 1985

Khatoon S, Grundke-Iqbal I, Iqbal K: Brain levels of microtubule-associated protein tau are elevated in Alzheimer's disease. J Neurochem 59:750–753, 1992

Killiany RJ, Moss MB, Albert MS, et al: Temporal lobe regions on magnetic resonance imaging identify patients with early onset Alzheimer's disease. Arch Neurol 50:949–954, 1993

Levy-Lahad E, Wasco W, Poorkaj P, et al: Candidate gene for the chromosome 1 familial Alzheimer's disease locus. Science 269:973–977, 1995

Mori H, Hosoda K, Matsubara E, et al: Tau in cerebrospinal fluids: establishment of the sandwich ELISA with antibody specific to the repeat sequence in tau. Neurosci Lett 186:181–183, 1995

Motter R, Vigo-Pelfrey C, Kholodenko D, et al: Reduction of β-amyloid peptide 42 in the cerebrospinal fluid of patients with Alzheimer's disease. Ann Neurol 38:643–648, 1995

Nitsch RM, Rebeck GW, Deng M, et al: Cerebrospinal fluid levels of amyloid β-protein in Alzheimer's disease: inverse correlation with severity of dementia and effect of apolipoprotein E genotype. Ann Neurol 37:512–518, 1995

Nixon RA, Cataldo AM, Paskevich PA, et al: The lysosomal system in neurons: involvement at multiple stages of Alzheimer's disease pathogenesis. Ann N Y Acad Sci 674:65–88, 1992

Parnetti L, Palumbo B, Cardinali L, et al: Cerebrospinal fluid neuron-specific enolase in Alzheimer's disease and vascular dementia. Neurosci Lett 183:43–45, 1995

Percy ME: Peripheral biological markers as confirmatory or predictive tests for Alzheimer's disease in the general population and in Down's syndrome, in Alzheimer's Disease and Down's Syndrome. Edited by Berg JM, Karlinsky H, Holland AJ. New York, Oxford University Press, 1993, pp 199–223

Pettigrew JW, Kanagasabai P, Moossy J, et al: Correlation of phosphorus-31 magnetic resonance spectroscopy and morphological findings in Alzheimer's disease. Arch Neurol 45:1093–1096, 1988

Pirozzolo FJ, Inbody SB, Sims PA, et al: Neuropathological and neuropsychological changes in Alzheimer's disease: relationship of biological markers to behavioral markers. Clin Geriatr Med 5:425–440, 1989

Pirttila T, Kim KS, Mehta PD, et al: Soluble amyloid β-protein in the cerebrospinal fluid from patients with Alzheimer's disease, vascular dementia and controls. J Neurol Sci 127:90–95, 1994

Reiman EM, Caselli RJ, Yun LS, et al: Preclinical evidence of Alzheimer's disease in persons homozygous for the epsilon 4 allele for apolipoprotein E. N Engl J Med 334:752–758, 1996

Relkin N: Apolipoprotein E genotyping in Alzheimer's disease. Lancet 347: 1091–1095, 1996

Roses A: Apolipoprotein E in the differential diagnosis, not prediction, of Alzheimer's disease. Ann Neurol 38:6–14, 1995

Roses A, Strittmatter WJ, Pericak-Vance MA, et al: Clinical application of apolipoprotein E genotyping to Alzheimer's disease. Lancet 343: 1564–1565, 1994

Schatzkin A, Freedman L, Schiffman M: An epidemiological perspective on biomarkers. J Intern Med 233:75–79, 1993

Schwagerl AL, Mohan PS, Cataldo AM, et al: Elevated levels of the endosomal-lysosomal proteinase cathepsin D in the cerebrospinal fluid in Alzheimer disease. J Neurochem 64:443–446, 1995

Scinto LFM, Daffner KR, Dressler D, et al: A potential noninvasive neurobiological test for Alzheimer's disease. Science 266:1051–1054, 1994

Scott RB: Extraneuronal manifestations of Alzheimer's disease. J Am Geriatr Soc 41:268–276, 1993

Sherrington R, Rogaev E, Liang Y, et al: Cloning of a novel gene bearing missense mutations in early onset familial Alzheimer's disease. Nature 375:754–760, 1995

Shonk TK, Moats RA, Gifford P, et al: Probable Alzheimer's disease: diagnosis with proton MR spectroscopy. Radiology 195:65–72, 1995

Small GW, Mazziota JC, Collins MT, et al: Apolipoprotein E type 4 allele and cerebral glucose metabolism in relatives at risk for familial Alzheimer's disease. JAMA 273:492–497, 1995

Strittmatter WJ, Saunders AM, Schmechel D, et al: Apolipoprotein E: high-avidity binding to beta-amyloid and increased frequency of type 4 allele in late-onset familial Alzheimer disease. Proc Nat Acad Sci U S A 90:1977–1981, 1993

Tabaton M, Nunzi MG, Xue R, et al: Soluble amyloid β-protein is a marker of Alzheimer amyloid in brain but not in cerebrospinal fluid. Biochem Biophys Res Commun 200:1598–1603, 1994

Tato RE, Frank A, Hernanz A: Tau protein concentrations in cerebrospinal fluid of patients with dementia of the Alzheimer's type. J Neurol Neurosurg Psychiatry 59:280–283, 1995

Thal LJ, Davies P: Detection of antigens in Alzheimer cerebrospinal fluid by monoclonal antibodies. J Am Geriatr Soc 35:1047–1050, 1987

Trojanowski JQ, Schmidt ML, Shin RW, et al: Altered tau and neurofilament proteins in neurodegenerative diseases: diagnostic implications for Alzheimer's disease and Lewy body dementias. Brain Pathol 3:45–54, 1993

Urenjak J, Williams SR, Gadian DG, et al: Proton nuclear magnetic resonance spectroscopy unambiguously identifies different neuronal cell types. J Neurosci 13:981–989, 1993

Vandermeeren M, Mercken M, Vanmechelen E, et al: Detection of τ proteins in normal and Alzheimer's disease cerebrospinal fluid with a sensitive sandwich enzyme-linked immunosorbent assay. J Neurochem 61:1828–1834, 1993

van Gool WA, Bolhius PA: Cerebrospinal fluid markers of Alzheimer's disease. J Am Geriatr Soc 39:1025–1039, 1991

van Gool WA, Hijdra A: Diagnosis of Alzheimer's disease by apolipoprotein E genotyping (letter). Lancet 344:275, 1994

van Gool WA, Kuiper MA, Walstra GJ, et al: Concentrations of amyloid beta protein in cerebrospinal fluid of patients with Alzheimer's disease. Ann Neurol 37:277–278, 1995

Van Nostrand WE, Wagner SL, Shankle W, et al: Decreased levels of soluble amyloid β-protein precursor in cerebrospinal fluid of live Alzheimer disease patients. Proc Nat Acad Sci U S A 89:2551–2555, 1992

Vigo-Pelfrey C, Suebert P, Barbour R, et al: Elevation of microtubule-associated protein tau in the cerebrospinal fluid of patients with Alzheimer's disease. Neurology 45:788–793, 1995

Vitiello B, Veith RC, Molchan SE, et al: Autonomic dysfunction in patients with dementia of the Alzheimer type. Biol Psychol 34:428–433, 1993

Wolozin BL, Pruchnicki A, Dickson DW, et al: A neuronal antigen in the brains of Alzheimer patients. Science 232:648–650, 1986

CHAPTER

14

Pharmacotherapy Past and Future

Leon J. Thal, M.D.

Diseases of the elderly are a major public health concern largely because of increased life expectancy. As of 1990, 12.5% of the U.S. population was over the age of 65. This percentage will change dramatically over the next 50 years so that by the year 2040, 22.5% of the U.S. population will exceed 65 years of age. Approximately 15% of people over the age of 65 suffer from some form of acquired cognitive deficit and of these two-thirds have dementia secondary to Alzheimer's disease (AD). Thus, by 2040, approximately 6 million Americans will be afflicted with this disorder. The economic consequences are considerable, with an estimated cost of $80 billion in 1990 and double that within the next 50 years. These demographic and economic factors coupled with our expanding scientific knowledge base have prompted a major focus on developing effective treatments for AD.

This work was supported by NIH Grants AGO 5131 and 10483.

Biological Considerations in AD Clinical Trials

Numerous problems are associated with the development of medications for AD. These issues range from the accuracy of clinical diagnosis to variability of the rate of decline.

Diagnostic Accuracy

At present, there is no biological marker for AD during life. Clinical criteria, such as DSM-IV (American Psychiatric Association 1994) for dementia and the National Institute of Communicative Disorders and Stroke–Alzheimer's Disease and Related Disorders Association (NINCDS-ADRDA) criteria for AD, are utilized to define the disorder. Using these criteria, diagnostic accuracy for AD is approximately 85% in large clinical series with autopsy verification (Galasko et al. 1994; Jellinger et al. 1990; Mölsa et al. 1985; Wade et al. 1987). More importantly, clinical criteria allow for the exclusion of unusual or atypical patients so that patients enrolled in clinical drug trials are probably correctly diagnosed with accuracy that exceeds 90%. Nevertheless, approximately 10% of individuals enrolled in clinical drug trials are likely to have another etiological explanation for their dementia. In addition, diagnosis of individuals in the very earliest stages of the disease is less certain. The development of a unique biological marker would be most useful for identifying very early or at-risk subjects. Although many biological markers have been proposed during the last decade, none have demonstrated adequate sensitivity and specificity to be clinically useful. Recently, dilatation of the pupil in response to a low dose of a cholinergic antagonist has been suggested as a possible diagnostic marker for AD. Preliminary data indicate that early and middle-stage AD patients are more sensitive than controls to the pupil-dilating effects of this agent (Scinto et al. 1994). However, the procedure was tested only in very well-diagnosed subjects, and it will require verification in larger series of patients with AD, as well as in individuals whose dementia is due to other etiologies, to verify its sensitivity and specificity. The development of a sensitive and specific biological marker would be extraordinarily useful, particularly to recruit patients for clinical drug trials designed to treat subjects at risk for the development of AD.

Biological Differences and Rate of Change of Dementia

Normal subjects have widely varying cognitive skills including differences in memory, language, intelligence, abstract thinking, and judgment; this variance is both innate and acquired. In addition, during the course of AD, difficulties with language, visuospatial relations, mood, and behavioral changes occur at different stages of disease and progress at different rates. For these reasons, a group of AD patients enrolled in a study will show heterogeneity in their clinical features. Therefore, considerable attention must be paid to the symptom complex that is targeted for treatment in AD. Should drug development be limited to the treatment of the cognitive disorder that is the hallmark of the disease? Alternately, should drug development also address the issue of behavioral disturbance, which is a common accompaniment of this disorder?

While it has long been recognized that all individuals with AD decline over time, the rate of decline is highly variable. Decline can be assessed in many ways. The simplest and most obvious method utilizes cognitive scales. Four global cognitive scales are widely employed. These are the Blessed Information Memory Concentration Test (BIMC) (Blessed et al. 1968), the Dementia Rating Scale (DRS) (Mattis 1976), the Mini-Mental State Examination (MMSE) (Folstein et al. 1975), and the Alzheimer Disease Assessment Scale (ADAS) (Rosen et al. 1984), particularly its cognitive subcomponent (ADAS-Cog). These instruments are generally suitable for monitoring patients with mild to moderate dementia. They are limited by both ceiling and floor effects and are not sensitive to change during either the very early or very late stages of the disorder. For these instruments, the average 1-year rate of change of AD patients is approximately equal to the standard deviation of the 1-year rate of change (Table 14–1). More recent studies have indicated that

Table 14–1.   Annual rate of change in Alzheimer's disease

Scale	Study	Number	Rate of change
BIMC	Katzman et al. 1988	161	4.4 ± 3.6
	Thal et al. 1988	40	4.5 ± 3.1
	Ortof and Crystal 1989	54	4.1 ± 3.0
	Salmon et al. 1990	50	3.2 ± 3.0
DRS	Salmon et al. 1990	55	11.4 ± 11.1
MMSE	Uhlman et al. 1986	120	2.2 ± 5.0
	Salmon et al. 1990	55	2.8 ± 4.3
	Teri et al. 1990	106	2.8 ± 4.6
ADAS	Kramer-Ginsberg et al. 1988	60	9.3 ± 9.8
	Stern et al. 1994	93	9.1 ± 8.4

greater precision can be obtained in estimating cognitive change by increasing the period of observation beyond 1 year (Morris et al. 1993). In addition, the rate of cognitive change is not linear over the entire course of the dementia. The most rapid change occurs in the middle stages of the disease, with slower change in mild and severe patients, indicating that the initial degree of dementia has an important effect on the observed rate of decline (Morris et al. 1993; Stern et al. 1994). Despite these limitations, rate of change is quite predictable for groups of patients, allowing for the accurate computation of sample size for AD clinical trials. In addition to measuring decline on cognitive scales, some work has been carried out measuring decline on global staging systems (Berg et al. 1988) and on activities of daily living (Green et al. 1993). Unfortunately, much less data exist for these noncognitive scales.

The Lewy Body Variant of AD

Many clinical features have been examined to determine whether they affect the rate of decline. Common clinical features such as psychotic behavior, myoclonus, and extrapyramidal features have all been found to be associated with a more rapid rate of decline

(Mayeux et al. 1985; Mortimer et al. 1992; Stern et al. 1987). Recently, approximately 15%–20% of AD patients have been found to have cortical Lewy bodies at autopsy. These individuals frequently present with mild extrapyramidal features such as masked facies, bradykinesia, slowing of rapidly alternating movements, and gait difficulty (Hansen et al. 1990). They generally do not have some of the classical features of parkinsonism such as flexed posture or resting tremor. In addition, many of these individuals have an essential or action tremor. At autopsy, these patients show AD pathology along with both cortical and subcortical Lewy bodies. There is often vacuolization in the entorhinal cortex and abundant senile plaques but only a small number of neurofibrillary tangles. This constellation of findings has been named the Lewy body variant of AD, senile dementia of the Lewy body type, or various other appellations. In a study of 44 patients clinically identified as having the Lewy body variant, compared to 207 AD subjects without the Lewy body variant, it was found that the Lewy body variant group exhibited approximately a 50% greater annual rate of decline on the MMSE, DRS, and Physical Self Maintenance Scale (PSMS) (Klauber et al. 1992), a measure of activities of daily living. Neurochemical analyses performed on the brains of patients with Lewy body variant indicate that they have a much greater depletion of dopamine in the basal ganglia than is seen in classical AD. In addition, cortical choline acetyltransferase levels are even lower than those seen in classic AD (Langlais et al. 1993). Whether this subgroup will respond differentially to treatment remains to be answered.

The Role of the Federal Government in AD Drug Research

The National Institute on Aging (NIA) is currently the major supporter of AD research along with the National Institute of Mental Health (NIMH) and the National Institute of Neurologic Disorders and Stroke (NINDS). The NIA has committed more than one-half of its research budget to AD. Initially, support was primarily directed toward investigator-sponsored grants to support basic biomedical research in dementia. In 1984 the NIA established the first five Alzheimer Disease Research Centers. Subsequently, the Alzheimer center program expanded to more than 20 centers and more than two dozen satellites. These centers were developed to identify and study cohorts of subjects with AD, to derive common nosology and diagnostic criteria, and to carry out clinicopathologic studies. In 1991 the NIA also funded six basic drug discovery groups and the Alzheimer Disease Cooperative Study (ADCS). The ADCS was developed to

1. Develop the organizational structure to carry out clinical drug trials.
2. Establish an independent data coordinating center.
3. Evaluate and improve on existing instruments for drug testing in AD.
4. Conduct clinical drug trials of promising agents.

The ADCS currently has 31 participating sites, most of which are colocated with existing Alzheimer Disease Centers. The ADCS both develops new instruments and carries out clinical drug trials. As of March 1996, more than 1,000 subjects had entered clinical drug trials sponsored by the ADCS.

Potential Treatments for AD

There are many approaches to considering potential treatments for AD. One conceptualization divides them into five primary foci which include 1) treatment of behavioral symptoms, 2) treatment of cognitive symptoms, 3) preventing decline, 4) delaying the onset of appearance, and 5) disease prevention.

1. Treatment of Behavioral Symptoms

A wide variety of behavioral symptoms occur in AD. However, five types of symptoms occur with great frequency, namely depression, anxiety, insomnia, agitation, and psychotic symptoms. In general, the treatment of these symptoms is based on treatments tested and used in non-AD populations. Unfortunately, treatment by analogy suffers from significant drawbacks in that behavioral symptoms in AD manifest differently than in patients without dementia. For example, loss of interest, apathy, and frequent complaints of depression are present in more than 50% of AD subjects. Thus, diagnostic criteria for depression in subjects with dementia are different than in individuals without dementia. Since the symptom complexes vary, response to treatment might also differ. Very few clinical trials have been carried out to empirically demonstrate whether dementia patients with behavioral disturbances respond in the same fashion as subjects without dementia.

Agitation is an important behavioral symptom in AD. Since disruptive agitated behaviors in AD are a common precipitant of institutionalization, investigation of more effective treatments for agitation are needed. Effective treatment is particularly important because between 70% and 90% of patients with dementia develop disruptive behavior at some time during the course of their illness (Swearer et al. 1988). Neuroleptics are widely used for managing agitation in AD. A recent meta-analysis of double-blind placebo-controlled trials of neuroleptics in agitated patients with dementia showed that these medications had a significant, although small, symptomatic effect (Schneider et al. 1990). Unfortunately, treatment with neuroleptics often produces significant side effects on the motor system, such as parkinsonism and tardive dyskinesia. Many clinicians also use sedating antidepressants such as trazodone to control agitated AD patients. However, clinicians are uncertain of the benefit-risk ratio of these treatments in AD.

To address this issue, the ADCS has recently initiated a controlled clinical trial of haloperidol, trazodone, and behavioral management techniques in AD patients with disruptive agitated behaviors. The specific aims of this trial are to

1. Determine whether haloperidol, trazodone, or behavioral management is more effective than placebo in the treatment of disruptive agitated behaviors.
2. Determine whether subtypes of disruptive agitated behaviors respond differentially to these three treatments.
3. Determine the side effect profile of each intervention.

In addition to this study of agitated behavior, many additional studies of behavioral disturbances in AD are needed.

2. Treatment of Cognitive Symptoms

Attempts to improve cognition in AD have been pursued for more than three decades. However, it was not until the demonstration of cholinergic abnormalities in AD in 1976 that rational drug therapy became possible. Over the past two decades, cognitive drug trials in AD have largely focused on augmenting cholinergic neurotransmission based on the well-established deficiencies in cortical choline acetyltransferase in AD (Davies and Maloney 1976), the decrease in synthesis of cortical acetylcholine (Francis et al. 1985), and the strong association between degree of dementia and decrease in cortical choline acetyltransferase levels (Perry et al. 1978). This line of research has resulted in the development of clinically useful cholinesterase inhibitors and in the approval of tetrahydroaminoacridine, first under a treatment investigational new drug (IND) application (Davis et al. 1992), followed by release of this agent in 1993 for the treatment of cognitive dysfunction in mildly to moderately impaired AD patients (Farlow et al. 1992; Knapp et al. 1994). Unfortunately, the use of tetrahydroaminoacridine produces only a small degree of cognitive improvement in a subset of AD patients. In addition, significant hepatotoxicity is encountered in clinical use. Numerous additional cholinesterase inhibitors are in development, many of which are likely to be free of hepatotoxicity. Nevertheless, neurotransmitter replacement therapy is likely to produce only small and temporary improvement in patients with AD. At present, there is no available evidence suggesting that the use of such agents will alter the inevitable downhill course. Use of symptomatic therapy should therefore result in a shift effect, where the slope representing rate of progression of AD does not change but cognitive test scores are temporarily improved (Figure 14–1A).

3. Preventing Decline in AD

Altering the rate of decline in AD would have a profound effect on the course of the disease. If a truly neuroprotective agent was developed and it continued to work throughout the course of the disease, then application of such a treatment should decrease the slope of decline. Over time, the effect size would increase with continued drug administration (Figure 14–1B). Ideally, one would wish to apply such a treatment early in the course of disease and slow the rate of decline to zero. Practical considerations, however, dictate that even a modest slowing in the downhill course by 20% would be clinically useful if the agent were nontoxic and reasonably priced. There are many clues currently available suggesting treatments that might prevent progression.

Anti-Inflammatory Drugs

Although AD has classically been considered to be a degenerative disease of uncertain etiology, recent evidence points to the involvement of inflammatory and immune mechanisms in the degenerative process. Acute-phase reactants such as C-reactive protein and alpha-1-antichymotrypsin are elevated in the serum of AD patients compared to age-matched controls (Matsubara et al. 1990). The increased levels of alpha-1-antichymotrypsin are particularly intriguing because it is a major component of the amyloid plaque (Abraham et al. 1988). Cytokines, including tumor necrosis factor, interleukin-1, and interleukin-6, are also elevated either in the serum (Fillit et al. 1991) or brain (Bauer et al. 1991; Griffin et al. 1989) of AD patients. A cellular immune response is present in AD

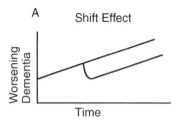 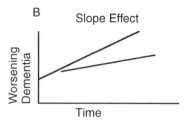

Figure 14–1. *A.* Symptomatic treatment should cause short-term improvement, but it should not change the slope of decline. This results in a shift effect. *B.* Treatment with a neuroprotective agent should alter the slope of decline, providing a progressively larger effect.

brains, as indicated by the presence of T8 and T4 lymphocytes and reactive microglia (McGeer et al. 1987; Rogers et al. 1988). Finally, complement is present in senile plaques (Eikelenboom and Stam 1982).

Epidemiological data obtained from twins discordant for the development of AD suggest that the use of either steroidal or non-steroidal anti-inflammatory drugs may delay the clinical onset of AD (Breitner et al. 1994). A 6-month controlled clinical trial of indomethacin, a nonsteroidal anti-inflammatory drug, suggested that cognitive stabilization occurred in a small cohort of AD subjects (Rogers et al. 1993). However, these results are preliminary and based on a very small sample size (only 14 patients in each group completed the study). Additionally, a high incidence of adverse events were reported. Nevertheless, the scientific rationale and these preliminary data are sufficiently provocative that the ADCS has initiated a multicenter controlled clinical trial of prednisone in AD to determine whether this form of therapy can slow the rate of decline.

Monoamine Oxidase Inhibitors and Antioxidants in AD

In AD, there is a significant increase in monoamine oxidase B (MAO-B) activity in brain (Oreland and Gottfries 1986) that exceeds the MAO-B increase associated with aging (Alexopoulos et al. 1984). The increase in brain MAO-B may result in an increase in the oxidative deamination of monoamines, with subsequent formation of hydrogen peroxide and other free radicals resulting in lipid peroxidation and predisposing toward cell injury. By reducing oxidative deamination, MAO inhibitors (MAOI) may prevent the formation of these free radicals and thereby preserve neuronal integrity (Smith et al. 1991). The largest increases in MAO-B in AD are found in the hippocampus (Oreland and Gottfries 1986), a key structure for processing memory. Inhibition of MAO-B may produce a selective augmentation of monoaminergic transmission that can improve cognitive functions mediated by catecholaminergic neurons.

Antioxidants may also be useful in the treatment of AD. The central nervous system is particularly vulnerable to lipid peroxidation because of its high lipid content (Halliwell and Gutteridge 1985). Vitamin E, or alpha-tocopherol, is a lipid-soluble vitamin capable of blocking lipid peroxidation. In cell culture systems, alpha-tocopherol has been shown to attenuate excitatory amino acid induced toxicity in neuroblastoma cells (Murphy et al. 1990), and it was further shown to attenuate the death of PC12 cells exposed to amyloid peptide (Behl et al. 1992).

Clinical trials using alpha-tocopherol in AD patients have not been carried out. There are, however, numerous small clinical trials using MAOI in AD (for review, see Corey-Bloom and Thal 1994). In general, these studies have demonstrated modest improvement in behavior on such measures as the Brief Psychiatric Rating Scale (Overall and Gorham 1962) and the Cornell Scale for Depression in Dementia (Alexopoulos et al. 1988). In addition, some studies have shown small cognitive effects on a variety of verbal learning tasks. A single 15-month study has been carried out examining the effects of selegiline, a MAOI, on the rate of decline in AD (Burke et al. 1993). Although the selegiline subjects declined at one-half the rate of the placebo-treated patients on the MMSE, the overall result was negative because of the very small sample size (16 placebo- and 17 drug-treated patients completed the trial).

The ADCS has initiated a double-blind, placebo-controlled multicenter study to examine the safety and efficacy of selegiline and alpha-tocopherol in the treatment of AD. The specific aims of this study are to

1. Determine whether the administration of selegiline, alpha-tocopherol, or a combination of the two will delay progression of symptoms and signs of AD.
2. Characterize the disease progression in a longitudinal manner using novel outcome measures that capture clinically important milestones.
3. Determine the feasibility of using survival analysis to evaluate drugs for the treatment of AD.

The study is a 2 × 2 factorial design examining selegiline alone, alpha-tocopherol alone, a combination of the two agents, or placebo in a cohort of AD subjects with moderate dementia followed for 2 years. Primary end points include death, institutionalization, loss of two out of three activities of daily living, and progression from moderate to severe dementia. This trial is unique in many respects. It is the first U.S. AD trial to be carried out for 2 years using concurrent placebo. It is also the first AD trial using survival analysis for these unique, highly clinically relevant end points.

Results from this trial have recently been published (Sano et al. 1997) and demonstrate that both agents delay the time to the primary end point by about 6 months.

Amyloid

Substantial evidence supports the role of beta amyloid in the pathogenesis of AD. This evidence is presented elsewhere in this volume (see Chapters 3 and 4). Evidence supporting beta amyloid in the pathogenesis of AD includes the role of mutations in the beta amyloid region of the amyloid precursor protein (APP) encoded on chromosome 21 in promoting early-onset familial AD and the neurotoxicity of beta amyloid in cell culture and in vivo (see Selkoe 1991 for review). The processing of APP and beta amyloid has not

been completely resolved. Present evidence suggests that secretases are responsible for cleaving the beta amyloid moiety from its
precursor protein. Since beta and gamma secretases are believed
to be responsible for cleaving beta amyloid from its precursor, the
development of selective secretase inhibitors is being pursued in
an effort to decrease the production of this amyloidogenic molecule.

Estrogens

Estrogens may play an important role in cognitive functioning.
Estrogen-sensitive neurons are found in both male and female
brains in specific locations. Receptors for circulating estradiol have
been localized to the nuclei of the basal forebrain, which degen-
erate in AD. Estrogen receptors also colocalize with low-affinity
nerve growth factor (NGF) receptors on cholinergic neurons of the
basal forebrain (Toran-Allerand et al. 1990). Estrogen has also been
reported to regulate N-methyl D-aspertate (NMDA) receptors in hippocampus (Woolley and McEwen 1993). Thus, the age-associated
decrease in estrogens could compound ongoing neuronal loss and
result in a reduced threshold for the expression of clinical symptoms.

Psychological symptoms in postmenopausal women include
difficulties in attention, concentration, and memory, as well as
emotional disturbances such as irritability and depression. Various
studies have demonstrated the beneficial effects of estrogen in reversing depressive symptoms in postmenopausal women (de-
Lignieres and Vincens 1982). Sherwin (1988) also studied the effect of hormone therapy and cognition after surgically induced
menopause. Improvements in digit span, paragraph recall, abstract
reasoning, and performance speed were demonstrated in these
women when they took estrogens.

Only three small trials of estrogen therapy in AD have been
reported (Fillit et al. 1986; Honjo et al. 1989; Ohkura et al. 1994).
Each of these studies reported improvement in some areas of emotional or cognitive functioning. However, the inclusion of depressed

women, small sample size, and problems with study design do not allow firm conclusions to be drawn from these data. In addition to the limited clinical trial data, epidemiological data from a case-control study suggest that the risk of AD is significantly less for those taking estrogen compared to those not taking it (Paginini-Hill and Henderson 1994; Paginini-Hill et al. 1993). In view of these suggestive results, a clinical trial of estrogen replacement therapy in patients with mild to moderate AD appears warranted.

Neurotropic Factors

NGF, the best-characterized neurotrophic factor, has a profound effect on cholinergic neurons. Three animal models have been employed to study its central nervous system cholinergic pharmacological effects. In the first model, cholinergic neurons located in the medial septum die after axotomy by transection of the fimbria fornix in the rat or primate. Intraventricular administration of NGF can prevent this axotomy-induced loss of cholinergic neurons (Gage et al. 1988; Hefti 1986; Tuszynski et al. 1990). In the second model, rats that are lesioned in the cholinergic neurons of the nucleus basalis have difficulty locating a submerged platform in the Morris water maze. Intraventricular administration of NGF to nucleus basalis–lesioned rats can improve performance in this water maze task (Dekker et al. 1992) and increase the release of acetylcholine from the cortex (Dekker et al. 1991). In the third model, deficits in water maze performance and shrinkage of basal forebrain cholinergic neurons can be demonstrated in aged rodents. This behavioral deficit can be partially reversed by intraventricular administration of NGF (Fisher et al. 1987).

At present, there is very little human experience with NGF. NGF is currently under investigation for peripheral neuropathy in the United States. In a Swedish study, three AD patients have received intraventricular NGF. After the infusion of high-dose NGF extracted from mouse salivary glands, significant cognitive improvement has not been reported in these subjects (Olson 1993). Significant toxicity occurred, including the development of pain and herpes zoster. The intraventricular infusion of NGF into rats has been reported to induce Schwann cell hyperplasia in the subarachnoid spaces surrounding the brain stem and spinal cord (Stewart et al. 1995; Winkler at al. 1995). Human clinical trials using this route of administration are unlikely to be attempted.

In addition to NGF, numerous additional neurotrophic factors have recently been identified and proposed for use in a wide variety of neurodegenerative disorders (for review, see Winkler and Thal 1994). The prospect of utilizing these agents in the treatment of neurodegenerative disorders is quite exciting since they are likely to not only slow the loss of cell populations but may be able to stimulate axonal growth and the development of new synapses in both the central and peripheral nervous systems.

4. Delaying the Onset of Disease Appearance

Available data indicate that the prevalence of AD doubles with every 5-year epoch beginning at age 65. Thus, a treatment that delays the appearance of disease by 5 years would halve its prevalence in one generation. Similarly, if disease appearance could be delayed by 10 years, its prevalence would diminish by 75% in one generation. Development of such a treatment would have far-reaching medical, economic, and ethical consequences.

Clinical prevention trials in AD have not yet occurred, which is in contradistinction to other fields of medicine, such as heart disease and stroke. Dementia trials in AD would require treatment of either a large segment of the elderly population or individuals who are recognized to be at high risk for the development of AD based on identification of risk factors. At present, the risk factors most important for predicting AD include older age, positive family history of AD, and apolipoprotein E (APOE) 4 status. Prevention trials could be targeted to either the older age population as a whole or to individuals who fall into these high-risk categories. As with cardiovascular trials, large numbers of subjects would be required since the incidence of AD in the over-age-65 population is less than 2% per annum.

Numerous agents might be considered for such a trial. However, in all cases, safety must be the primary consideration since the agent will be administered to thousands of normal individuals, many of whom will never develop the disease. Classes of compounds that might be considered for study include antioxidants, estrogens, anti-inflammatory drugs, drugs designed to alter APOE ε4 metabolism, and compounds that block the deposition of amyloid.

5. Disease Prevention

At present, there is insufficient information regarding the pathogenesis of AD to recommend strategies designed to prevent the disorder. These treatment strategies will therefore depend on further advances in understanding the neurobiology of the disorder. For example, if amyloid is ultimately proven to be central to the development of AD, then strategies to block its deposition or enhance its removal might be initiated early in life.

Future Considerations

At present, more than 60 agents are in clinical drug trials for AD. Although only one compound has been approved for use in AD to date, other agents are rapidly being developed. Additional cholinesterase inhibitors are most likely to be marketed first based on the success of tetrahydroaminoacridine. The cost of development for each agent is high. The pharmaceutical industry estimates costs to be $150 to $300 million for each successfully marketed agent. In addition, thousands of subjects need to be enrolled in controlled clinical trials before a drug can be proven to be both effective and safe. In the future, considerations other than simply safety and efficacy are likely to influence drug development. The most important of these issues are effect size, quality of life, and pharmacoeconomics. At present, there are no federal regulations specifying the effect size needed before a drug can be marketed. As third-party payers, the Health Care Financing Administration, and hospital and health maintenance organization formularies attempt to deal with the costs of medications, the issues of effect size and influence on quality of life will assume increasing importance. The issue of pharmacoeconomics is likely to play an increasing role in decisions regarding reimbursement for drugs. Future clinical drug trials are likely to consider the areas of activities of daily living, quality of life, and pharmacoeconomics as worthy of measuring.

References

Abraham CR, Selkoe DJ, Potter H: Immunohistochemical identification of the serine protease inhibitor alpha-1-antichymotrypsin in the brain amyloid deposits of Alzheimer's disease. Cell 52:487–501, 1988

Alexopoulos GS, Lieberman KW, Young RC: Platelet MAO activity in primary degenerative dementia. Am J Psychiatry 141:97–99, 1984

Alexopoulos GS, Abrams RC, Young RC, et al: Cornell Scale for Depression in dementia. Biol Psychiatr 23:271–284, 1988

American Psychiatric Association: Diagnostic and Statistical Manual of Mental Disorders, 3rd Edition, Revised. Washington, DC, American Psychiatric Association, 1987

American Psychiatric Association: Diagnostic and Statistical Manual of Mental Disorders, 4th Edition. Washington, DC, American Psychiatric Association, 1994

Bauer J, Strauss S, Schreiter-Gasser U, et al: Interleukin-6 and alpha-2-macroglobulin indicate an acute phase response in Alzheimer's disease cortices. FEBS Lett 285:111–114, 1991

Behl C, Davis J, Cole GM, et al: Vitamin E protects nerve cells from amyloid β protein toxicity. Biochem Biophys Res Commun 186:944–950, 1992

Berg L, Miller JP, Storandt M, et al: Mild senile dementia of the Alzheimer type 2: longitudinal assessment. Ann Neurol 23:477–484, 1988

Blessed G, Tomlinson BE, Roth M: The association between quantitative measures of dementia and of senile change in the cerebral grey matter of elderly subjects. Br J Psychiatry 114:797–822, 1968

Breitner JC, Gau BA, Welsh KA, et al: Inverse association of anti-inflammatory treatments and Alzheimer's disease: initial results of a co-twin control study. Neurology 44:227–232, 1994

Burke WJ, Roccaforte WH, Wengel SP, et al: L-Deprenyl in the treatment of mild dementia of the Alzheimer type: results of a 15-month trial. J Am Geriatr Soc 41:1219–1225, 1993

Corey-Bloom J, Thal LJ: Monoamine oxidase inhibitors in Alzheimer's disease, in Monoamine Oxidase Inhibitors in Neurological Diseases. Edited by Lieberman A, Olanow CW, Youdim MBH, Tipton K. New York, Chapman & Hall Medical, 1994, pp 279–294

Davies P, Maloney AJF: Selective loss of central cholinergic neurons in Alzheimer's disease (letter). Lancet 2:1403, 1976

Davis K, Thal L. Gamzu E, et al: A double-blind, placebo-controlled multicenter study of tacrine for Alzheimer's disease. N Engl J Med 327: 1253–1259, 1992

Dekker AJ, Langdon DJ, Gage FH, et al: NGF increases cortical acetylcholine release in rats with lesions of the nucleus basalis. Neuroreport 2:577–580, 1991

Dekker AJ, Gage FH, Thal LJ: Delayed treatment with nerve growth factor improves acquisition of a spatial task in rats with lesions of the nucleus basalis magnocellularis: evaluation of involvement of different neurotransmitter systems. Neuroscience 48:111–119, 1992

deLignieres B, Vincens M: Differential effects of exogenous oestradiol and progesterone on mood in postmenopausal women: individual dose effect relationship. Maturitas 4:67–72, 1982

Eikelenboom P, Stam FC: Immunoglobulins and complement factors in senile plaques: an immunohistochemical study. Acta Neuropathol (Berl) 57:239–242, 1982

Farlow M, Gracon S, Hershey L, et al: A controlled trial of tacrine in Alzheimer's disease. JAMA 268:2523–2529, 1992

Fillit H, Weinreb H, Cholst I, et al: Observations in a preliminary open trial of estradiol therapy for senile dementia-Alzheimer's type. Psychoneuroendocrinology 11:337–345, 1986

Fillit H, Ding W, Buee L, et al: Elevated circulating tumor necrosis factor levels in Alzheimer's disease. Neurosci Lett 129:318–320, 1991

Fisher W, Wictorin K, Bjorklund A, et al: Amelioration of cholinergic neuron atrophy and spatial memory impairment in aged rats by nerve growth factor. Nature 329:65–68, 1987

Folstein MF, Folstein SE, McHugh PR: Mini-Mental State: a practical method for grading the cognitive status of patients for the clinician. J Psychiatr Res 12:189–198, 1975

Francis PT, Palmer AM, Sims NR, et al: Neurochemical studies of early-onset Alzheimer's disease: possible influence on treatment. N Engl J Med 313:7–11, 1985

Gage FH, Armstrong DM, Williams LR, et al: Morphological response of axotomized septal neurons to nerve growth factor. J Comp Neurol 269:147–155, 1988

Galasko D, Hansen LA, Katzman R, et al: Clinical-neuropathological correlations in Alzheimer's disease and related dementias. Arch Neurol 51:888–895, 1994

Green CR, Mohs RC, Schmeidler J, et al: Functional decline in Alzheimer's disease: a longitudinal study. J Am Geriatr Soc 41:654–661, 1993

Griffin WS, Stanley LC, Ling C, et al: Brain interleukin 1 and S-100 immunoreactivity are elevated in Down syndrome and Alzheimer disease. Proc Natl Acad Sci U S A 86:7611–7615, 1989

Halliwell B, Gutteridge JMC: Oxygen radicals in the nervous system. Trends Neurosci 8:22–26, 1985

Hansen L, Salmon D, Galasko D, et al: The Lewy body variant of Alzheimer's disease: a clinical and pathological entity. Neurology 40:1–8, 1990

Hefti F: Nerve growth factor promotes survival of septal cholinergic neurons after fimbrial transections. J Neurosci 14:2155–2162, 1986

Honjo H, Ogino Y, Naitoh K, et al: In vivo effects by estrone sulfate on the central nervous system-senile dementia (Alzheimer's type). J Steroid Biochem Mol Biol 34:521–525, 1989

Jellinger K, Danielczyk W, Fischer P, et al: Clinicopathological analysis of dementia disorders in the elderly. J Neurol Sci 95:239–258, 1990

Katzman R, Brown T, Thal LJ, et al: Comparison of rate of annual change of mental status score in four independent studies of patients with Alzheimer's disease. Ann Neurol 24:384–389, 1988

Klauber MR, Hofstetter CR, Hill LR, et al: Patterns of decline in the Lewy body variant of Alzheimer's disease. Shanghai Archives of Psychiatry 4:50–53, 1992

Knapp MJ, Knopman DS, Solomon PR, et al: A 30-week randomized controlled trial of high-dose tacrine in patients with Alzheimer's disease. JAMA 271:985–991, 1994

Kramer-Ginsberg E, Mohs RC, Aryan M, et al: Clinical predictors of course for Alzheimer patients in a longitudinal study: a preliminary report. Psychopharmacol Bull 24:458–462, 1988

Langlais PJ, Thal L, Hansen L, et al: Neurotransmitters in basal ganglia and cortex of Alzheimer's disease with and without Lewy bodies. Neurology 43:1927–1934, 1993

Matsubara E, Hirai S, Amari M, et al: Alpha-1-antichymotrypsin as a possible biochemical marker for Alzheimer-type dementia. Ann Neurol 28:561–567, 1990

Mattis S: Mental status examination for organic mental syndrome in the elderly patient, in Geriatric Psychiatry: A Handbook for Psychiatrists and Primary Care Physicians. Edited by Bellak L, Karasu TE. New York, Grune & Stratton, 1976, pp 77–121

Mayeux R, Stern Y, Spanton S: Heterogeneity in dementia of the Alzheimer type: evidence of subgroups. Neurology 35:453–461, 1985

McGeer PL, Itagaki S, Tago H, et al: Reactive microglia in patients with senile dementia of the Alzheimer type are positive for the histocompatibility glycoprotein HLA-DR. Neurosci Lett 79:195–200, 1987

Mölsa PK, Paljarvi L, Rinne JO, et al: Validity of clinical diagnosis in dementia: a prospective clinico-pathological study. J Neurol Neurosurg Psychiatry 48:1085–1090, 1985

Morris JC, Edland S, Clark C, et al: The consortium to establish a registry for Alzheimer's disease (CERAD), IV: rates of cognitive change in the longitudinal assessment of probable Alzheimer's disease. Neurology 43:2457–2465, 1993

Mortimer JA, Ebbitt B, Jun SP, et al: Predictors of cognitive and functional progression in patients with probable Alzheimer's disease. Neurology 42:1689–1696, 1992

Murphy TH, Schnaar RI, Coyl JT: Immature cortical neurons are uniquely sensitive to glutamate toxicity by inhibition of cystine uptake. FASEB J 4:1624–1633, 1990

Ohkura T, Isse K, Akazawa K, et al: Evaluation of estrogen treatment in female patients with dementia of the Alzheimer type. Endocr J 41:361–371, 1994

Olson L: NGF and the treatment of Alzheimer's disease. Exp Neurol 124:5–15, 1993

Oreland L, Gottfries CG: Brain and brain monoamine oxidase in aging and in dementia of Alzheimer's type. Prog Neuropsychopharmacol Biol Psychiatry 10:533–540, 1986

Ortof E, Crystal HA: Rate of progression of Alzheimer's disease. J Am Geriatr Soc 37:511–514, 1989.

Overall JE, Gorham DR: The Brief Psychiatric Rating Scale. Psychol Rep 10:799–812, 1962

Paginini-Hill A, Henderson VW: Estrogen deficiency and risk of Alzheimer's disease. Am J Epidemiol 140:256–261, 1994

Paginini-Hill A, Buckwalter JG, Logan CG, et al: Estrogen replacement and Alzheimer's disease (abstract). Society for Neuroscience Abstracts 19:1046, 1993

Perry EK, Tomlinson BE, Blessed G, et al: Correlation of cholinergic abnormalities with senile plaques and mental test scores in senile dementia. Br Med J 2:1457–1459, 1978

Rogers J, Luber-Narod J, Styren SD, et al: Expression of immune-system-associated antigens by cells of the human central nervous system: relationship to the pathology of Alzheimer's disease. Neurobiol Aging 9:339–349, 1988

Rogers J, Kirby LC, Hempelman SR, et al: Clinical trial of indomethacin in Alzheimer's disease. Neurology 43:1609–1611, 1993

Rosen WG, Mohs RC, Davis KL: A new rating scale for Alzheimer's disease. Am J Psychiatry 141:1356–1364, 1984

Salmon DP, Thal LJ, Butters N, Heindel WC: Longitudinal evaluation of dementia of the Alzheimer type: a comparison of 3 standardized mental status examinations. Neurology 40:1225–1230, 1990

Sano M, Ernesto C, Thomas RG, et al: A controlled trial of selegiline, alpha-tocopherol, or both as treatment for Alzheimer's disease. N Engl J Med 336:1216–1222, 1997

Schneider LS, Pollock VE, Lyness SA: A meta-analysis of controlled trials of neuroleptic treatment in dementia. J Am Geriatr Soc 38:553–563, 1990

Scinto LFM, Daffner KR, Dressler D, et al: A potential noninvasive neurobiological test for Alzheimer's disease. Science 266:1051–1054, 1994

Selkoe DJ: Amyloid protein and Alzheimer's disease. Sci Am 265:68–71, 1991

Sherwin B: Estrogen and/or androgen replacement therapy and cognitive functioning in surgically menopausal women. Psychoneuroendocrinology 13:345–357, 1988

Smith CD, Carney JM, Starke-Reed PE, et al: Excess brain protein oxidation and enzyme dysfunction in normal aging and Alzheimer's disease. Proc Natl Acad Sci U S A 88:10540–10543, 1991

Stern Y, Mayeux R, Sano M, et al: Predictors of disease course in patients with probable Alzheimer's disease. Neurology 37:1649–1653, 1987

Stern RG, Mohs RC, Davidson M, et al: A longitudinal study of Alzheimer's disease: measurement, rate, and predictors of cognitive deterioration. Am J Psychiatry 151:390–396, 1994

Stewart GR, Day-Lollini PA, Taylor MJ, et al: Hyperplastic changes within the leptomeninges in response to chronic ICV infusion of nerve growth factor (abstract). Society for Neuroscience 21:278, 1995

Swearer JN, Drachman DA, O'Donnell BF, et al: Troublesome and disruptive behaviors in dementia: relationships to diagnosis and disease severity. J Am Geriatr Soc 36:784–790, 1988

Teri L, Hughes JP, Larson EB: Cognitive deterioration in Alzheimer's disease: behavioral and health factors. J Gerontol 45:P58–P63, 1990

Thal LJ, Grundman M, Klauber MR: Dementia: characteristics of a referral population and factors associated with progression. Neurology 38: 1083–1090, 1988

Toran-Allerand CD, Miranda RC, Bentham WDL, et al: Estrogen receptors co-localize with low-affinity nerve growth factor receptors in cholinergic neurons of the basal forebrain. Proc Natl Acad Sci U S A 89: 4668–4672, 1990

Tuszynski MH, U HS, Amaral DG, et al: Nerve growth factor infusion in primate brain reduces lesion-induced cholinergic neuronal degeneration. J Neurosci 10:3604–3614, 1990

Uhlman RF, Larson EB, Koepsell TD: Hearing impairment and cognitive decline in senile dementia of the Alzheimer's type. J Am Geriatr Soc 34:207–210, 1986

Wade JPH, Mirsen TR, Hachinski VC, et al: The clinical diagnosis of Alzheimer's disease. Arch Neurol 44:24–29, 1987

Winkler J, Thal LJ: Clinical potential of growth factors in neurological disorders. CNS Drugs 2:465–478, 1994

Winkler J, Ramirez GA, Kuhn HG, et al: Induction of Schwann cell hyperplasia in vivo after intracerebroventricular administration of nerve growth factor (abstract). Society for Neuroscience 21:178, 1995

Woolley CS, McEwen BS: Estradiol regulates hippocampal dendritic spine density via an NMDA receptors dependent mechanism (abstract). Society for Neuroscience Abstracts 379:15, 1993

CHAPTER

15

Practical Management of Alzheimer's Disease

Murray A. Raskind, M.D.

Introduction

Alzheimer's disease (AD) afflicts millions of older persons in the United States and is the most common dementing disorder of later life. Although the core signs and symptoms of AD are acquired impairment of memory and other intellectual functions, this disorder is often complicated by noncognitive behavioral problems, particularly disruptive agitated behaviors and depressive signs and symptoms. Disruptive agitated behaviors are the most troublesome noncognitive problems for caregivers. These disruptive agitated behaviors include physical and verbal aggression, uncooperativeness with personal care activities necessary for hygiene and safety, wandering and motoric hyperactivity, and psychotic delusions and hallucinations. Depressed mood and demoralization also frequently occur in the course of AD. The practical management of these noncognitive behavioral problems has been approached both psychopharmacologically and by psychosocial interventions. In this chapter I focus on the results of controlled studies evaluating psychopharmacologic and psychosocial therapies used in the practical management of behavioral problems complicating AD. Because well-designed and adequately controlled studies are scarce, despite the extensive use of both pharmacologic and nonpharmacologic treatments for agitated disruptive behaviors and depressive signs and symptoms in AD, the results from uncontrolled but heuristically useful studies also are discussed.

Psychopharmacologic Management of Disruptive Agitated Behaviors: Epidemiology

The majority of AD patients experience disruptive agitated behaviors at some point during the course of their illness. These signs and symptoms are frequently managed psychopharmacologically (Salzman 1987). That prescription of psychotropic drugs to AD patients is widespread is best documented in long-term care settings. Beers et al. (1988) studied psychotropic medication use in long-term facility residents in Massachusetts. To ensure that these facilities represented typical community geriatric nursing homes rather than facilities caring for deinstitutionalized chronic mental hospital patients with lifelong schizophrenia or other chronic psychiatric disorders, facilities were not included in the sample if they had greater than 20% of residents admitted from inpatient psychiatric hospitals. In this study, more than half of all elderly residents were receiving a psychotropic medication. Twenty-six percent were receiving antipsychotic medication, and 28% were receiving a benzodiazepine or other medication with primarily sedative or hypnotic activity. A similar pattern of psychotropic medication use in long-term care facilities was demonstrated by Buck (1988) in a group of elderly Medicaid recipients in nursing homes in Illinois. Of these residents, 60% received at least one psychotropic medication during the year of study. Again, antipsychotic drugs (particularly haloperidol and thioridazine) and sedative or hypnotic drugs (particularly the benzodiazepine flurazepam) were frequently prescribed. Avorn et al. (1989) found an even higher prevalence of antipsychotic medication use in a random sample of 55 long-term care facilities in Massachusetts. Thirty-nine percent of the patients were being administered an antipsychotic medication. Furthermore, this study documented that approximately half of the residents in nursing homes with particularly high levels of antipsychotic drug use were lacking participation by a physician in decisions about management of psychiatric problems.

Since the Omnibus Budget Reconciliation Act (OBRA)-1987 regulations for psychotropic drug use in long-term care facilities have been instituted, there is suggestion that the use of psychotropic drugs has been reduced. Garrard et al. (1992) documented antipsychotic medication use in 17% of elderly nursing home residents (mean age 83), most of whom were suffering from AD. He also found that trial discontinuations of antipsychotic medication were common among his sample. This important study suggests that physicians and other health care providers are attempting to reduce prescription of psychotropic medications to behaviorally disturbed AD patients. Slater and Glazer (1995) reported a reduction of mean antipsychotic drug dose in a community nursing home following implementation of OBRA standards.

Antipsychotic Drugs

The rationale for the widespread use of antipsychotic drugs in AD patients is at least partially based on the phenomenologic similarities between some of their disruptive agitated behaviors and the behaviors observed in subjects with "functional" schizophrenia but without dementia. The nonspecific sedative effects of the antipsychotic drugs may also play a role in their popularity for the treatment of disruptive agitated behaviors complicating AD. It is technically correct that signs and symptoms that meet the definition of delusions and hallucinations occur commonly in AD (Cummings et al. 1987; Wragg and Jeste 1989). It must be pointed out, however, that the delusions and hallucinations occurring in the context of AD often are qualitatively different from the bizarre and complex symptoms occurring in schizophrenia. In AD, the most common psychotic symptoms are of simple delusions of theft. It is likely that the memory defect in AD contributes to the genesis of these delusional beliefs. If a patient with AD forgets where he or she has placed an item and cannot locate it, it may not be unreasonable for him or her to assume that the item has been stolen. Similarly, when an article of clothing discarded many years earlier now cannot be located by the forgetful patient, the belief that it has been stolen is quite common. Because many AD patients have little insight concerning their memory impairments, reassuring explanations often are of no avail. That these false beliefs meet formal criteria for delusions cannot be contested, but in many ways they are dissimilar from the elaborate and bizarre delusions frequently encountered in schizophrenia for which the antipsychotic drugs have been demonstrated so effective. The quality of hallucinations also differs frequently from that in schizophrenia. Visual hallucinations are common in AD, but schizophrenia-like auditory hallucinations of voices communicating with the patient are uncommon. It should also be mentioned that disruptive behaviors without clear evidence of any type of delusions or hallucinations frequently are treated with antipsychotic medications. Resistance and uncooperativeness to care, motor restlessness and pacing, and verbal and physical aggression often are assumed (rightly or wrongly) to be related to an underlying psychotic process that is not overtly evident because of the patient's dysphasia or other communication disturbances.

Treatment Outcome Trials of Antipsychotic Drugs

Although clinical outcome trials of antipsychotic drugs in dementia patients with disruptive agitated behaviors are more numerous than for any other class of psychotropic medications, placebo-controlled well-designed studies providing interpretable data remain scarce. Clinicians also should be cautioned that many of these studies were performed before the introduction of DSM-III (American Psychiatric Association 1980) and National Institute of Communicative Disorders and Stroke (NINCDS) criteria for AD and thus often use confusing diagnostic nomenclature and occasionally use the term *psychotic* to connote severe cognitive impairment rather than the presence of delusions or hallucinations. Furthermore, the earlier studies were frequently performed in state hospital populations that included both patients with AD and other degenerative neurologic dementing disorders and patients with chronic schizophrenia who had grown old.

Despite these caveats, studies of antipsychotic drugs performed before the introduction of current diagnostic criteria for AD still provide some useful information. Placebo-controlled trials of chlorpromazine (Seager 1955), acetophenazine (Hamilton and Bennett 1962a), and haloperidol (Sugarman et al. 1964) indicate that antipsychotic drugs are more effective than placebo for global ratings of disturbed behavior, assaultiveness, hyperexcitability, hostility, and hallucinations. However, in each of these studies the subjects receiving antipsychotic medications had frequent adverse effects, including excessive sedation, unsteady gait, pseudoparkinsonian rigidity, and falls. Several studies that failed to demonstrate an advantage for antipsychotic medications compared to placebo in AD and other late-life dementing disorders shared a common feature. That is, they did not include patients with disruptive agitated behaviors as target symptoms. Rather, antipsychotic drugs were assessed for efficacy in the management of cognitive and activities-of-daily-living deterioration. Hamilton and Bennett (1962b) compared trifluoparazine to placebo for the management of apathy, withdrawal, cognitive impairment, incontinence, loss of ambulation, and severe disorientation. Trifluoperazine did not improve these symptoms more than placebo and induced problematic sedation and rigidity in the majority of active medication patients. Rada and Kellner (1976) assessed the effects of thiothixene compared to placebo for amelioration of cognitive deficits in AD patients. Interestingly, global improvement was noted in both the thiothixene and placebo groups, and the percentage of improved patients did not differ between treatments. The substantial placebo response in this latter study was notable.

In the only study using modern diagnostic criteria carried out in a typical community nursing home population (mean age of subjects 83), Barnes et al. (1982) compared thioridazine, loxapine, and placebo for the treatment of disruptive agitated behaviors in patients with AD. Overall results favored antipsychotic drugs over placebo, but differences among treatment groups were modest and not always what the investigators predicted. Ratings of excitement and uncooperativeness improved significantly more with antipsychotic drug than with placebo. Although suspiciousness and hostility improved with antipsychotic medication, these parameters also improved with placebo; the differences between active drug and placebo did not reach statistical significance. These results suggest real but limited efficacy for antipsychotic drugs in the management of disruptive agitated behaviors in AD patients. They also point out the surprising strength of the placebo effect in this population with dementia. Petrie et al. (1982) studied the effects of haloperidol and loxapine compared to placebo in a younger sample (mean age 73) of patients with either AD or multi-infarct dementia who were residents of a large state psychiatric hospital. Their results were similar to those of Barnes et al. (1982). Global ratings were moderately or markedly improved in approximately one-third of active drug patients compared to 9% of patients who had been assigned to the placebo group. Active medications were significantly more effective than placebo in treating suspiciousness, hallucinatory behavior, excitement, hostility, and uncooperativeness. The younger mean age of the patients in this sample suggests that the results of Barnes et al. (1982) are more applicable to the typical community nursing home population. Not surprisingly, both of these studies demonstrated a high prevalence of parkinsonian rigidity and other adverse effects of antipsychotic medications.

One study (Monane et al. 1991) evaluated the frequency of parkinsonian side effects associated with haloperidol use in an elderly nursing home population. In this sample, antipsychotic drug use occurred in 40% of patients. Haloperidol was the most commonly prescribed agent. Increased muscle tone was significantly more prevalent in haloperidol users, although residents taking less than 1 mg haloperidol per day had muscle tone ratings similar to residents on no antipsychotic drugs. Bradykinesia, cogwheel rigidity, and masked facies were noted in 43% of the entire sample and were significantly more prevalent in haloperidol users. Monane et al. (1991) concluded that parkinsonian adverse effects are commonly associated with haloperidol use in the elderly nursing home population, particularly in residents receiving greater than 1 mg haloperidol per day.

AD outpatients in earlier stages of the disease have received less attention in clinical outcome trials of antipsychotic drugs, despite the observation that disruptive agitated behaviors are major precipitants of long-term care placement (Steele et al. 1990). Reisberg et al. (1987) reported that disruptive agitated behaviors in AD were effectively managed with thioridazine in AD outpatients, but this study did not include a placebo control group and must be considered anecdotal. Devanand et al. (1989) performed a placebo-controlled crossover design study comparing haloperidol to placebo in nine AD outpatients who had clear psychotic behaviors, as defined by delusions, hallucinations, and disruptive agitated behaviors. Haloperidol was significantly superior to placebo, with five of nine patients showing clinically substantial improvement with haloperidol compared to placebo. However, cognitive deterioration and extrapyramidal rigidity tempered the behavioral gains of subjects in the haloperidol group. This study is important because it addresses outpatients in the earlier stages of disease and is the only study to date in which the AD subject sample was restricted to those who manifested clear delusions or hallucinations. A meta-analysis of studies evaluating antipsychotic drugs in patients with AD and related disorders (Schneider et al. 1990) concluded that antipsychotics are more effective than placebo, but the effect size is small and one antipsychotic drug is equivalent to any other.

The OBRA regulation for time-limited use of antipsychotic drugs in AD patients has received some support from Risse and colleague's (1987) evaluation of the response of AD patients to withdrawal of antipsychotic medications. These dementia patients were selected for having apparently benefited from antipsychotic medication administration and for chronic antipsychotic maintenance (longer than 6 months). Nine male dementia patients maintained on antipsychotic drugs were switched in a double-blind manner to placebo over a 6-week period. At the end of the 6-week placebo period, only one patient had developed disruptive behavior severe enough to warrant reinstitution of antipsychotic medication. Of the remaining eight patients, one was rated as more agitated, two were unchanged, and five actually were rated as less agitated than they had been before substitution of placebo for the antipsychotic medication. This result supports periodic trials of antipsychotic medication tapering and, if possible, discontinuation in patients chronically maintained on antipsychotic medication.

Trazodone

A number of anecdotal reports suggest that the antidepressant trazodone may be useful in the management of disruptive agitated behaviors in AD. Simpson and Foster (1986) treated four elderly dementia patients with trazodone after antipsychotic drug therapy had proved ineffective. In these four subjects, doses of trazodone ranging from 250 to 500 mg daily decreased agitation, combative behavior, and violent outbursts. Similarly, Pinner and Rich (1988) treated seven elderly dementia patients with trazodone for symptomatic aggressive behavior. All patients had failed to show a therapeutic response to prior treatment with antipsychotic drugs. Three of seven patients demonstrated marked decreases in aggressive behavior following 4 to 6 weeks of trazodone treatment at 200 to 300 mg per day. In both of these studies, patients were relatively young (in their sixth or seventh decades), and results of these anecdotal studies should be extrapolated with caution to the average nursing home patient in the ninth decade of life. In contrast to the antipsychotics, trazodone does not produce extrapyramidal adverse effects but is a sedating drug and can produce orthostatic hypotension. Placebo-controlled trials of trazodone for disruptive agitated behavior in AD and related disorders appear warranted.

Buspirone

Buspirone is an antianxiety drug with a benign adverse effect profile. Colenda (1988) anecdotally reported that buspirone, at 45 mg per day, produced marked improvement in angry outbursts and oppositional behavior in a 74-year-old AD patient who had failed to respond to haloperidol. Sakauye et al. (1993) administered open label buspirone (30 to 40 mg per day) to 10 patients with AD complicated by disruptive agitated behaviors. They reported a modest (22%) but significant overall reduction in disruptive behaviors. Response was variable in these subjects, and no placebo condition was studied. Because of its benign adverse effect profile, however, placebo-controlled trials of buspirone for the management of disruptive agitated behaviors in AD appear warranted.

Anticonvulsant Drugs

The anticonvulsants carbamazepine and valproate have received anecdotal support as effective in the management of disruptive agitated behaviors in AD. Marin and Greenwald (1989) reported that two AD patients and one multi-infarct dementia patient who had failed to respond to haloperidol showed marked reduction in combative agitated behaviors within 2 weeks of instituting carbamazepine at doses ranging from 100 to 300 mg per day. Gleason and Schneider (1990) studied nine AD patients with disruptive agitated behaviors who had failed to respond to antipsychotic drugs. They noted symptomatic improvement in hostility, agitation, and uncooperativeness in five of nine patients. However, ataxia and confusion mitigated the therapeutic gains of two of these patients. Mean dose of carbamazepine in this study was 480 mg per day, and mean plasma carbamazepine level was 6.5 μg/ml. A negative study of carbamazepine in elderly dementia patients given doses of 100 to 300 mg per day or placebo in a crossover design was reported in 1982 by Chambers et al. This latter study may have been handicapped by too low a dose of medication, but the use of a placebo group is to be applauded and again underlies the necessity for placebo control in any studies of disruptive agitated behaviors in AD. Mervis et al. (1991) compared carbamazepine to trazodone in reduction of behavioral problems associated with dementia in patients not satisfactorily managed with antipsychotic drugs. Trazodone but not carbamazepine was associated with decreased wandering, agitation, and aggression in this small pilot study. Valproate has been reported anecdotally to improve AD complicated by disruptive agitated behaviors. Mellow et al. (1993) prescribed sodium valproate at doses ranging from 500 mg bid to 500 mg tid to four AD patients with disruptive agitated behaviors and noted substantial behavioral improvement in two of these patients.

Benzodiazepines

The epidemiologic studies noted previously (Beers et al. 1988; Buck 1988; Garrard et al. 1992) document that benzodiazepines are the second most commonly prescribed class of drugs (after the antipsychotics) for disruptive agitated behaviors complicating AD in the long-term care setting. The use of benzodiazepines in dementia patients has been reviewed (Stern et al. 1991). Sanders (1965) compared oxazepam to placebo in elderly (mean age 81) "emotionally disturbed" patients. Although oxazepam was superior to placebo after 6 weeks of treatment, there was no difference in placebo and oxazepam at the end of the treatment period. Symptoms of anxiety and agitation showed the most favorable albeit transient response to active treatment. Kirven and Montero (1973) compared thioridazine to diazepam in a non-placebo-controlled comparison study for behavioral symptoms associated with senility. Symptomatic improvement occurred in both treatment conditions, but there was a trend for greater improvement in the thioridazine subjects. Tolerance to benzodiazepine appeared to be developing by the end of the treatment protocol.

Coccaro et al. (1990) compared haloperidol, oxazepam, and the sedating antihistamine diphenhydramine in a group of elderly institutionalized patients, most of whom met criteria for AD and manifested agitated behaviors. A placebo group was not included in this study. Disruptive agitated behaviors decreased in all treatment groups over the 8-week treatment period, but there was no differential response among the drugs. There was an apparent trend for superiority of haloperidol and diphenhydramine compared to oxazepam. Given the development of tolerance to oxazepam in several of the previously discussed studies and the tendency for oxazepam to be less effective than either diphenhydramine or haloperidol in the study of Coccaro et al. (1990), the widespread use of benzodiazepines in long-term care settings may be inappropriate. The likelihood that benzodiazepines will produce excessive sedation and ataxia in a substantial number of elderly patients prescribed these agents also supports caution in using benzodiazepines to treat AD complicated by disruptive agitated behaviors.

Psychosocial Therapies in the Management of Disruptive Behaviors in AD

It appears to many clinicians that environmental and interpersonal factors contribute to the genesis, timing, and modification of disruptive agitated behaviors in AD patients. These observations have prompted the following questions: What is the best environment for eliminating disruptive agitated behaviors in AD? Do interpersonal factors exacerbate or ameliorate disruptive agitated behaviors in AD? Can classic or modified behavioral interventions reduce the frequency or intensity of disruptive agitated behaviors in AD? Although much has been written in response to these questions, well-designed outcome trials evaluating environmental, interpersonal, and behavioral treatments of AD are even more scarce than for pharmacologic interventions. A few representative studies will be described to emphasize the importance of these issues.

In response to concerns that typical nursing home staff members may not be knowledgeable about effective ways of responding to behavioral symptoms in residents with AD, that inappropriate staff responses may exacerbate behavioral symptoms, and that psychotropic medications and physical restraints are used inappropriately to manage behavioral symptoms, special care units (SCUs) for persons with dementia have been established in many nursing homes around the country (Maslow 1994). Despite the proliferation of these units, little is known about their effectiveness. Common sense suggests that an SCU with controlled access and egress would be helpful in the management of wandering and that an SCU with selected staff motivated and enthusiastic toward providing excellent care for AD patients would prove beneficial. However, SCUs are probably more costly than standard nursing home care, and further research is needed to justify these expenditures and determine exactly what components of an SCU are involved in effective reduction of behavioral symptoms (Maslow 1994).

In an important recent study, Mittelman et al. (1993) evaluated the effect of psychosocial therapy for spouse caregivers of AD patients on eventual nursing home placement. Psychosocial therapy consisted of individual and family counseling, support group participation, and ad hoc consultation. A control group received routine support as requested. At 12 months the treatment group had less than half as many nursing home placements as did the control group, a statistically significant and clinically meaningful result.

Interpersonal variables may contribute to disruptive agitated behaviors in AD patients. For example, Burgener et al. (1992) examined the relationships between caregivers and elderly residents with dementia in long-term care. They found that residents' problematic behaviors varied according to the type of activity of daily living in which they were involved. The most disruptive behaviors occurred during bathing. Significant relationships during both dressing and toileting emerged between caregivers' relaxed and smiling behavior and residents' calm and functional behaviors. This type of study does not establish a cause-and-effect relationship between caregiver and resident behaviors but opens new lines of research. Cohen-Mansfield et al. (1990) studied screaming in nursing home residents. They noted that nursing home residents with dementia screamed more often when alone in their rooms during the evening hours. Although a cause-and-effect relationship was not established, that reduction of social isolation decreases screaming behavior is an experimentally testable hypothesis.

Classic behavior modification approaches to disruptive agitated behaviors in AD have been discussed by McGovern and Koss (1994). They acknowledged that empiric studies evaluating the efficacy of such behavior modification strategies in AD patients have not yet been performed but noted that anecdotal reports demonstrate reductions in such behaviors as urinary and fecal incontinence (Burgio et al. 1988) and socially inappropriate behaviors (Haley 1983; Hussian 1982). They advocate clear identification of target behaviors that need to be modified, the use of distraction to avert management problems, the use of primary reinforcers such as food and liquids, a continuous reinforcement schedule for specific behaviors, and the availability of the clinician as coach and troubleshooter for the caregiver. Again, controlled outcome studies of such behavioral approaches have yet to be performed for the management of agitated behaviors in AD patients. Gwyther (1994) approaches the behavioral management of disruptive behaviors in AD in a somewhat different manner. She has observed that patients with AD do more to modify the behavior of their caregivers than vice versa. She advocates changing the ways caregivers communicate with patients and urges them to understand and use nonverbal approaches. Gwyther suggests that indirect approaches are more effective and feasible than classic behavioral modifications because they do not rely on the patient's use of experience or new learning. Her approaches stress changing the behavior of the caregiver, which secondarily will produce positive changes in the behavior of the AD patient.

Depressive Signs and Symptoms Complicating AD

Because depression adversely affects quality of life and may impair cognitive function, the recognition and effective management of depressive signs and symptoms complicating AD are important. The diagnosis of major depressive disorder is complicated in the AD patient by the confounding of the accepted clinical diagnostic criteria for major depressive disorder with signs and symptoms of AD per se. Common to both disorders are loss of interest in previously interesting activities, agitation, sleep disturbances, weight change, and inability to concentrate. However, even depressive signs and symptoms that may not be clearly part of a major depressive episode can be associated with added functional impairment in AD patients (Pearson et al. 1989).

Although anecdotal case reports (Jenike 1985) and open label trials of standard antidepressant pharmacotherapy in hospitalized AD patients with coexisting depressive signs and symptoms (Greenwald et al. 1989; Reynolds et al. 1987; Zubenko and Moossy 1988) have been interpreted as supporting the efficacy of antidepressant drugs in AD patients with concurrent depressive signs and symptoms, the only placebo-controlled treatment trial reported in the literature (Reifler et al. 1989) raises serious concerns about the interpretability of uncontrolled studies. Reifler et al. (1989) compared imipramine to placebo in a double-blind outcome study of depressive signs complicating AD. Subjects in this study were outpatients who met clinical criteria for both AD and major depressive episode, had a mean Mini-Mental State Exam (MMSE) (Folstein et al., 1975) score of 17, and were suffering from depressive signs and symptoms of mild to moderate severity. Substantial and highly significant improvement over time in depressive signs and symptoms was documented in both the imipramine and the placebo groups, but the amount of improvement in both groups was almost identical. The magnitude of improvement in this study was almost identical to that reported in the open clinical trials of Reynolds et al. (1987), Greenwald et al. (1989), and Zubenko and Moossy (1988). Although newer antidepressants such as the selective serotonin reuptake inhibitor drugs and venlafaxine may be useful for treatment of depressive signs and symptoms in AD and do not cause orthostatic hypotension or anticholinergic adverse effects, these and other newer antidepressants have not been evaluated in AD patients suffering from depressive signs and symptoms. Such studies would be welcome additions to the psychopharmacologic database.

The results of the study by Reifler et al. (1989) suggest that nonpharmacologic aspects of the treatment milieu of the AD patients participating in that study accounted for the reduction in severity of depressive signs and symptoms. Although a simple time duration effect cannot be excluded, it is likely that interactions between the research team and the patient caregiver dyad, as well as increased activity associated with attending weekly evaluation and dosage adjustment visits, contributed to symptom amelioration. Based on these findings, Teri (1994) has developed a behavioral management treatment protocol for depressive signs and symptoms complicating AD that stresses training the caregiver to increase the AD patient's pleasurable activities. Preliminary results suggest that a behavioral management approach to depressive signs and symptoms complicating AD is effective. Further studies of behavioral management therapy of depressive signs and symptoms in AD are under way.

References

Avorn J, Dreyer P, Connelly MA, Soumerai SB: Use of psychoactive medication and the quality of care in rest homes. New Engl J Med 320: 227–232, 1989

Barnes R, Veith R, Okimoto J, et al: Efficacy of antipsychotic medications in behaviorally disturbed dementia patients. Am J Psychiatry 139: 1170–1174, 1982

Beers M, Avorn J, Soumerai SB, et al: Psychoactive medication use in intermediate-care facility residents. JAMA 260:3016–3020, 1988

Buck JA: Psychotropic drug practice in nursing homes. J Am Geriatr Soc 36:409–418, 1988

Burgener SC, Jirovec M, Murrell L, Barton D: Caregiver and environmental variables related to difficult behaviors in institutionalized, demented elderly persons. J Gerontol 47:P242–P249, 1992

Burgio KL, Whitehead WE, Engel BT: Urinary incontinence in elderly patients: initial attempts to modify prompting and toileting procedures. Behav Ther 19:345–357, 1988

Chambers CA, Bain J, Rosbottom R, et al: Carbamazepine in senile dementia and overactivity: a placebo controlled double blind trial. IRCS Medical Science 10:505–506, 1982

Coccaro EF, Kramer E, Zemishlany Z, et al: Pharmacologic treatment of noncognitive behavioral disturbances in elderly demented patients. Am J Psychiatry 147:1640–1656, 1990

Cohen-Mansfield J, Werner P, Marx MS: Screaming in nursing home residents. J Am Geriatr Soc 38:785–792, 1990

Colenda CC: Buspirone in treatment of agitated demented patients (letter). Lancet 1:1169, 1988

Cummings JL, Miller B, Hill MA, Neshkes R: Neuropsychiatric aspects of multi-infarct dementia and dementia of the Alzheimer type. Arch Neurol 44:389–393, 1987

Devanand DP, Sackheim HA, Brown RP, et al: A pilot study of haloperidol treatment of psychosis and behavioral disturbance in Alzheimer's disease. Arch Neurol 46:854–857, 1989

Folstein MF, Folstein SE, McHugh PR: Mini-Mental State: a practical method for grading the cognitive state of patients for the clinician. J Psychiatr Res 12:189–198, 1975

Garrard J, Dunham T, Makris L, et al: Longitudinal study of psychotropic drug use by elderly nursing home residents. J Gerontol 47:M183–M188, 1992

Gleason RP, Schneider LS: Carbamazepine treatment of agitation in Alzheimer's outpatients refractory to neuroleptics. J Clin Psychiatry 51:115–118, 1990

Greenwald BS, Kramer-Ginsberg E, Martin DB, et al: Dementia with coexistent major depression. Am J Psychiatry 146:1472–1478, 1989

Gwyther L: Managing challenging behaviors at home. Alzheimer Dis Assoc Disord 8(suppl 3):110–112, 1994

Haley WE: Behavioral self-management: application to a case of agitation in an elderly chronic psychiatric patient. Clinical Gerontologist 1:45–51, 1983

Hamilton LD, Bennett JL: Acetophenazine for hyperactive geriatric patients. Geriatrics 17:596–601, 1962a

Hamilton LD, Bennett JL: The use of trifluoperazine in geriatric patients with chronic brain syndrome. J Am Geriatr Soc 10:140–147, 1962b

Hussian RA: Stimulus control in the modification of problematic behavior in elderly institutionalized patients. International Journal of Behavioral Geriatrics 1:33–46, 1982

Jenike MA: Monoamine oxidase inhibitors as treatment for depressed patients with primary degenerative dementia (Alzheimer's disease). Am J Psychiatry 162:763–764, 1985

Kirven LE, Montero EF: Comparison of thioridazine and diazepam in the control of nonpsychotic symptoms associated with senility: double-blind study. J Am Geriatr Soc 21:546–551, 1973

Marin DB, Greenwald BS: Carbamazepine for aggressive agitation in demented patients (letter). Am J Psychiatry 146:805, 1989

Maslow K: Special care units for persons with dementia: expected and observed effects on behavioral symptoms. Alzheimer Dis Assoc Disord 8(suppl 3):122–137, 1994

McGovern RJ, Koss E: The use of behavior modification with Alzheimer patients: values and limitations. Alzheimer Dis Assoc Disord 8(suppl 3):82–91, 1994

Mellow AM, Solano-Lopez C, Davis S: Sodium valproate in the treatment of behavioral disturbance in dementia. J Geriatr Psychiatry Neurol 6: 28–32, 1993

Mervis JR, Ganzell S, Fitten LJ, et al: Comparison of carbamazepine and trazodone in the control of aggression/agitation in demented, institutionalized patients: a randomized double blind parallel study (abstract). J Am Geriatr Soc 39:A75, 1991

Mittelman MS, Ferris SH, Steinberg G, et al: An intervention that delays institutionalization of Alzheimer's disease patients: treatment of spouse-caregivers. Gerontologist 33:730–740, 1993

Monane M, Avorn J, Everitt D, et al: Haloperidol use in the nursing home: frequency of parkinsonian side effects (abstract). J Am Geriatr Soc 39:A42, 1991

Pearson JL, Teri L, Reifler BV, Raskind MA: Functional status and cognitive impairment in Alzheimer's disease patients with and without depression. J Am Geriatr Soc 37:1117–1121, 1989

Petrie WM, Ban TA, Berney S, et al: Loxapine in psychogeriatrics: a placebo- and standard-controlled clinical investigation. J Clin Psychopharmacol 2:122–126, 1982

Pinner E, Rich CL: Effects of trazodone on aggressive behavior in seven patients with organic mental disorders. Am J Psychiatry 145:1295–1296, 1988

Rada RT, Kellner R: Thiothixene in the treatment of geriatric patients with chronic organic brain syndrome. J Am Geriatr Soc 24:105–107, 1976

Reifler BV, Teri L, Raskind M, et al: Double-blind study of imipramine in Alzheimer's disease patients with and without depression. Am J Psychiatry 146:45–49, 1989

Reisberg B, Borenstein J, Salob SP, et al: Behavioral symptoms in Alzheimer's disease: phenomenology and treatment. J Clin Psychiatry 48(suppl 5):9–15, 1987

Reynolds CF III, Perel JM, Kupfer DJ, et al: Open-trial response to antidepressant treatment in elderly patients with mixed depression and cognitive impairment. Psychiatry Res 21:111–122, 1987

Risse SC, Cubberly L, Lampe TH, et al: Acute effects of neuroleptic withdrawal in elderly dementia patients. Journal of Geriatric Drug Therapy 2:65–67, 1987

Sakauye KM, Camp CJ, Ford PA: Effects of buspirone on agitation associated with dementia. Am J Geriatr Psychiatry 1:82–84, 1993

Salzman C: Treatment of the elderly agitated patient. J Clin Psychiatry 48(suppl 5):19–22, 1987

Sanders JF: Evaluation of oxazepam and placebo in emotionally disturbed aged patients. Geriatrics 20:739–746, 1965

Schneider LS, Pollock VE, Lyness SA: A metaanalysis of controlled trials of neuroleptic treatment in dementia. J Am Geriatr Soc 38:553–563, 1990

Seager CP: Chlorpromazine in treatment of elderly psychotic women. Br Med J 1:882–885, 1955

Simpson DM, Foster D: Improvement in organically disturbed behavior with trazodone treatment. J Clin Psychiatry 47:191–193, 1986

Slater EJ, Glazer W: Use of OBRA-87 guidelines for prescribing neuroleptics in a VA nursing home. Psychiatric Serv 46:119–121, 1995

Steele C, Rovner B, Chase GA, Folstein M: Psychiatric symptoms and nursing home placement of patients with Alzheimer's disease. Am J Psychiatry 147:1049–1051, 1990

Stern RG, Duffelmeyer ME, Zemishlani Z, Davidson M: The use of benzodiazepines in the management of behavioral symptoms in dementia patients. Psychiatr Clin North Am 14:375–384, 1991

Sugarman AA, Williams BH, Adlerstein AM: Haloperidol in the psychiatric disorders of old age. Am J Psychiatry 120:1190–1192, 1964

Teri L: Behavioral treatment of depression in patients with dementia. Alzheimer Dis Assoc Disord 8(suppl 3):66–74, 1994

Wragg RE, Jeste DV: Overview of depression and psychosis in Alzheimer's disease. Am J Psychiatry 146:577–587, 1989

Zubenko GS, Moossy J: Major depression in primary dementia. Arch Neurol 45:1182–1186, 1988

CHAPTER

16

Genetic Counseling in Alzheimer's Disease and Huntington's Disease: Principles and Practice

Susan E. Folstein, M.D., and
Marshal F. Folstein, M.D.

Introduction

Genetic counseling is the education of a patient or client, called a consultand, who believes he or she is at increased risk for a disorder and requests information about the genetic risk and burden of that particular disorder (Murphy and Chase 1975). *Consultand* is a term coined by Murphy and Chase to designate the person in a family, often someone not affected with the disorder in question, who consults a genetic counselor.

In this chapter, we discuss the general principles of genetic counseling and the implementation of these principles for Hun-

Supported in part by NIMH Grant #R01 MH39936.

tington's disease (HD) and Alzheimer's disease (AD), two dementia disorders with very different clinical and genetic features.

Definitions and Principles in Genetic Counseling

Genetic Counseling

Genetic counseling is the process of acquiring and giving information (by the counselor) to a person (the consultand) who requests information about the genetic risk for a particular disorder for himself or herself or a child or fetus. The counselor collects the data needed and provides the information requested about risk and disease burden to the consultand. The consultand usually requests counseling to aid in making life decisions about childbearing, education, job choice, or insurance. For disorders that become manifest at or shortly after birth, such as the autistic syndrome, the fragile X mutation, or tuberous sclerosis, the consultand is usually a parent requesting information about unborn children. For disorders that begin later in life, such as manic-depressive disorder, schizophrenia, HD, or AD, the consultand may be requesting information about himself or herself or about children.

Information about risk is quite specific for HD, where the vast majority of cases are caused by mutation in only one gene, which is more or less fully penetrant; that is, nearly all persons with the disease gene will express the phenotype. However, for many genetic disorders, including AD, we do not know how many genes may be involved, by what mechanism they are transmitted, how many people with the genes will fall ill, or how the genetic risk factors interact with nongenetic factors. For these reasons, risk estimates given to consultands are often approximate and vary upward from 10%; they approach 50% only in rare families in which symptoms begin in the fifth and sixth decades.

It is most important that the counselor remain neutral with regard to the range of decisions that the consultand might make using the information given in genetic counseling. The goal of genetic counseling is to provide information and, through counseling, to help the consultand sort through the pros and cons of options; its goal is not to advise against childbearing with the intent to reduce the prevalence of diseases. Taking such a neutral stance is not always the instinctive human response, particularly when considering disorders known to have high risks of recurrence and a high burden, such as Tay-Sachs disease or HD. Consequently, genetic counseling carries special risks for the consultand and his or her family. The abuses of individuals—not only in Nazi Germany—based on speculated genetic differences illustrate the dangers of this type of information falling into the wrong hands. For example, it would be more difficult for some individuals to obtain health and life insurance if their risk for certain genetic diseases were known. Therefore, genetic counseling must be carried out with care and with the consultand's full understanding of its risks and benefits.

Genetic Testing

Genetic testing involves testing a particular individual for the presence of a specific disease gene or nearby marker. Genetic counseling should be a part of the process of genetic testing, encouraging the consultand to consider the possible consequences of knowing that he or she has a detrimental gene. In contrast to traditional genetic counseling, much more specific information is given to the consultand about his or her probability of having the disease gene in question. In genetic counseling, the risk estimate rarely exceeds 50% (for having a dominant disorder with early onset), but when the gene itself can be tested for, probabilities given are either very high to certainly present or very low to certainly absent. Genetic testing, like genetic counseling, is provided only at the request of the consultand and puts him or her at risk for being denied life and health insurance and employment.

There are two general types of genetic testing. One involves amniocentesis or chorionic villus sampling (CVS) of a fetus known to be at high risk for a particular disorder because of a previously affected sibling or other relative or because of advanced maternal age. However, many women now request genetic testing via CVS for Down's syndrome (DS) and other disorders that can be detected through a karyotype or ultrasound, even though their risk is not elevated over that of the general population. Prenatal genetic testing is usually requested for recessive disorders that become manifest at early ages, such as inborn errors of metabolism (Weaver 1992). This testing often involves testing samples for gene products, but useful markers for the genes themselves are becoming available. Examples include phenylketonuria (PKU) and adrenoleukodystrophy. Prenatal genetic testing can be done for HD and a few other disorders where there can be a long period of normal life before the disease is manifested. Parents who know they have the disease gene can be told whether the fetus has the gene.

The other general type of genetic testing is presymptomatic testing for subjects who wish to find out if they themselves (rather than their fetus) have a disease gene. For this type of genetic testing, it is most important that genetic counseling accompany the testing because of the psychological stigmatization risks involved. Presymptomatic testing will be considered in more detail as it applies to HD and AD.

Genetic Screening

In contrast to genetic counseling and genetic testing, genetic screening is carried out for some public health purpose either in the population as a whole or in a population at high risk for the disorder in question. In the case of PKU, in which treatment is effective if instituted shortly after birth, the goal is to decrease disease cost and burden in persons who are homozygous for the genetic defect. The treatment is so effective that society has decided to make testing obligatory by law. It is important to note that the public health goal here is not eugenic (i.e., to decrease the gene frequency) but rather directed at easing the burden of disease on the patient, family, and economy. (Prenatal genetic testing is also available for PKU, but this is a voluntary undertaking by parents who have had another affected child.) Genetic screening for Tay-Sachs disease has been carried out in Ashkenazi Jewish populations, where the gene frequency is high, with the purpose of preventing the birth of affected babies by detecting asymptomatic carriers who then would have the option to refrain from childbearing or abort affected fetuses. That screening effort was different from genetic counseling because it was advertised and promoted, but unlike testing for PKU it has always been voluntary. The screening effort has resulted in a decreased incidence of Tay-Sachs disease, and it now occurs mostly in non-Ashkenazi families (Kaback et al. 1993).

However, there are also problems in screening high-risk populations: it must be acceptable to the targeted community (Fost 1992; Markel 1992). Acceptability may depend on cultural factors (Wooldridge and Murray 1984) but also on the uniformity of severity of the disease burden. For example, programs to screen African-American populations for adult carriers of the recessive mutation for sickle-cell anemia were not well accepted, partly because of concerns about racism but also because not everyone with sickle-cell disease is affected severely.

Genetic screening can also be carried out anonymously, often using blood samples collected for other purposes, to estimate the frequency of particular genetic alleles or mutations in populations. The information can be used to estimate disease prevalence, mutation patterns, or frequency and number of various alleles of a particular gene.

In screening programs, the geneticist is an investigator or administrator who has no therapeutic relationship with any of the individuals screened. When the purpose is to uncover individuals with disease (such as PKU screening), the geneticist informs the family's physician who then conveys the information and takes the appropriate action. In programs aimed at establishing gene frequencies in populations or for other experimental purposes, samples drawn for another purpose (e.g., from blood banks) are sometimes used. In this case, all identifiers are removed because the stored information could otherwise be used to the detriment of the individuals involved. For example, insurance companies could use the screening results to draw up lists of people who are more likely to die early or use more health services.

Also, subjects often do not wish to know about detrimental genes they may have; their having given consent to have their blood drawn for donation or for a scientific study does not imply a wish to know the results. Most participants who volunteered for our study on genetic linkage in HD indicated that they did not wish to have the linkage information, and many questioned the level of confidentiality of the stored genotype information. The informed consent for the linkage study described the steps taken to assure confidentiality and made it clear that no data would be distributed since blood was drawn with the purpose of finding the HD gene rather than in the clinical context of genetic counseling and testing (Folstein et al. 1985).

Eugenics

Any activity with the goal of improving the quality of human genes is eugenic in nature. One dictionary defines *eugenics* as "the study of hereditary improvement, especially human improvement, by genetic control" (Morris 1979). However, eugenics is not just a study but an attitude of mind and intent. Although genetic counseling, screening, and testing are not eugenic by nature, they are sometimes carried out by eugenicists—individuals who feel that it would be beneficial to society for persons carrying disease genes or other genes not to reproduce. The barbaric human behaviors that can occur as a consequence of eugenic intent are well-known, but it is worth recalling that people with abnormal cognition and behaviors and psychiatric patients are most often singled out. In the United States, such individuals were involuntarily sterilized as recently as the 1950s (Ludmerer 1972).

Physicians often have eugenic thoughts; to advise persons at high risk for a very high burden disease, such as HD, to refrain from having children can seem appropriate to a physician who has watched many patients deteriorate and die from the disease. However, many families with HD recount with resentment their inter-actions with clinicians who advised them not to have children; they point out the personal nature of childbearing decisions, as well as that subjects may have many years of normal life before the disease begins.

Even if eugenic practices were ethically acceptable to human society, prevention of reproduction by persons with most geneti-cally mediated disorders would not be effective in decreasing the frequency of the disorders. New mutations occur constantly and account for varying, and sometimes large, proportions of cases of nearly all genetic disorders so far investigated. One likely reason for some sporadic (nonfamilial) cases of AD is new mutation. Also, some disorders are probably caused by the interaction of several genes, each one of which may be valuable in other ways, so that attempts to decrease the gene frequencies might be detrimental.

Principles of Giving Genetic Information

Giving genetic information about neuropsychiatric conditions to those requesting it is guided by the principles of providing infor-mation for any medical condition but is modified in two ways. First, the special characteristics of some disorders place patients at risk for suicide and stigma and may also affect their ability to under-stand the information provided. Second, to obtain the necessary data needed to provide accurate genetic counseling, diagnostic in-formation must often be obtained from or about relatives of the consultand who did not request any information. This necessity poses a threat to confidentiality for both the consultand and the relatives who give information.

Balancing Neutrality With Support

Although the physician must remain neutral with respect to giving advice about childbearing and other life decisions, a supportive, therapeutic approach is needed to help the consultand articulate those aspects of the risk and burden information that are personally important to him or her in the decision-making process. Genetic counseling is more than simple textbook genetic teaching. Studies have shown that subjects who have had genetic counseling are most satisfied with the process when they perceive the relationship as therapeutic or as enhancing their well-being and hope. The transaction between the consultand and counselor is individual and, ideally, is based on an understanding of that individual's unique life story and circumstances. The same facts about magnitude of recurrence risk and disease burden have different meanings to different individuals in different families and cultures. For this reason, consultands do not find a cookbook approach helpful.

This supportive approach needs to be used by an individual who is highly knowledgeable about the principles of genetic counseling and experienced with the particular disorder in question, so that questions can be answered accurately based on a background of experience with many families who have faced similar decisions. Sometimes families find it useful to talk to other families with the same disorder to gain perspective on their own situations. Support groups or contact with individuals who have weathered similar experiences may help families struggling to understand the reality of the disorder.

Confirming the Diagnosis

People who seek genetic counseling are often not patients themselves but the parents, siblings, or offspring of someone with the disorder. They often come with no diagnostic information except the name of the disorder, which is frequently incorrect. It is almost always necessary to get a history from an affected family member or knowledgeable informant and to examine personally the patient or—ideally—patients. Sometimes the only identified patient in the family who can conveniently be examined has not been diagnosed and may not wish to be. In our experience, this situation has occurred in both bipolar disorder and HD families. Therefore, the consultand rather than the physician must decide how best to ne-gotiate these family and confidentiality issues. Sometimes patients express willingness to be examined on the condition that they are not given any information. In AD, the problem is often that the patient who was thought to have AD is deceased. Unless there was an autopsy, information may need to be gathered from several in-formants to acquire adequate diagnostic information.

Even if only one affected member in the family can be person-ally examined, it is important to develop as extensive a pedigree as possible by obtaining family history information on all first-degree (parents, siblings, and offspring of the proband) and second-degree relatives (grandparents, aunts, and uncles), as well as first cousins. The information may indicate patterns of inheritance that can aid in diagnosis. For example, for X-linked disorders such as fragile X, there are often no other affected first-degree relatives, and the X-linked pattern may only be discerned by asking about second- and third-degree relatives. The acquisition of information needed to develop a detailed pedigree is a major task for genetic counseling. In our experience, clinicians must be trained to obtain this infor-mation. The names, birth and death dates, and descriptions of any illnesses must be obtained from each family member. Too often the consultand is asked whether anyone else has a psychiatric or other disorder. This approach always leads to underestimates of illness in the family. Consequently, family histories found in medical rec-ords are of limited value. Although the family history method is insensitive for milder expressions of the illness and can thereby lead to underestimation of genetic risk, it is still useful for obtaining diagnostic information about the phenotypes in the family and a minimum estimate of the density of disorder.

Obtaining these data necessitates certain procedures, which are sometimes cumbersome, to maintain confidentiality through-out the family. There is a tremendous amount of secrecy in families having several members with psychiatric or neuropsychiatric dis-orders. Family relationships may be fragile or fragmented. The con-sultand must obtain permission from each member from whom information is needed before the counselor contacts that family member. Also, each family member needs to be assured that all information that he or she gives will be kept confidential from any other family members contacted.

It is also important to explore the possibility that the consultand is himself or herself affected with the illness. Usually the consultand expects to be examined but occasionally does not wish to be given the diagnostic information. Under these conditions, the consultand needs to understand that it is not possible to estimate personal risk with much accuracy.

People requesting information about illnesses often anonymously telephone genetics clinics. They may not divulge the reason for their request, but usually they have heard that the illness is present in their families, acquaintances, or prospective spouses of their children. There are many reasons that genetic information should not be given over the telephone, including confidentiality, as well as the uncertainty about the diagnosis of the proband and the emotional and threatening nature of some genetic illnesses.

Deciding What, How, and When to Give Genetic Information

Before transmitting any information to a consultand, it is important to understand who he or she is. First, what prompted the request for information? Is the individual asking for help in explaining to a prospective spouse the impact of schizophrenia on the family? Is a couple making childbearing decisions or contemplating purchasing nursing home insurance? Is the consultand concerned that another family member may be affected and so wishes to discuss how to persuade him or her to seek diagnosis and treatment? Is advice being sought about how to give genetic information to nieces and nephews whose at-risk or affected parent has not done so?

Second, what does the consultand already know about the illness and what further information is desired? Some people at risk for HD request genetic counseling about burden and risk but do not wish to be examined themselves. Others are very knowledgeable about their family illness and want a research update. Still others need an explanation that starts from the beginning.

Third, what impact has the illness had on the consultand's life? Some people have cared for parents with serious chronic illness and others may be at risk but have never experienced the illness firsthand. Such patients, along with spouses of at-risk family members, have only an abstract appreciation of the burden of the illness. A consultand who has experienced it firsthand may wish the counselor to convince a spouse that this illness is too burdensome to take even a small risk that offspring will be affected.

Fourth, how much does the consultand know about genetic risk and transmission? A surprising number of well-educated people believe that if a parent has AD, they are certain to get it. Risk is very complicated to explain, even for HD. Consultands may believe that their risk cannot be 40%—they either have the disease or they do not. For AD, the challenge is to explain that although the genetic risk may be high, the probability of living through the age of risk is much lower.

Finally, what is the cognitive and emotional state of the consultand? Is the consultand so anxious as to be unlikely to adequately remember the information? Is the person affected by an illness that may impair the capacity to understand or to judge? For example, providing genetic information to someone who is currently depressed may best be delayed or at least provided in the presence of a spouse or another person with whom the consultand has a close, trusting relationship.

Methods of Transmitting Information

Several studies have demonstrated that physicians are generally very poor at communicating medical information to their patients. Patients often feel that the information given is not sufficient but are afraid to ask questions. Their anxiety may also decrease their ability to formulate their questions and to assimilate information. By following several simple rules, information can be transmitted effectively (Bradshaw et al. 1975; Ley 1973, 1979, 1982).

First, the sessions must be adequate in length and patients encouraged to ask questions. The physician should quiz patients on the most salient points to assure comprehension and to correct misunderstanding.

Second, the physician should use topic sentences to introduce a subject. For example, say, "Now I am going to tell you about the symptoms of Alzheimer's disease" or "Now we shall talk about your chances of getting Alzheimer's disease." Physicians should also provide a summary sentence at the end of the session.

Third, the physician should tailor both vocabulary level and the type of information transmitted to the particular patient. Patients' levels of education and—independently—knowledge about the illness vary greatly.

Fourth, material that summarizes the main points and addresses questions that commonly arise should be written at the appropriate reading level and provided for the patient to take home. The best-written newspapers try to approach an eighth-grade reading level, but most medical documents are well above college level. Inexpensive computer programs are now available to grade any text for reading level and to make suggestions for simplification. Some evidence suggests that giving patients a tape of the interview is particularly helpful (Hogbin and Fallowfield 1989).

Fifth, provide opportunity for a follow-up visit or scheduled telephone consultation so that further questions can be asked and previously offered information clarified.

Genetic Counseling and Testing

Huntington's Disease

HD is an autosomal dominant disorder, with a point prevalence of about 5 to 6 per 100,000, although the prevalence in adults is about 12 per 100,000 (Folstein 1989). The onset is delayed, usually until middle adult life, but symptoms and signs can begin at any time from early childhood to old age. The three clinical features of the disease are dyskinesia, dementia, and a variety of psychiatric features, in particular depression, irritability, and apathy. The illness may present with any of these features, but depression, when present, always occurs early on in the illness. Dementia begins with cognitive inefficiency: difficulties in thinking quickly, formulating a problem, and changing from one task or thought to another. Later, the dementia is more global, but patients never have a Wernicke's aphasia, as in AD. The average duration of illness is about 16 years, but there is wide variation. Some patients die early in the course of the disease from suicide or accidents, and other patients seem to have a slow progression, with survival as long as 40 years. Patients with very early onset seldom survive for more than 14 years after onset. The neuropathological hallmark is atrophy and neuronal loss in the neostriatum, caudate nucleus, and putamen, but after many years of illness there is some loss of cortical neurons in certain lamina.

Genetic Counseling for HD

Even though patients at risk for HD now have the opportunity to know with nearly 100% accuracy whether they will get the disease, most do not choose testing. In fact, most subjects who know they are at risk do not seek any information from experts but learn about HD from their relatives and make their own assessment of risk and burden of disease. Those who seek professional advice usually do so in one of two contexts. Some are well-educated individuals who are anxious and like to plan their futures well in advance. They may schedule regular neurologic examinations to get a more precise estimate of their risk. Others who seek counseling have just learned that HD is present in their families and are frantically seeking information (Folstein 1989).

The risk that an asymptomatic individual will get HD depends on his or her age. Someone age 40 has already lived through about 40% of the risk period. That is, by age 40, about 40% of subjects with the gene will have become symptomatic, so the risk to those who are still asymptomatic is adjusted downward. The remaining risk is also related to the age at onset of their affected family members. Asymptomatic 40-year-old siblings of juvenile-onset subjects have little remaining risk, whereas those whose family members become symptomatic in their 50s and 60s have lived through only a small portion of their risk. Finally, remaining risk is modestly altered by the gender of the affected parent. Offspring of affected males, on average, have a somewhat earlier age at onset than offspring of affected females (Folstein 1989). This risk is an example of anticipation and is associated with an increased number of trimeric repeats in the mutation (Stine et al. 1993).

Once this information is given, genetic counseling for HD is an entirely psychological undertaking. Most of the encounter is spent in supporting the consultand as he or she begins to comprehend the impact HD may have on his or her life, should the patient become affected. Some people never return for further visits; others return frequently and may require supportive psychotherapy. Most commonly, subjects maintain intermittent contact to stay abreast of research advances. Genetic counseling is emotionally draining, and professional training is needed.

Genetic Testing for HD

HD is similar in several ways to the major psychoses, and thus our experience with presymptomatic testing for persons at risk for HD can provide a partial model for genetic counseling and testing for other neuropsychiatric conditions. Like the major psychoses, the clinical onset of HD occurs in early to middle adult life. Second, the features of the disease include problems in thinking and can present as major mood disorder (sometimes bipolar) or a schizophrenia-like psychosis. Third, persons at risk for HD, like others from families with major psychiatric disorders, are often afraid to acknowledge their risk because they fear social and occupational prejudice (Folstein 1989). The major difference is that there are effective treatments, if not cures, for affective disorders and schizophrenia, whereas HD is fatal. Thus, it could be said that HD provides the worst-case scenario for genetic testing; that is, it might be considered very risky to tell people who are at risk for HD that they are almost certain to get the illness later in life.

Once it was established that there was only one genetic locus for HD, it was possible to test asymptomatic family members for the gene based on linkage analysis without yet knowing which gene was responsible. The question then arose as to whether testing should be done, because there is no treatment for HD. After much discussion, a few centers that serve large HD populations and have experience with the disorder decided to proceed with presymptomatic testing (Brandt et al. 1989; Meissen et al. 1988). Currently, a fair number of clinics in North America and Europe provide testing. The decision was made to go forward despite the absence of an effective treatment, in part because many young at-risk adults said they wanted the information. Half or more of those surveyed thought they would want to be tested (Tyler and Harper 1983). They felt that knowing would help them in making life decisions concerning insurance, education, job choice, and childbearing.

The testing protocol eventually adopted by most centers has several requirements (Huntington's Disease Society of America 1994). To ensure that persons requesting testing can give informed consent, applicants are screened for cognitive and serious emotional impairment. So that we can be made aware of any clinical situations that might arise during or after testing, all patients are required to have a confidant or advocate who comes to some of the pretest counseling and to the session at which the test results are disclosed. During the first 2 years of the Johns Hopkins presymptomatic testing program, we accepted only subjects living within 150 miles of Baltimore so that we could be easily available should the need arise and trips for pretest counseling and follow-up would not be unduly burdensome. Later it was clear that most subjects who chose to be tested, even those testing positive, did not require or request frequent follow-up. As a result, we expanded our catchment area to the entire mid-Atlantic region and required those living more than 150 miles from Baltimore to identify a local therapist before receiving the test results. Now that the gene itself has been found and can be used for testing, the only difference in the test protocol is that fewer family members are needed to provide an informative test.

Although knowing which gene is involved eliminates the complex psychological issues that arose when persons wishing to be tested had to ask for many relatives' participation and makes testing possible for most subjects with no living affected relatives, the psychological issues surrounding the consultand remain unchanged. When the number of trimeric repeats exceeds 38, it indicates that the person will become affected; fewer than 34 repeats is normal. Because the number of trimeric repeats is occasionally between 34 and 38, an ambiguous number, it is useful to have DNA from the consultand's parents. For example, if the affected parent's two Huntington alleles contained 19 and 36 repeats and the unaffected parent had 10 and 18 repeats, a consultand with 10 and 36 alleles would have inherited the parent's affected gene. Very often the number of repeats changes as it is passed from parent to child. Occasionally, the number dips back into the unaffected range. When the gene is passed from mother to child, the number of repeats is equally likely to increase or decrease, usually by 1 to 4 repeats (Ranen et al. 1995). When the gene is passed from father to child, the repeat size is more likely to increase, sometimes by a large amount. This increase in repeats is one of the reasons for anticipation: the earlier onset of symptoms in the subsequent generation.

Each applicant is examined neurologically and psychiatrically. Subjects are cleared for pretest counseling who, at screening, 1) are neurologically well and have no major mental illness, 2) deny suicidal intent, and 3) have no other personal problems that would interfere with their ability to make a considered decision about testing.

All subjects who are accepted and choose to enter the testing program are seen for several counseling sessions with a clinical psychologist who has experience with HD. At these sessions, the test and the technical features that limit its accuracy are explained. The persons' motivations for testing are discussed at length, and the counselor ascertains whether patients are aware of the nature of HD. Possible social, marital, insurance, and psychological consequences of positive or negative test outcomes are also discussed. Considerable emphasis is placed on ensuring that subjects have clearly faced the fact that the test could be positive for HD; before counseling, many persons have allowed themselves to consider only a good outcome. At all times during the course of testing, subjects are reminded that testing is entirely voluntary and that they may change their minds at any time until the genetic information is disclosed. After disclosure, subjects are seen as often as we and they feel necessary. During the first year, however, patients are evaluated psychiatrically and neurologically at least every 3 months. After the first year they are seen at least every 6 months.

As of January 1, 1995, the Hopkins group had tested 142 persons at 50% risk for HD; 131 have had informative tests, and 14 were uninformative using linkage analysis. Of the 131 with informative tests, 44 (34%) had test results suggesting that they are highly likely to have the HD gene (A. Codori, personal communication, March 1995). Very few of those tested, including subjects with a high risk for developing HD, have exhibited serious psychological problems during posttest follow-up (Brandt et al. 1989; Codori and Brandt 1994). The number is probably low because those who choose testing are self-selected for the belief that they are able to deal with emotional stress (Codori et al. 1994). Also, many potential difficulties are rehearsed by subject and physician, either before or during pretest counseling.

Numerous ethical (Brandt 1994), psychological (Codori and Brandt 1994), and psychiatric issues have arisen in the course of screening and testing. These issues are discussed weekly by the testing team (a psychiatrist, social worker, nurse, psychologist, and geneticist). For example, about 15% of persons who present for testing are already affected with HD. The team decides, based on what is known of the subject and his or her family, whether and how to tell the patient about the diagnosis. (Interestingly, it is not uncommon for people to say that they want to know if they will have HD in the *future* but would not like to know if they have signs currently.) Another issue commonly discussed at the weekly staff meeting involves the decision to offer testing to subjects exhibiting minor neurological signs that could represent early manifestation of HD but are below threshold for diagnosis. Testing persons with psychiatric disorders is another issue raised. Although most persons who request testing are psychiatrically well, several have had depressive syndromes, ongoing substance abuse, or a severe personality disorder. Such subjects are examined by a psychiatrist who, in consultation with the rest of the team, decides whether testing will be offered at this time. On some occasions, testing has been delayed until the disorder (particularly depression) is successfully treated. Another difficult issue is to decide whether a person is being coerced into testing by others. Sometimes this is obvious ("I was sent by my family doctor, but I do not really want to do this"); other times, the issue is not so clear. If a couple has several children who may be at risk, or if the at-risk member of the pair wants to have children, the spouse's request that the at-risk member have testing needs to be addressed in joint counseling.

Codori and Brandt (1994) surveyed 68 subjects who had completed testing from 1 to 6 years earlier. All felt there were positive aspects to testing, and 15 of the 17 who had high-risk outcomes said they would do it again; 49 of the 52 with low-risk tests shared that opinion. There were a number of minor but important psychological sequelae, but only two were experienced differentially by the high- and low-risk groups. First, only 14% of high-risk patients had told their children about their risk, whereas 80% of those with low-risk tests had done so. Second, high-risk testers were more likely to endorse the statement that they now realized what was important in life, and they were also more likely to travel. Nevertheless, it cannot be emphasized enough that fewer than 10% of persons at 50% risk for HD who could take the test have actually chosen to do so. Interestingly, only 30% of those tested using linkage wished to have their blood retested using the gene test, illustrating the magnitude of the testing process's emotional impact (A. Codori, unpublished data, March 1995).

There are a number of ways in which involvement of the psychiatrists on the team has been beneficial to the process of genetic testing for HD. Contributions have been made in psychiatric diagnosis and appraisal of the severity of depressive symptoms or personality features, in the discussion of ethical principles and their implementation in particular cases, and in providing psychiatric consultation and treatment before or after testing. Psychiatric input has also been helpful in maintaining the cohesiveness of the team and in providing support for team members who are involved in disclosing genetic information to persons who have had test results positive for the HD gene.

Alzheimer's Disease

AD is a clinicopathologic entity characterized by cortical dementia with amnesia, aphasia, apraxia, and agnosia; it is characterized neuropathologically by neuronal loss resulting in atrophy, with amyloid plaques and fibrillary tangles in the cerebral cortex and brain stem. AD is the most common cause of dementia in late adult life. The disorder is fatal after an average of 8 to 10 years of illness. The prevalence rises from 1% of 65-year-olds to 20% of 85-year-olds (Katzman and Kawas 1994).

The proportion of cases of AD that are inherited is under study. Most analyses of AD populations suggest that the majority of cases that manifest the classical features of aphasia, apraxia, and agnosia are inherited as an autosomal dominant trait (Breitner and Folstein 1984; Powell and Folstein 1984). However, the actual risk for a relative of a patient who became affected very late in life is not much greater than the risk to the general population, because the relative is more likely to die of some other cause before reaching the age at which AD would become symptomatic. It has been difficult to establish clearly what proportion of Alzheimer's cases are inherited because the disorder manifests late in life; thus, there are few large pedigrees of living, affected individuals whose diagnoses can be verified. In addition to genetic causes, there is evidence that head trauma in earlier life and chronic exposure to high levels of aluminum are possibly risk factors for AD (Katzman and Kawas 1994; Rifat et al. 1990).

Genetic Counseling for AD

Many family members ask for information about their at-risk status. Many others are worried about their status but do not ask unless the clinician questions them directly about their concerns about developing the disorder. Such persons have not come for genetic counseling themselves; rather, they are being seen in the context of their role as a caregiver for an affected parent.

Very often adult children who have witnessed the disease in their parents become concerned about their own cognition as they age. They come to physicians complaining about difficulties with concentration and word finding. In all such individuals we have seen so far, no cognitive impairment has been found on testing. They have all been far younger than the age at which their parents became ill and so are not yet even at any substantial risk for disease expression. Rather, they are anxious and vigilant about their risk.

In the absence of known genes in a particular family, counseling can be given based on the presence or absence of a family history and the age at onset of the other affected members. It is not always easy to determine whether there are other affected family members. We have defined a family history as negative when both the proband's parents lived to be at least as old as the proband was at onset of illness. On the other hand, when there is a history of other family members who have suffered late-life cognitive impairment, it is usually not possible to be certain (i.e., to have neuropathological confirmation) that they had AD. However, a report of the typical onset, symptoms, and course of illness can often be obtained from relatives who witnessed the illness.

The risk to offspring is also related to the age at which their parents became affected, since age at onset tends to run in families (Powell and Folstein 1984). If the parent had an onset at age 85 (at which age the prevalence of AD is 20%), offspring can be told that their risk for having AD is only slightly higher than the general population. Presuming that only one copy of any AD gene is needed for expression (which is not yet known for most genetic forms), such persons would have a 50% risk of inheriting the gene (genotypic risk), but the probability of their reaching age 85 is approximately 30%. Therefore, the risk of expressing the symptoms (phenotypic risk) would be 15%. The children of early-onset cases are at greater risk for having symptoms than persons from late-onset families. These individuals can be told that their risk is somewhat higher than average, but they have less than a 50% chance of developing the genetic form of the disease. Heston et al. (1981) report a recurrence risk of 40% for siblings of early-onset subjects who had an affected parent. The issue of anticipation has not yet been studied in families with AD.

Genetic Testing for AD

Genetic testing is now possible in principle but would be highly expensive for large families in which the onset is very early. Most of the early-onset families (keeping in mind that not all early-onset cases are familial) have a gene at one of three loci (Table 16–1). A few point mutations have been discovered in the apolipoprotein (APP) gene, but the gene accounts for only a tiny fraction of early-onset AD (reviewed in Schellenberg 1995a). A much more common genetic locus for early-onset AD, on chromosome 14, was discovered by genetic linkage analysis in 1992 (Mullan et al. 1992), and the gene has now been cloned (Zhao et al. 1995). It is found in a number of different ethnic groups (Schellenberg 1995b) and accounts for the majority of cases of early-onset familial AD (Mullan and Crawford 1994), although not necessarily for the majority of early-onset cases in general. The protein coded for by the gene has

Table 16–1.   Classification of genetic variants

Variant	Duke	Seattle	London-Swedish	Down's syndrome	Idiopathic
% of all AD	50%	Most early-onset cases	<1%	<1%	20%–50%
Onset	Late	Early	Early	Early	?
Amyloid production	?	Incr	Incr	Incr	?
Family history	+ or −	+	+	−	+ or −
Locus	19	14, 1	21	21	?
Genes	APOE	Presenilin 1 Presenilin 2	APP	APP	?

been identified and named presenilin 1. It has a number of trans-membrane domains (Sherrington et al. 1995), but how it causes AD is still under investigation. A variety of mutations have been found in different families (Zhao et al. 1995). Immediately after the gene for presenilin 1 was characterized, it was used to search for other genes of similar structure, and one was promptly found on chromosome 1, dubbed presenilin 2, in several of the Volga German families (Levy-Lahad et al. 1995a,b; Rogaev et al. 1995). The Volga German families are a group of AD kindreds living in various coun-tries who trace their ancestry to the Germans living on the Volga River in Russia (Bird et al. 1988).

The problem with genetic testing is that there are so many different mutations within these genes. For presenilin 1 on chro-mosome 14, there are almost as many different mutations as there are families. Consequently, to do genetic testing for at-risk family members, it would be necessary to carry out a genetic linkage study on that particular family to determine whether it is linked to one of the three known loci. Then the particular mutation for the gene in that family would have to be found. Obviously, genetic linkage could be done only if the family was large enough, with at least five or six affected members from whom blood could be ob-tained.

The genes on chromosomes 14 and 1 account for most of the early-onset AD families, but there remain a few that do not link to either of these genes. It should be mentioned that one of the origi-nal reports describing a kindred with early-onset AD was discov-ered to have antibody staining for prion protein, suggesting that the gene on chromosome 20 coding for the prion protein may occa-sionally cause the AD phenotype (DeArmond 1993), although it is usually associated with the Creutzfeld-Jakob phenotype.

In 1991, Pericak-Vance and colleagues (1991) reported an as-sociation between AD and the ε4 allele of the gene coding for apolipoprotein E (APOE). There is no evidence that this gene is sufficient to cause late-onset AD; it is not linked to the gene (Schel-lenberg et al. 1992) but rather seems to function as a risk factor.

Apolipoprotein E, a member of the apolipoprotein lipid trans-porter family, is coded for by a gene, APOE, on chromosome 19.

The gene has several alleles, the most common of which are ε2, ε3, and ε4. Those individuals with two copies of the APOE ε4 allele (ε4 homozygotes) are at greatly increased risk for developing AD by age 85. Individuals with one copy of ε4 are at intermediate risk, and those with at least one copy of the ε2 allele are at decreased risk, relative to the general population. These risks are independent of whether the patient has a positive family history of dementia and appear to be important for both early and late-onset forms (Chartier-Harlin et al. 1994). Similar risk estimates have been described in multiple racial groups, including African-Americans (Hendrie et al. 1995), although a community-based sample suggests that the relationship to the APOE alleles may be more complicated in African-Americans (Maestre et al. 1995). The association with APOE ε4 has been demonstrated in several different European ethnic groups (Kuusisto et al. 1994; van Duijn et al. 1994b) and in Japanese subjects (Muramatsu et al. 1994). One study reported that APOE ε4 increased risk for early-onset AD only when there was a positive family history (van Duijn et al. 1994). Among patients with onset after age 65, homozygosity for the ε4 allele seems to lower the age at onset of symptoms (Corder et al. 1993; Poirier et al. 1993).

Studies of the influence of APOE ε4 on AD have so far been limited to the comparison of patients who already have AD with persons of the same age without any dementia. While the rates vary somewhat from study to study, about half the AD patients have at least one APOE ε4 allele, compared with about 20% of age-matched controls. Prospective studies that estimate how having an APOE ε4 allele influences the risk for someone developing AD have not yet been reported.

APOE alleles are of little use in the diagnosis of AD because dementias of other etiologies may be found in persons with APOE ε4 alleles and because half the patients who get AD do not have the ε4 allele. Similarly, it is not possible to use APOE alleles to predict that an asymptomatic person will develop AD. Some individuals with ε4 alleles, even homozygotes with two ε4 alleles, have been found to live to old age without developing the disease. A thorough history, examination of the clinical features, and appropriate laboratory tests are still essential for clinical diagnosis. (Bird 1995; Farrer et al. 1995).

Thus, AD displays locus heterogeneity: Different families have mutations for genes on different chromosomes. AD is probably also etiologically heterogeneous—not all patients have a genetic cause and thus, from a genetic perspective, represent phenocopies. The result is that, unlike in HD, genetic testing cannot be based on genetic linkage to a single locus. Individuals can be tested if a parent with AD has been demonstrated to have one of the known mutations; however, until all the mutations are known, the failure to find a particular mutation in persons at risk will not imply that the individual is at low risk for AD. At this writing, no centers are yet undertaking AD presymptomatic testing because the two clearly known genetic loci are rare, each family may have its own mutation, and the predictive value of having an APOE ε3 or ε4 allele is not at all certain.

It seems likely at this time that genetic testing for late-onset AD may not ever be as simple as testing for the presence of one specific mutation. A number of nongenetic risk factors appear to interact with genetic ones (Table 16–2). As studies are designed that incorporate all these factors simultaneously (including APOE) in following a variety of populations, more precise risk estimates to be used in genetic counseling will be developed. Table 16–2 also includes estimates of odds ratios for AD, relative to matched controls who did not have the risk factor. Much of the data presented come from the European Dementia Consortium (EURODEM) Risk Factors Research Group (Katzman and Kawas 1994; van Duijn et al. 1994a). This group reanalyzed seven case-control studies, comprising a total of 814 AD patients and 894 control subjects. Most of the factors are equally relevant to persons with and without a family history of dementia, but some interact with family history.

Family history of dementia.   As described previously, a positive family history of dementia is a powerful risk factor for developing AD. In the EURODEM study, the odds ratio was 3.5; in the Canadian Study of Health and Aging (1994), it was 2.6.

Table 16–2.   Risk factors for Alzheimer's disease

Risk factor	Odds ratio: European Dementia Consortium (EURODEM) analysis of 11 case-control studies	Odds ratio: EURODEM for positive versus negative family history	Odds ratio: Canadian Study of Health and Aging
Family history of dementia	3.5	—	2.6
Family history of Parkinson's disease	2.4	Higher when family history is negative but difs. ns	Same as column 2
Head injury	1.8	Same???	
Head injury, sporadic cases	2.3		
Maternal age >40	1.7	Same	
Hypothyroidism	2.3		
Down's syndrome	2.7	Higher when family history is negative but difs. ns	
Depression in late-onset cases	2.4	Same	
Ever smoked	0.78	Protective when family history is positive	Same as column 2
Education			<6 versus ?10: odds ratio = 4
Arthritis			0.54
Anti-inflammatory drugs			Lower
Exposure to pesticides, fertilizers, glue			Higher
Estrogen	Lower risk		

Age.   AD is rare in subjects under age 65, and the incidence (new cases per year) rises with age. In the East Boston study, incidence rates were as follows: age 65–69, 0.6%; 70–74, 1%; 75–79, 2%; 80–84, 3.3%; and 85 and older 8.4% (Hebert et al. 1995). Very likely there are internal cellular processes that become more susceptible with age. Possible external mechanisms that accrue with age are increased exposure to environmental agents, accumulation of DNA repair defects, or a protective effect of some AD gene against other common causes of death such as heart disease or cancer.

Head injury. A head injury, even a mild one, earlier in life (Rasmusson et al. 1995) clearly increases the risk for the later development of AD. Both Rasmusson and the EURODEM analysis suggested that it is a more powerful factor in patients without a family history of dementia. Two other reports have shown a clear interaction between head injury and the APOE ε4 allele, with the risk being additive (Mayeux et al. 1995; Nicoll et al. 1995).

Aluminum. Several epidemiological studies indicate that risk for AD is increased by exposure to aluminum in the air or water (Jacqmin et al. 1994; Martyn 1992). Some authors suggest that the effect of aluminum will vary locally, depending on other elements in the water and air, such as silicate and fluorine (Forbes and Agwani 1994). However, not all studies have confirmed the finding. Similarly, several studies report the presence of increased aluminum in AD brains (Perl and Good 1992; reviewed by McLachlan et al. 1992), but others do not (Lovell et al. 1993). Although the effect of aluminum is still uncertain, some laboratory studies support its plausibility. In vitro experiments suggest that both aluminum and calcium salts can cause conformational changes in phosphorylated neurofilament fragments that result in precipitation of beta pleated sheets (Shen et al. 1994). In one single-blind trial, the trivalent chelating agent desferrioxamine (DFO) was given to AD patients. In the treated group, measures of severity worsened at half the rate of the controls (McLachlan et al. 1993).

Down's syndrome. All brains of individuals with trisomy 21 who die at or after age 45 have neuropathology AD (Holland and Oliver 1995); these changes are not found in other individuals with mental retardation (Cole et al. 1994). There may also be an increased risk for AD in the mothers of persons with DS (Henderson et al. 1994). The ε2 allele is associated with longevity (Royston et al. 1994). In another study, ε4 was related to earlier age at death but had no effect on the extent of the pathology (Mann et al. 1995).

Education.   Several studies have now reported higher rates of AD in persons with lower levels of education (Canadian Health Study 1994; Katzman 1993; Mortel et al. 1995; Ott et al. 1995; Powell et al. 1994; Stern et al. 1994; Zhang 1990). Whether less education is associated with an earlier onset of symptoms in persons already at risk for other reasons or represents an independent risk factor for disease is unknown. Several studies that have demonstrated this phenomenon are reviewed in Katzman and Kawas (1994).

Parental age.   In some autosomal dominant disorders, new mutations are associated with advanced paternal age (e.g., achondroplastic dwarfism [McKusick et al. 1994]). One chart review that tested this hypothesis found that patients with a negative family history had older fathers than those with a positive family history (Powell and Folstein 1984). A similar effect of advanced maternal age was detected in the EURODEM analyses. Since maternal and paternal age are correlated, it is sometimes difficult to distinguish which parent is exerting the effect.

Pesticides and fertilizers.   An unexpected finding in the Canadian Study of Health and Aging (1994) was that risk for AD was increased by exposure to glues, pesticides, and fertilizer. This provocative finding has not been replicated.

Protective Factors

Smoking.   The EURODEM analysis of seven case-control studies strongly suggests that smoking decreases risk for AD (van Duijn et al. 1994a). This finding applies to both early- and late-onset disease and those with both a positive and negative family history. The finding does not appear to be related to a decreased probability of smokers with the ε4 allele surviving to the age of risk for AD (van Duijn et al. 1995).

Nonsteroidal anti-inflammatory agents.   At least three studies now point to a protective effect of anti-inflammatory agents, both on age at onset (Breitner et al. 1994) and rate of progression of illness for persons already affected (Rich et al. 1995). It also may actually decrease the risk for becoming affected (Andersen et al. 1995). One controlled trial reports beneficial effects of nonsteroidals (Rogers et al. 1993).

Arthritis.   The Canadian Study of Health and Aging (1994) found that reduced risk was associated with arthritis, with an odds ratio of .54. In this study, nonsteroidal intake was also protective, but the interaction of arthritis with said intake was not reported. This finding also has not yet been replicated.

Estrogen.   In vitro studies indicate that estrogen is an antioxidant that protects against oxidative stress and regulates the production of the soluble form of beta A4, suggesting that estrogen may be protective in vivo (Cotton 1994; Jaffe et al. 1994). Two epidemiological studies (Henderson et al. 1994; Paganini-Hill and Henderson 1994) and a third unpublished one suggest that estrogen replacement is associated with a decreased risk for disease and a dose-related effect on severity, such that Alzheimer patients taking estrogen had better cognitive function than those not taking estrogen. One case series (Ohkura et al. 1995) reports improvement in cognition and social function of individuals taking estrogen, but double-blind clinical trials have not yet been conducted.

Clinically Detectable Changes in Persons at Risk

Now that a number of risk factors have been detected by the study of affected individuals, prospective case-control studies of these risks are being undertaken in unaffected persons. Snowdon et al. (1996) demonstrated that, compared to age-matched controls, nuns who went on to have AD had lower cognitive achievement many years before onset of AD. In another study, 50% of first-degree relatives of AD subjects, compared with 20% of controls, had impaired cognitive function across several domains (Hom et al. 1994). These studies indicate that eventual victims of disease suffer from greater cognitive abnormalities than controls who subsequently do not develop disease but that these deficits are not clinically apparent.

Some biological differences between at-risk relatives of AD patients and controls have also been noted. Serra et al. (1994) found that relatives of subjects with AD have increased red blood cell copper-zinc superoxide dismutase activity relative to age-matched controls without a family history of AD. In a flurodioxyglucose (fdg) positron-emission tomography (PET) study, asymptomatic at-risk persons in their 50s with the APOE ε4 allele were compared with at-risk persons without ε4 (Small et al. 1995). Those with the ε4 allele had temporoparietal hypometabolism, whereas those without the allele did not.

Conclusions

Hofman et al. (1993) reported on the results of a survey in which primary care physicians and psychiatrists were asked several questions about genetic counseling, screening, and testing. On average, these physicians had less than 75% of the knowledge they needed to provide accurate genetic information for disorders for which they might be called on to provide information. In a similar survey (Holtzman 1992), physicians were asked if they would offer an inexpensive test for cystic fibrosis. The proportion who said yes decreased from 72% to 46% after the physicians were informed about the sensitivity of the test and the implications for genetic discrimination. Other surveys of physicians (Wertz and Fletcher 1989) suggest that physicians have not considered carefully all the implications of providing genetic information to persons who have not requested it.

Psychiatric practice of the next decade will certainly be more firmly based on the emerging knowledge of genetics and how genes are expressed in the nervous system. Since such information is now quickly disseminated through television and print media, patients and their families will learn about the relationship between their symptoms and their genes and will turn to their doctors for education and support (Stancer and Wagener 1984). If psychiatrists are to properly serve their patients, they will need to learn the principles of genetics and how to transmit this information effectively.

References

Andersen K, Launer LJ, Ott A, et al: Do nonsteroidal anti-inflammatory drugs decrease the risk for Alzheimer's disease? the Rotterdam study. Neurology 45:1441–1445, 1995

Bird TD: Apolipoprotein E genotyping in the diagnosis of Alzheimer's disease: a cautionary view. Ann Neurol 38:2–4, 1995

Bird T, Lampe T, Nemens E, et al: Familial Alzheimer disease in descendants of Volga Germans: probable genetic founder effect. Ann Neurol 23:25–31, 1988

Bradshaw PW, Ley P, Kincey JA: Recall of medical advice: comprehensibility and specificity. British Journal of Social & Clinical Psychology 14:55–62, 1975

Brandt J: Ethical considerations in genetic testing with examples from presymptomatic diagnosis of Huntington's disease in medicine and moral reasoning, in Medicine and Moral Reasoning. Edited by Fulford KWM, Soskice J, Gillet G. Cambridge, Cambridge University Press, 1994

Brandt J, Quaid KA, Folstein SE, et al: Presymptomatic diagnosis of delayed-onset disease with linked DNA markers: the experience in Huntington's disease [see comments]. JAMA 261:3108–3114, 1989

Breitner JC, Folstein MF: Familial Alzheimer dementia: a prevalent disorder with specific clinical features. Psychol Med 14:63–80, 1984

Breitner JC, Gau BA, Welsh KA, et al: Inverse association of anti-inflammatory treatments and Alzheimer's disease: initial results of a co-twin control study. Neurology 44:227–232, 1994

Canadian Study of Health and Aging: Risk factors for Alzheimer's disease in Canada. Neurology 44:2073–2080, 1994

Chartier-Harlin MC, Parfitt M, Legrain S, et al: Apolipoprotein E, epsilon 4 allele as a major risk factor for sporadic early and late-onset forms of Alzheimer's disease: analysis of the 19q13.2 chromosomal region. Hum Mol Genet 3:569–574, 1994

Codori AM, Brandt J: Psychological costs and benefits of predictive testing for Huntington's disease. Am J Med Genet 54:174–184, 1994

Codori AM, Hanson R, Brandt J: Self-selection in predictive testing for Huntington's disease. Am J Med Genet 54:167–173, 1994

Cole G, Neal JW, Fraser WI, et al: Autopsy findings in patients with mental handicap. J Intellect Disabil Res 38:9–26, 1994

Corder EH, Saunders AM, Strittmatter WJ, et al: Gene dose of apolipoprotein E type 4 allele and the risk of Alzheimer's disease in late onset families. Science 261:921–923, 1993

Cotton P: Constellation of risks and processes seen in search for Alzheimer's clues. JAMA 271:89–91, 1994

DeArmond SJ: Alzheimer's disease and Creutzfeldt-Jakob disease: overlap of pathogenic mechanisms. Curr Opin Neurol 6:872–881, 1993

Farrer LA, Brin MF, Elsas L, et al: Statement on use of apolipoprotein E testing for Alzheimer disease. JAMA 22:1627–1629, 1995

Folstein MF: Heterogeneity in Alzheimer's disease. Neurobiol Aging 10: 434–435, 1989

Folstein M, Anthony JC, Parhad I, et al: The meaning of cognitive impairment in the elderly. J Am Geriatr Soc 33:228–235, 1985

Forbes WF, Agwani N: A suggested mechanism for aluminum biotoxicity. J Theor Biol 171:207–214, 1994

Fost N: Ethical implications of screening asymptomatic individuals. FASEB J 6:2813–2817, 1992

Hebert LE, Scherr PA, Beckett LA, et al: Age-specific incidence of Alzheimer's disease in a community population. JAMA 273:1354–1359, 1995

Henderson VW, Paganini-Hill A, Emanuel CK, et al: Estrogen replacement therapy in older women: comparisons between Alzheimer's disease cases and nondemented control subjects. Arch Neurol 51:896–900, 1994

Hendrie HC, Hall KS, Hui S, et al: Apolipoprotein E genotypes and Alzheimer's disease in a community study of elderly African Americans. Ann Neurol 37:118–120, 1995

Heston LL, Mastri AR, Anderson VE, et al: Dementia of the Alzheimer type: clinical genetics, natural history, and associated conditions. Arch Gen Psychiatry 38:1085–1090, 1981

Hofman KJ, Tambor ES, Chase GA, et al: Physicians' knowledge of genetics and genetic tests. Acad Med 68:625–632, 1993

Hogbin B, Fallowfield L: Getting it taped: the 'bad news' consultation with cancer patients. Br J Hosp Med 41:330–333, 1989

Holland AJ, Oliver C: Down's syndrome and the links with Alzheimer's disease. J Neurol Neurosurg Psychiatry 59:111–114, 1995

Holtzman NA: The diffusion of new genetic tests for predicting disease (review). FASEB J 6:2806–2812, 1992

Hom J, Turner MB, Risser R, et al: Cognitive deficits in asymptomatic first-degree relatives of Alzheimer's disease patients. J Clin Exp Neuropsychol 16:568–576, 1994

Huntington's Disease Society of America: Guidelines for Genetic Testing for Huntington's Disease. New York, Huntington's Disease Society of America, 1994

Jacqmin H, Commenges D, Letenneur L, et al: Components of drinking water and risk of cognitive impairment in the elderly. Am J Epidemiol 139:48–57, 1994

Jaffe AB, Toran-Allerand CD, Greengard P, et al: Estrogen regulates metabolism of Alzheimer amyloid beta precursor protein. J Biol Chem 269:13065–13068, 1994

Kaback M, Lim-Steele J, Dabholkar D, et al: Tay-Sachs disease–carrier screening, prenatal diagnosis, and the molecular era: an international perspective, 1970 to 1993. The International TSD Data Collection Network. JAMA 270:2307–2315, 1993

Katzman R: Education and the prevalence of dementia and Alzheimer's disease. Neurology 43:13–20, 1993

Katzman R, Kawas CH: The epidemiology of dementia and Alzheimer disease, in Alzheimer Disease. Edited by Terry R, Katzman R, Bick K. New York, Raven, 1994, pp 105–122

Kuusisto J, Koivisto K, Kervinen K, et al: Association of apolipoprotein E phenotypes with late onset Alzheimer's disease: population based study. BMJ 309:636–638, 1994

Levy-Lahad E, Wasco W, Poorkaj P, et al: Candidate gene for the chromosome 1 familial Alzheimer's disease locus. Science 269:973–977, 1995a

Levy-Lahad E, Wijsman EM, Nemens E, et al: A familial Alzheimer's disease locus on chromosome 1. Science 269:970–973, 1995b

Ley P: Memory for medical information. British Journal of Social & Clinical Psychology 18:245–255, 1979

Ley P: Satisfaction, compliance and communication. Br J Clin Psychol 21: 241–254, 1982

Ley P, Bradshaw PW, Eaves D, et al: A method for increasing patients' recall of information presented by doctors. Psychol Med 3:217–220, 1973

Lovell MA, Ehmann WD, Markesbery WR: Laser microprobe analysis of brain aluminum in Alzheimer's disease. Ann Neurol 33:36–42, 1993

Ludmerer KM: Genetics, eugenics, and the Immigration Restriction Act of 1924. Bull Hist Med 46:59–81, 1972

Maestre G, Ottman R, Stern Y, et al: Apolipoprotein E and Alzheimer's disease: ethnic variation in genotypic risks. Ann Neurol 37:254–259, 1995

Mann DM, Pickering-Brown SM, Siddons MA, et al: The extent of amyloid deposition in brain in patients with Down's syndrome does not depend upon the apolipoprotein E genotype. Neurosci Lett 196:105–108, 1995

Markel H: The stigma of disease: implications of genetic screening. Am J Med 93:209–215, 1992

Martyn CN: The epidemiology of Alzheimer's disease in relation to aluminum. Ciba Found Symp 169:69–79, 1992

Mayeux R, Ottman R, Maestre G, et al: Synergistic effects of traumatic head injury and apolipoprotein-epsilon 4 in patients with Alzheimer's disease. Neurology 45:555–557, 1995

McKusick V, et al: Mendelian Inheritance in Man: A Catalog of Human Genes and Genetic Disorders. Baltimore, MD, Johns Hopkins University Press, 1994

McLachlan DR, Fraser PE, Dalton AJ: Aluminum and the pathogenesis of Alzheimer's disease: a summary of evidence. Ciba Found Symp 169: 87–98, 1992

McLachlan DR, Smith WL, Kruck TP: Desferrioxamine and Alzheimer's disease: video home behavior assessment of clinical course and measures of brain aluminum. Ther Drug Monit 15:602–607, 1993

Meissen GJ, Myers RH, Mastromauro CA, et al: Predictive testing for Huntington's disease with use of a linked DNA marker. N Engl J Med 318: 535–542, 1988

Morris W (ed): The American Heritage Dictionary of English Language. Boston, MA, Houghton Mifflin, 1979

Mortel KF, Meyer JS, Herod B, et al: Education and occupation as risk factors for dementias of the Alzheimer and ischemic vascular types. Dementia 6:55–62, 1995

Mullan M, Crawford F: The molecular genetics of Alzheimer's disease. Mol Neurobiol 9:15–22, 1994

Mullan M, Houlden H, Windelspecht M, et al: A locus for familial early-onset Alzheimer's disease on the long arm of chromosome 14, proximal to the alpha 1-antichymotrypsin gene. Nat Genet 2:340–342, 1992

Muramatsu T, Higuchi S, Arai H, et al: Apolipoprotein E epsilon 4 allele distribution in alcoholic dementia and in Alzheimer's disease in Japan. Ann Neurol 36:797–799, 1994

Murphy E, Chase G: Principles of Genetic Counseling. Chicago, IL, Year Book Medical, 1975

Nicoll JA, Roberts GW, Graham DI: Apolipoprotein E epsilon 4 allele is associated with deposition of amyloid beta-protein following head injury. Nat Med 1:135–137, 1995

Ohkura T, Isse K, Akazawa K, et al: Long-term estrogen replacement therapy in female patients with dementia of the Alzheimer type: 7 case reports. Dementia 6:99–107, 1995

Ott A, Breteler MM, van Harskamp F, et al: Prevalence of Alzheimer's disease and vascular dementia: association with education. The Rotterdam study. BMJ 310:970–973, 1995

Paganini-Hill A, Henderson VW: Estrogen deficiency and risk of Alzheimer's disease in women. Am J Epidemiol 140:256–261, 1994

Pericak-Vance MA, Bebout JL, Gaskell PC Jr, et al: Linkage studies in familial Alzheimer disease: evidence for chromosome 19 linkage. Am J Hum Genet 48:1034–1050, 1991

Perl DP, Good PF: Aluminum and the neurofibrillary tangle: results of tissue microprobe studies. Ciba Found Symp 169:217–227, 1992

Poirier J, Davignon J, Bouthillier D, et al: Apolipoprotein E polymorphism and Alzheimer's disease. Lancet 342:697–699, 1993

Powell AL, Brooks J, Zahner DA, et al: Education, occupation, and Alzheimer's disease. JAMA 272:1405–1406, 1994

Powell D, Folstein MF: Pedigree study of familial Alzheimer disease. J Neurogenet 1:189–197, 1984

Ranen NG, Stine OC, Abbott MH, et al: Anticipation and instability of IT-15 (CAG)n repeats in parent-offspring pairs with Huntington disease. Am J Hum Genet 57:593–602, 1995

Rasmusson DX, Brandt J, Martin DB, et al: Head injury as a risk factor in Alzheimer's disease. Brain Inj 9:213–219, 1995

Rich JB, Rasmusson DX, Folstein MF, et al: Nonsteroidal anti-inflammatory drugs in Alzheimer's disease. Neurology 45:51–55, 1995

Rifat SL, Eastwood MR, McLachlan DR, et al: Effect of exposure of miners to aluminum powder. Lancet 336:1162–1165, 1990

Rogaev EI, Sherrington R, Rogaeva EA, et al: Familial Alzheimer's disease in kindreds with missense mutations in a gene on chromosome 1 related to the Alzheimer's disease type 3 gene. Nature 376:775–778, 1995

Rogers J, Kirby LC, Hempelman SR, et al: Clinical trial of indomethacin in Alzheimer's disease. Neurology 43:1609–1611, 1993

Royston MC, Mann D, Pickering-Brown S, et al: Apolipoprotein E epsilon 2 allele promotes longevity and protects patients with Down's syndrome from dementia. Neuroreport 5:2583–2585, 1994

Schellenberg GD: Genetic dissection of Alzheimer disease: a heterogeneous disorder. Proc Natl Acad Sci U S A 92:8552–8559, 1995a

Schellenberg GD: Molecular genetics of familial Alzheimer's disease. Arzneimittelforschung 45:418–424, 1995b

Schellenberg GD, Boehnke M, Wijsman EM, et al: Genetic association and linkage analysis of the apolipoprotein CII locus and familial Alzheimer's disease. Ann Neurol 31:223–227, 1992

Serra JA, Famulari AL, Kohan S, et al: Copper-zinc superoxide dismutase activity in red blood cells in probable Alzheimer's patients and their first-degree relatives. J Neurol Sci 122:179–188, 1994

Shen ZM, Perczel A, Hollosi M, et al: Study of Al3 + binding and conformational properties of the alanine-substituted C-terminal domain of the NF-M protein and its relevance to Alzheimer's disease. Biochemistry 33:9627–9636, 1994

Sherrington R, Rogaev EI, Liang Y, et al: Cloning of a gene bearing missense mutations in early-onset familial Alzheimer's disease. Nature 375:754–760, 1995

Small GW, Mazziotta JC, Collins MT, et al: Apolipoprotein E type 4 allele and cerebral glucose metabolism in relatives at risk for familial Alzheimer disease. JAMA 273:942–947, 1995

Snowdon DA, Kemper SJ, Mortimer JA, et al: Linguistic ability in early life and cognitive function and Alzheimer's disease in late life: findings from the Nun Study. JAMA 275:528–532, 1996

Stancer HC, Wagener DK: Genetic counselling: its need in psychiatry and the directions it gives for future research. Can J Psychiatry 29:289–294, 1984

Stern Y, Gurland B, Tatemichi TK, et al: Influence of education and occupation on the incidence of Alzheimer's disease. JAMA 271:1004–1010, 1994

Stine OC, Pleasant N, Franz ML, et al: Correlation between the onset age of Huntington's disease and length of the trinucleotide repeat in IT-15. Hum Mol Genet 2:1547–1549, 1993

Tyler A, Harper PS: Attitudes of subjects at risk and their relatives towards genetic counselling in Huntington's chorea. J Med Genet 20:179–188, 1983

van Duijn CM, Clayton DG, Chandra V, et al: Interaction between genetic and environmental risk factors for Alzheimer's disease: a reanalysis of case-control studies. EURODEM Risk Factors Research Group. Genet Epidemiol 11:539–551, 1994a

van Duijn CM, de Knijff P, Cruts M, et al: Apolipoprotein ε4 allele in a population-based study of early-onset Alzheimer's disease. Nat Genet 7:74–78, 1994b

van Duijn CM, Havekes LM, Van Broeckhoven C, et al: Apolipoprotein E genotype and association between smoking and early onset Alzheimer's disease. BMJ 310:627–631, 1995

Weaver D: Catalog of Prenatally Diagnosed Conditions, 2nd Edition. Baltimore, MD, Johns Hopkins University Press, 1992

Wertz DC, Fletcher JC: An international survey of attitudes of medical geneticists toward mass screening and access to results. Public Health Rep 104:35–44, 1989

Wooldridge EQ, Murray RF Jr: The psychodynamics associated with sickle cell gene carrier status. Birth Defects: Original Article Series 20:169–186, 1984

Zhang M: Prevalence study on dementia and Alzheimer disease. Chung Hua I Hsueh Tsa Chih 70:424–428, 1990

Zhao B, Sisodia SS, Kusiak JW: Altered processing of a mutant amyloid precursor protein in neuronal and endothelial cells. J Neurosci Res 40:261–268, 1995

17

Ethical Issues in Dementia: Bioethics, Autonomy, and the Experience of Persons With Dementia

Thomas H. Murray, Ph.D.

Introduction

Dementia has proven to be a special challenge for bioethics, a challenge rooted both in the particular characteristics of dementia as a slow but inexorable deterioration of one's mental capacities and in the kinds of solutions that have proven particularly attractive and robust in bioethics.

Dementia's slow, ineluctable course makes it a persistent challenge. In a crisis, we may choose rightly or wrongly, but then the crisis is over. We learn from our mistakes, cope with our guilt, and move on. Living with or treating a person with dementia is a prospect that may last a decade or longer. For subjects with dementia and their primary caregivers, the dementia can easily become the defining characteristic of those years.

The particular nature of the decline—forgetfulness, loss of self-identity, and ultimately failure to recognize those you have loved—is a series of grave blows to what we value most in our close and enduring human relationships. These same manifestations of the loss of one's capacity for rational thought and deliberation also pose a quandary for bioethics.

Dementia and Bioethics

A Practical Syllogism

It is possible to think of dementia's challenge to bioethics in terms of a rough, practical syllogism:

1. One of dementia's primary manifestations is a defect in reasoning that results in impairment and loss of autonomy—literally, reasoned self-direction.
2. Autonomy has served as the linchpin for many of the consensus solutions bioethics has achieved. Examples include the centrality of informed consent in research and treatment and the obligation physicians have to tell the truth to their patients about diagnosis and prognosis, even when the truth may be difficult and unwelcome. It is not much of an exaggeration to say that for certain theorists autonomy has become something close to a universal moral solvent—a concept that dissolves all moral dilemmas. Bioethicists have used it to deal with an enormous variety of moral problems, at times with great success and at other times less so.
3. The most robust tool we have in bioethics—the appeal to individual autonomy—is poorly adapted to many of the problems posed by dementia, resulting in an erosion and eventual ablation of precisely those human capacities that underpin autonomy and that give it its moral force. Applying autonomy to

the often subtle and complex moral problems arising in the care of persons with dementia is like dusting priceless family china with a sledgehammer: It is a sturdy tool, tremendously useful for certain tasks and wholly unsuited for others.

Despite the disadvantages of autonomy as a means for understanding and resolving moral problems in dementia, bioethicists' familiarity with this tool has led them to try to push its use as far as they can as a possible solution. Certainly, for some problems in dementia, autonomy remains a useful approach. Early in the course of the disease, persons with dementia may well retain sufficient capacities for reason, memory, and judgment that the same considerations that lead us to have such great respect for autonomous decisions in competent adults without dementia hold with almost the same force for persons with mild, sporadic dementia.

The focus on autonomy, for all of its usefulness, also has its limitations. For one thing, it has contributed to a relative lack of attention to the *experience of dementia*—what life is like for persons with dementia. For another, it has disposed us to grasp proffered solutions to knotty problems a bit too hastily. One example of such a premature solution is the promotion of advance directives in health care to make end-of-life decisions for persons with dementia.

Advance Directives

There are two basic forms of advance directives for health care decision making: living wills and durable powers of attorney for health care (Avila 1993; English and Meisel 1993). Both living wills and durable powers of attorney are intended to be used once the individual is no longer competent to make decisions for himself or herself. Living wills are documents specifying what health care interventions an individual would desire or reject given certain medical circumstances. They vary from precise tables or checklists to vague statements refusing heroic measures if one becomes terminally ill. (See, for example, Ind. Code §16, §8, §11, §12 [Burns Supp. 1988]; Uniform Rights of Terminally Ill Act [URTIA] §2, 9B U.L.A. 609 [1989]; Omnibus Reconciliation Act, 42 U.S.C. §§1395cc, 1395i-3, 13951, 1396a [1990].) Durable powers of attorney for health care appoint another individual to decide on behalf of the patient once he or she is incompetent. Although others may lack specific information about the person's preferences for treatment options, they have the virtue of flexibility: the person executing the durable power of attorney does not have to anticipate either what the person's precise condition might be or what treatment options might then exist (Gilfix 1994). Some advance directives are hybrids, appointing someone with durable power of attorney and also making statements about the individual's preferences for treatment or nontreatment (English and Meisel 1994).

In 1990 advance directives were given a legal boost by the creation of a new federal law, the Patient Self Determination Act. This law placed a legal obligation on certain health care facilities, including hospitals and long-term care institutions, to inform their patients about advance directives, to inquire whether patients have one, and to offer them an opportunity to execute one if they so wished (Omnibus Reconciliation Act 1990; Roach 1991).

It is not difficult to see why advance directives have such appeal. To persons who are now competent and who fear the loss of control over their medical fate should they lapse into incompetence, advance directives offer the promise that their current wishes could direct their future treatment. The advance directive would be relevant whether the individual feared unwanted life-prolonging treatment, in which case the advance directive could forestall such interventions, or whether the person feared that treatment would be ended before she or he would have wanted. In the latter event, the person could request, through an advance directive, that aggressive treatment be pursued up to the moment of death. To health professionals, advance directives can provide reassurance that the decisions that have to be made, especially potentially end-of-life decisions, are in accordance with the no-longer-competent patient's own preferences. Given the often enormous emotional difficulty of such decisions, to say nothing of their moral and legal ramifications, advance directives as manifestations of autonomy can offer substantial comfort. We feel better acting in the sincere belief that what we now do is what the patient himself or herself wanted.

Three Problems With Advance Directives for Persons With Dementia

For all of their merits, advance directives encounter three problems as possible solutions to end-of-life decision making for persons with dementia. First, despite all of the publicity about advance directives, and despite the Patient Self Determination Act's promotion of advance directives, few people have them (Emanuel et al. 1991; Gamble et al. 1991).

Second, those advance directives that address the substance of what decisions the person would want to have made—living wills or the hybrid living wills or durable powers of attorney—require interpretation. Rarely is an individual fortunate or clairvoyant enough to anticipate the precise details of his or her medical condition or the interventions available. Even when people expressly refuse a certain intervention, interpretation is usually needed. Suppose a living will specified that no attempts at resuscitation should be made once the person was unlikely to regain full competency. Would this preclude cardioversion for an arrhythmia, which is a similar technology but applied for a different purpose? Whether or not physicians would agree that cardioversion is distinct from resuscitation, it is often not clear what patients meant when they wrote "no resuscitation" or something similar in their living wills. The specific examples here are not important. The central point is that substantive comments about end-of-life decisions are rarely self-interpreting; they almost always require interpretation at a time when the writer is not available to say which interpretation he or she prefers (Dresser and Whitehouse 1994; Emanuel et al. 1991).

Third, the premises that underlie advance directives as a solution to the problem of decision making for incompetent patients may not be so self-evidently correct as has been presumed. One of those premises is that people want and expect their advance directives to be followed exactly as they have written them. Yet at least one study has found that a group of patients—people on chronic renal dialysis—do not necessarily want their advance directives followed strictly (Seghal et al. 1992). Therefore, the meaning of a patient's advance directive may not be so obvious, even when the language itself seems abundantly clear.

For persons with dementia, an even more complex problem arises. The use of advance directives for persons with dementia depends, for its moral force, on either of two assumptions. Either we must presume that the preferences of the person before the loss of autonomous reason are morally more important than the interests of the person who now has dementia, or we must presume that those interests never change—that the interests of the person with dementia are identical with the interests of the same person before dementia interposed itself. The latter presumption seems highly implausible. A person who once abhorred idleness now, from all available evidence, may appear quite happy watching television or taking slow, apparently aimless walks. Dementia affects people in many ways. It is difficult to believe that those changes would fail to affect the interests an individual may have at various stages of the disease.

We are left then with the presumption that a person's preferences before dementia should trump their interests once dementia occurs. The belief is not self-evidently true. Certainly, there are instances in which a person accurately anticipates what life will be like with dementia, reflects on what he or she genuinely values, fears that such a life would destroy what he or she cares most about, and requests that once such a point is reached, no life-prolonging treatments be used. But there will be other instances in which people will not successfully anticipate what their lives may be like and make an advance directive out of ignorance or fear that requests a course of action at some future time that seems clearly at odds with the interests of the person who now has dementia. Is it clear that the morally preferable course is to ignore the person's current interests in favor of a declaration made years before when the person may have experienced the world quite differently than he or she now does (Dresser and Whitehouse 1994)?

Overall, advance directives at times may be useful aids in making difficult decisions for once-competent patients. Most patients do not have them. Even when they do, there are complexities of interpretation and ambiguities about the moral force of such directives for persons with dementia that limit their usefulness. Advance directives, that is, are not a panacea, certainly not for persons with dementia.

An Alternative Standard: The Patient's Best Interest

If individual autonomy and the advance directives meant to preserve its role in decision making for incompetent patients is not the answer, what then? Rebecca Dresser, a legal scholar, and Peter J. Whitehouse, a neurologist, identify three reasons why so little attention has been paid to the principal alternative to relying on the patient's own preferences—the standard of the best interest of the patient, also known as the objective, benefit-burden, or reasonable-person standard (Roach 1991).

The first reason for the preference for an autonomy-based standard was that the standard was created by people who were themselves competent and autonomous. It seems reasonable to suppose that such people were concerned about their own prospective interests as competent, autonomous persons without dementia. They were also unlikely to be attuned to the possible changes in interests that might accompany dementia.

Second, there is a genuine danger that healthy persons might devalue the life experiences of people with dementia. If we adopted a best-interests standard, people without dementia might impose on persons with dementia their prejudices about the poverty of life with dementia. Relying on the person's own preferences before dementia at least assures that it will not be someone else's irrational and indefensible prejudices that guide decisions about that individual. Of course, that leaves us with the uncomfortable possibility that the person (once competent, now having dementia) may have had prejudices every bit as irrational and indefensible as anyone else's. That their prejudice now affects primarily themselves is some reassurance, but not much.

The third reason behind the appeal of relying on some statement of the patient's own preferences is what philosophers call the problem of other minds. How can we ever know with certainty anything about the subjective mental experience of another person—an "other" mind? How much more uncertainty must there be when the other person suffers from an organic and functional brain disease such as dementia and cannot even describe his or her own experiences? One implication of the other-minds problem is to cast doubt on any possible effort to understand the mental experiences of persons with dementia (Dresser and Whitehouse 1994).

Without denying the philosophical complexity and durability of the problem of other minds, we can nevertheless observe that simple, everyday social interaction requires considerable skill at discerning what is going on in those other minds with which we interact continuously. Daily experience provides ample proof that we can understand with remarkable, though not perfect, accuracy what other people experience. The problem is more difficult concerning persons with dementia. But there remain a multitude of signs and signals for communicating and interpreting experience, even when language has been lost. Without underestimating the difficulty of the task, we can nonetheless affirm that the philosopher's other-minds problem no more disqualifies our efforts to understand the experience of persons with dementia than it renders impossible our everyday navigation of the social world.

Persons with dementia may no longer have the ability to make rational choices, but there is compelling reason to believe that most of them do have an experiential world, that that world is important and vivid to them, and that it should have some significance in making decisions that affect their future well-being. What is needed to give that experience its appropriate moral weight in our treatment of persons with dementia?

What a Best-Interest or Objective Standard Requires

Dresser and Whitehouse (1994) note that most legal and ethical analyses to date have focused almost exclusively on whatever physical sensations the person may be experiencing. This was clear in the *Conroy* decision, in which the New Jersey Supreme Court distinguished between cases in which there is "some trustworthy evidence" of a patient's wishes to refuse life-prolonging treatment and cases in which no such evidence is available. The Court in that case was willing to accept a reasonable balancing of life's pleasures against life's pains. When no information about the patient's own wishes is at hand, the Court would authorize foregoing treatment only if pain were so severe and unrelievable "that the effect of administering life-sustaining treatment would be inhumane" (Conroy, 486 A.2d 1209 [N.J. 1985], cited in Dresser and Whitehouse 1994).

Even a narrow focus on the experiential world of a person with dementia requires several moral and empirical judgments. Dresser and Whitehouse (1994, p. 7) note three principal ones: "(1) determining which positive and negative experiences (burdens and benefits) are relevant to the decision; (2) measuring the burdens and benefits experienced by an individual incompetent patient; and (3) deciding what balance of burdens and benefits indicates that continued life would confer sufficient benefit to mandate life-sustaining treatment." In any event, we need a richer understanding of the experiential world of persons with dementia.

The Experience of Dementia

We know too little about the experience of dementia. Granted, there will be difficulties trying to see the world as it is seen by someone with advanced Alzheimer's disease (AD). The philosophers who stress the obstacles to ever knowing what is in another person's mind do, after all, have a point. But we can enhance our ability to appreciate the experience, to enter the world, of persons with dementia. There are reports from sensitive and observant clinicians, such as Joseph M. Foley (1992). There are first-person accounts by subjects in the early stages of dementia (Davis 1989; Lerner 1984; McGowin 1993). And there are literary efforts to help us imagine what such a life might be like (Bernlef 1989). Together with clinical experience and other ways of knowing persons with AD, the growth of such materials could enhance enormously our understanding of the experiences of persons with the disease.

Questions about experience have important implications, especially as we take seriously the limitations of advance directives in making treatment decisions and begin to consider using objective or best-interest standards for those same decisions. Consider the case of a person whose treatment involves suffering, the purpose of which they cannot comprehend. A person with dementia is not spared other diseases. Suppose someone with moderately advanced dementia is found to have a type of cancer for which the treatment is successful in perhaps 30% of cases. Administering that treatment to someone who cannot understand why it is being given would require restraining him or her at times and would result in considerable suffering from the physical effects of the therapy. If we should base our treatment decision on whether, on the whole, the intervention is likely to benefit the individual patient, then we must do our best to understand how the patient is likely to experience that intervention. It is certainly plausible that a person with dementia who cannot understand why he or she is being restrained and subjected to painful procedures that create physical misery for weeks afterward would experience great distress—not just physical pain but a sense of betrayal at the mystifying behavior of his or her caregivers. The individuals who had constituted the patient's immediate social world, who provided care and solicitude, have now become torturers—or so the person with dementia might feel.

If we were to give greater consideration to what was in the best interests of persons with dementia, the answer would not be, in every case, to pursue aggressive, potentially life-prolonging treatment. In many cases, it would. But in other instances, such as the hypothetical cancer patient with dementia just mentioned, regard for the world of the person with dementia might well counsel us to forego such treatment if its net impact were to increase substantially the person's suffering.

Taking seriously the experience of persons with dementia would affect our response not only to life or death decisions but to more common and less dramatic ones as well. The Center for Biomedical Ethics at the School of Medicine, Case Western Reserve University, in collaboration with other organizations, sponsored a Community Dialogue on Ethics and the Progression of Dementia, led by Stephen G. Post. Forty-four people participated in the Dialogue's year-long deliberations. Participants included persons with AD and their caregivers, as well as nurses, physicians, home health workers, administrators, lawyers, and ethicists. The Dialogue's principal product—the "Fairhill Guidelines on Ethics and the Care of People with Alzheimer Disease"—addresses a range of issues confronted by persons with dementia and their caregivers, ranging from truthfulness in the disclosure of a diagnosis of AD, through issues of independence, such as limitations on driving, choosing where to live and whom to see for medical care, and the use of physical or chemical restraints, on to decisions of whether to forego life-prolonging interventions (Post and Whitehouse 1995).

For each topic, the experience of persons with dementia was represented; it proved important in shaping the group's recommendations. The Dialogue emphasized respecting the wishes of the person with AD as far as practicable and recognizing that Alzheimer's is a progressive disease with specific deficits rather than a global and immediate loss of all cognitive abilities.

Dementia and Public Policy: Managing the Deaths of Persons With Dementia

Despite its unpleasant connotations, *managing death* is an accurate description of how most people, certainly elderly persons in institutions, will perish. In contrast to just over half a century ago, when only 37% of those who died in America did so in an institution, today the number is between 80% and 85%. An estimated 70%

of all deaths in nursing homes and hospitals involve decisions to use or forego some potentially life-prolonging measure.

We should not assume that deaths that take place in the home are any less likely to involve decisions of whether to use or forego an intervention: A few years ago, when a group of primary care physicians was designing an ethics curriculum for a primary-care core clerkship, they insisted that it should include the topic of foregoing life-prolonging treatment. When I expressed puzzlement, because such treatments are usually provided in the hospital, one physician asked: "Who do you think decides whether they go to the hospital in the first place?"

Withholding and Withdrawing Treatments

It is by now a widely accepted conclusion in bioethics that withholding a life-prolonging treatment and withdrawing such a treatment are morally equivalent. An emerging consensus was solidified by the report of a presidential commission that reaffirmed that there was no moral distinction between withholding or withdrawing (President's Commission 1983). If there were good moral reasons to withhold some potentially life-prolonging treatment, those same reasons were equally cogent to a decision to withdraw that treatment. Conversely, when the moral case was compelling *against* withdrawing a treatment, it would be equally compelling against a failure to initiate the same treatment.

Certainly, health professionals may feel more responsible, more like they are doing something wrong, when a treatment is withdrawn rather than withheld. This psychological difference is important to acknowledge. However, it is just as important to realize that this emotional response does not reflect underlying sound moral reasons for regarding withholding as different from withdrawing.

Physician-Assisted Suicide

In contrast to the relatively settled nature of the question of whether there is any difference between withholding and withdrawing treatment, at this time a debate rages over whether there is any ethically significant difference between foregoing life-prolonging treatment on the one hand and accelerating death on the other, whether by aiding in a person's suicide or acting as the agent of death directly— so-called active euthanasia.

Jack Kevorkian has assured that the debate over physician-assisted suicide would encompass dementia. His very first "case"— Janet Adkins—was said to be in the early stages of a progressive dementia. Adkins's decision to seek death before her dementia robbed her completely of her capacity for autonomous choice suggests that she recognized the catch-22 AD presents for physician assistance in suicide. Whether one favors or opposes such physician assistance, it is easy to see that the strongest cases are those in which the person is fully competent and rational, where the person's suffering is severe and irremediable, and where death is imminent. For persons with AD, emotional distress may well be an important feature of the disease in its early stages. But this is not the kind of intense physical suffering many of the proponents of assisted suicide cite in its favor. Then there is the heart of the catch-22: Long before death is imminent, the person with dementia will have lost all capacity for rational, autonomous choice.

Oregon's law. The most recent effort to provide legal sanction for physician-assisted suicide is Ballot Measure 16 in the state of Oregon. Oregon voters approved the measure, known as the Oregon Death with Dignity Act, in November 1994. The act's legality was rapidly challenged. But even if it were approved it would have no direct impact whatsoever on the care of persons with dementia. In keeping with the emphasis on autonomy, the act requires two verbal and one written request from a competent patient who is acting voluntarily. Furthermore, at least two physicians must agree that the patient has a terminal illness and is likely to die within 6 months (Annas 1994). The catch-22 would surely hold. Recently, two federal courts concluded that states could not prosecute physicians who assisted terminally ill patients in taking their own lives. Significantly, the two courts—the United States Court of Appeals for the Ninth Circuit and the comparable court for the Second Circuit—reached their conclusions on quite different grounds. The

Ninth Circuit based its decision on an interpretation of the due process clause of the Fourteenth Amendment; the Second Circuit justified its decision by the equal protection clause of the same amendment. Legal scholars have expressed concern both about the different rationales utilized by the two courts and by the potentially far-reaching implications of the rulings (Capron 1996).

Active Euthanasia

Like physician-assisted suicide, active euthanasia is intensely controversial. There is no consensus among bioethicists as to either the morality or immorality of active euthanasia or to the wisdom of public policies permitting it. Proponents of active euthanasia stress the similarities between it and foregoing treatment when both lead to death. They argue that if preventing suffering is a justification for foregoing treatment, it is equally valid in justifying active euthanasia. They present cases in which they claim suffering cannot be adequately controlled by drugs and ask whether it is more compassionate to engage in active euthanasia than to forego treatment in which the person's suffering will be prolonged.

The case for active euthanasia is strongest under certain circumstances. Imagine a paradigmatically strong case for active euthanasia. In the case, the patient is a competent adult, not suffering from depression, thoughtful, calm, and well informed. Nonetheless, the patient is in extreme pain that is unresponsive to the most skillful efforts to relieve it. Death is near at hand. The physician and patient have enjoyed a long, open, and respectful relationship. The patient, fully conscious and in full knowledge of the implications of the choice, requests active euthanasia. The physician is acutely aware of the patient's severe suffering, the unsuccessful efforts to relieve it, and the absence of alternative means of reducing the suffering.

Opponents of active euthanasia, especially euthanasia by health professionals, can acknowledge the force of such a case without being persuaded that it would be good public policy to legalize it. They focus less on the burdens and benefits attending individual cases than on the likely consequences of generalizing the practice. They ask what kinds of people would use active euthanasia. Would it become the hospice of the poor? They point to the inevitability of errors, made without malice, and of abuses. They express concern for changes in the roles and images of physicians and health care institutions. Would the public's perception of physicians change? For the better or for the worse? Would people fear hospitals (more than they do now)? These sorts of policy concerns are the most prominent arguments used against legalizing active euthanasia.

What relevance does the active euthanasia debate have for the care of people with AD? Recall the paradigmatic case in favor of active euthanasia. Compare the particulars of that case with cases of people with advanced dementia. In contrast to the paradigm, AD patients' competence is profoundly impaired; they may be suffering, though the suffering is likely to be emotional more than physical. Furthermore, as the disease progresses, they may become less aware of what they have lost; and there is of course the catch-22 in operation once again—the closer to death, the farther from competence, rationality, and autonomy. In short, whatever one believes about active euthanasia, the case in its favor is weakest for persons with dementia.

Practical Considerations

Look for windows of lucidity.   Persons with AD differ in their insight and awareness as to the disease's impact on them. Though the disease's progression is inexorable, patients often experience good intervals in which their thoughts may be relatively clear and appropriate. Foley (1992, p. 41) notes many factors that can affect a person's current functioning, including "circadian rhythms, fatigue, fever, level of physical and social stimulation, biochemical and pharmacological changes of the internal environment, physical and social alterations of the external environment," as well as the severity of the disease itself. Such relative windows of lucidity afford opportunities to explore questions about what might be done with, for, and to the person with AD.

Decide in advance whenever possible.   Though we must remain mindful of the difficulties in extrapolating from the wishes of the once-competent person to the interests of the person who now has dementia, we should nonetheless take advantage of whatever lucidity appears in the early phases of the disease to discuss what the person would want done as the disease progresses. Whether such conversations are desirable and possible depends on several factors: how much insight the person has into his or her own disease; how far the disease has progressed; and whether the person is emotionally capable of considering his or her own demise. But we should not let our own reluctance to talk about such things rob patients and their families of opportunities to reflect on them and to ascertain the patient's wishes when that patient is still capable of deliberation.

Consider other ethical reasons for continuing or discontinuing life-prolonging treatment in the interests of the patient.   When the most widely accepted reason for foregoing life-prolonging treatment—that a competent, autonomous patient refuses the treatment—is not available, we must look at other standards to guide our decisions. One often expressed fear is that persons with dementia will have their deaths hastened because others perceive their lives to have less value than the lives of persons without dementia. This fear is not idle; there is ample historical precedent for such treatment of those with dementia. But not all reasons for considering the foregoing of life-prolonging treatment for a person with dementia involve denying the equal moral worth of persons with dementia. A focus on the experience of persons with dementia reveals a crucial distinction.

We should distinguish between nontreatment decisions based on a judgment that the individual's worth was diminished from nontreatment decisions that take into account the person's experience—his or her own perceptions and interests. An example would be a case in which the life of a person with dementia might be extended for a few weeks or months with a noxious therapy that will cause significant suffering. It is crucial to fix on the meaning of that experience for the person with dementia. If the person cannot understand the purpose of the therapy, if instead what that person experiences is suffering at the hands of those who had previously provided solicitous care, then the person may be baffled and frightened by the therapy, so that the last days may go on longer but be experienced by the person with dementia as laden with betrayal and suffering. To forego therapy under those circumstances would result in death coming a bit sooner but without the psychological suffering inflicted by painful therapies the purpose of which cannot be understood.

It is crucial to see the difference between this scenario, which is motivated by love for the person with dementia and sensitivity to the experience of persons with dementia, and an opposite scenario in which persons with dementia are allowed to die because their lives are deemed not worth living. The latter is the nightmarish echo of Nazi "racial hygiene" invoked by people suspicious of any decision to allow a person to die, especially a person disabled in any way (Proctor 1988). It would be a mistake, I believe, to dismiss such worries out of hand. People can and do devalue the lives of other people. But it would be an equally grievous mistake to suppose that all decisions to forego life-prolonging measures are morally wrong. Indeed, as the scenario described previously illustrates, there are times when decisions to employ potentially life-prolonging measures can be cruel and arbitrary, sacrificing the comfort and peace of mind of a person with dementia for an abstraction.

Given that our firmest moral warrant for foregoing medical treatment—the considered, voluntary, and informed judgment of the affected person—is either absent or diminished in persons with dementia, such decisions are likely to remain difficult and morally contested ones. With a better understanding of the experience of persons with dementia, we will have a firmer grasp on how our decisions affect the interests of such persons. Our best understanding of those interests will be short of perfect, but a serious effort to apprehend those interests and to ensure that they are considered in all important decisions about persons with dementia is a crucial step toward dealing ethically with the disorder.

Conclusion

In reflecting on ethical issues in dementia, it is useful to ponder the words of the eminent clinician, Joseph R. Foley:

> It is important to identify functions that are lost, but even more so to identify functions that are preserved. Dementia per se does not always deny patients the right to participation in decisions about their own care, their own life, or their own health. In the formulation of public and institutional policy we must beware of simplifications and generalizations; we must recognize that individual demented persons have their own unique attributes and that, despite metaphors loosely thrown around, they each remain a person, with their own gratifications and frustrations, their own unique background, and their own unique destiny. (Foley 1992, p. 42)

References

Annas GJ: Death by prescription: the Oregon initiative. N Engl J Med 331: 1240–1243, 1994

Avila D: Medical treatment rights of older persons with disabilities: 1991– 92 developments. Issues Law Med 8:429–466, 1993

Bernlef J: Out of Mind. Boston, David R. Godine, 1989

Capron AM: Liberty, equality, death! Hastings Cent Rep 26:23–24, 1996

Davis R: My Journey into Alzheimer's Disease. Wheaton, IL, Tyndale House, 1989

Dresser R, Whitehouse PJ: The incompetent patient on the slippery slope (ethical aspects of life-sustaining treatment for progressive dementia). Hastings Cent Rep 24:6–12, 1994

Emanuel LL, Barry MJ, Stoeckle JD, et al: Advance directives for health care: a case for greater use. N Engl J Med 324:889–895, 1991

English DM, Meisel A: Uniform health-care decisions act gives new guidance. Estate Planning 21:355–362, 1994

Foley JM: The experience of being demented, in Dementia and Aging: Ethics, Values, and Policy Choices. Edited by Binstock RH, Post S, Whitehouse PJ. Baltimore, Johns Hopkins University Press, 1992

Gamble ER, McDonald PJ, Lichstein PR, et al: Knowledge, attitudes, and behavior of elderly persons regarding living wills. Arch Intern Med 151:277–280, 1991

Gilfix MG: Client health care decision making: the role of the elder law attorney. Practising Law Institute. Estate Planning and Administration Course Handbook Series No. D-231:pp 317–354, 1994

Lerner AB: I've lost a kingdom: a victim's remarks on Alzheimer's disease. J Am Geriatr Soc 32:935, 1984

McGowin DF: Living in the Labyrinth. New York, Delacourt, 1993

Omnibus Reconciliation Act, 42 U.S.C. §§1395cc, 1395i-3, 13951, 1396a (1990)

Post SG, Whitehouse PJ: Fairhill guidelines on ethics of the care of people with Alzheimer disease: a clinical summary. J Am Geriatr Soc 43: 1423–1429, 1995

President's Commission for the Study of Ethical Problems in Medicine and Biomedical and Behavioral Research: Deciding to Forgo Life-Sustaining Treatment. Washington, DC, U.S. Government Printing Office, 1983

Proctor RN: Racial Hygiene: Medicine Under the Nazis. Cambridge, MA, Harvard University Press, 1988

Roach CA: Paradox and Pandora's box: the tragedy of current right-to-die jurisprudence. University of Michigan Journal of Law Reform 25:133–190, 1991–1992

Seghal A, Galbraith A, Chesney M, et al: How strictly do dialysis patients want their advance directives followed? JAMA 267:59–63, 1992

CHAPTER

18

Dementia and Health Care Reform

Robert H. Binstock, Ph.D.

Although research on the causes of dementias has progressed somewhat in the past few years, and treatment of symptoms can presently yield modest short-term benefits for some patients, the development of effective ways to prevent and cure dementias is not likely in the years immediately ahead. Yet, even at present, humane modes of care and services can be provided, both to lessen the suffering of people who are afflicted with irreversible dementia and to reduce the physical, emotional, and financial burdens of families and others who provide care for these patients.

As indicated in Table 18–1, a large range of medical, nursing, social, legal, financial, and other long-term care services that can be of value to dementia patients and their caregivers have been identified through program development and research. The service needs of dementia patients and their families are inextricably linked with the overlapping and parallel needs encountered by any of us—regardless of illness, disability, family situation, or age—who are faced with issues of long-term care. The essentiality of this linkage was reflected in the report of a national panel of experts that, though convened to consider the problems faced in locating

Table 18–1.   Services that may be needed for people with dementia and their families

Diagnosis	Protective services
Acute medical care	Supervision
Ongoing medical supervision	Home health aide
Treatment of coexisting medical conditions	Homemaker
	Personal care
Medication and elimination of drugs that cause excess disability	Paid companion/sitter
	Shopping
Multidimensional assessment	Home-delivered meals
Skilled nursing	Chore services
Physical therapy	Telephone reassurance
Occupational therapy	Personal emergency response system
Speech therapy	Recreation/exercise
Adult day care	Transportation
Respite care*	Escort service
Family/caregiver education and training	Special equipment (ramps, hospital beds, etc.)
Family/caregiver counseling	Vision care
Family support groups	Audiology
Patient counseling	Dental care
Legal services	Nutrition counseling
Financial/benefits counseling	Hospice
Mental health services	Autopsy

Note.   These services may be needed by and can be provided for persons who are living at home, in a nursing home, or in another care setting such as assisted living housing, a continuing care retirement community, a board and care facility, or an adult foster home.

*Respite care includes any service intended to provide temporary relief for the primary caregiver. When used for that purpose, homemaker, paid companion/sitter, adult day care, temporary nursing home care, and other services included on the list are regarded as respite care.

Source.   Office of Technology Assessment 1990, p. 16.

and arranging appropriate services for people with dementia, recommended overwhelmingly that Congress enact solutions that "serve people with dementia and people with other conditions and diseases as well" (Office of Technology Assessment 1990, p. 63).

Whether a dementia patient is living at home, in a nursing home, or in another type of residential setting, an ideal system of services would be amply available, of high quality, provided by well-trained personnel, easily located and arranged, and well funded through public and private resources. The present system, however, is far from ideal.

The supply of services is insufficient, service providers lack education and training, and the quality of many services is poor. Moreover, the system is so fragmented that even when high-quality services are sufficiently available, many patients and families do not know about them and require help in defining their service needs and in arranging for them to be provided (Office of Technology Assessment 1990).

Underlying each of these problems, in turn, is the issue of financing. As is the case with most aspects of the United States health care delivery system, the characteristics of long-term care services and access to them are substantially shaped by the nature and extent of policies for funding them. Indeed, attempts to reform long-term care services will largely lie in efforts to change the manner in which they are funded. And because dementia-related service needs are inextricably linked with the overlapping and parallel needs encountered by any of us who are faced with issues of long-term care, funding for services that will help dementia patients and their families will undoubtedly be incorporated in broader initiatives for reforming and financing long-term care in the United States.

In this chapter I assess the prospects for reform. First, I present an overview of the present mechanisms for financing long-term care services and the limitations of these mechanisms. Second, I discuss various experiments and demonstration projects in financing long-term care that are now under way in a limited number of communities. Third, I trace the development and status of recent major health care reform proposals affecting long-term care: the emergence of proposals to expand public funding for long-term care and proposals to turn Medicaid into a block grant program. And finally, I consider the outlook for the future, analyzing the politics of older and younger constituencies who might provide political support for expanded public funding of long-term care in the years ahead.

Present Financing for Long-Term Care

More than 80 federal programs and a plethora of state and local public and private agencies are sources of funding for long-term care services (Congressional Research Service 1988). But each source regulates the availability of funds with rules as to eligibility and breadth of service coverage and changes its rules frequently. Dementia patients are often ruled ineligible for funding through Medicare, Medicaid, the Veterans Administration, Title XX social services, the Older Americans Act, and other programs (Office of Technology Assessment 1987). Thus, despite the many sources of funding, specific patients and caregivers may find themselves ineligible for financial help and unable to pay out of pocket for needed services. In one study, about 75% of the informal caregivers for dementia patients reported that they did not use formal services because they were unable to pay for them (Eckert and Smyth 1988).

Paying the costs of long-term care out of pocket can be a catastrophic financial experience for patients and their families. The annual cost of a year's care in a nursing home averages $37,000 (Wiener and Illston 1996) and ranges higher than $100,000. Although the use of a limited number of services in a home- or other community-based setting is less expensive, noninstitutional care for patients who would otherwise be appropriately placed in a nursing home is not cheaper (Weissert 1990). Patients and their families paid more than $33.5 billion out of pocket for long-term care services in 1993 (Wiener et al. 1994). The total national expenditure for long-term care was $75.5 billion. Payments from all sources for nursing homes added up to $54.7 billion, and for home care the sum was $20.8 billion. Out-of-pocket payments accounted for 51% of nursing home costs and 26% of home care expenditures.

Private Insurance

Although Medicare pays for short-term, subacute nursing care, it does not reimburse patients for long-term care, either in nursing homes or at home. Private long-term care insurance, a relatively new product, is very expensive for the majority of older persons, and its benefits are limited in scope and duration. The best-quality policies—providing substantial benefits over a reasonable period of time—charged premiums in 1991 that averaged $2,525 for persons aged 65 and $7,675 for those aged 79 (Wiener and Illston 1996). About 4% to 5% of older persons have any private long-term care insurance, and only about 1% of nursing home costs are paid for by private insurance (Wiener et al. 1994). A number of analyses have suggested that even when the product becomes more refined, no more than 20% of older Americans will be able to afford it (Crown et al. 1992; Friedland 1990; Rivlin and Wiener 1988; Wiener et al 1994). Although some studies suggest a potential for a higher percentage of customers, they assume limited packages of benefit coverage (e.g., Cohen et al. 1987).

A variation on the private insurance policy approach to financing long-term care is continuing care retirement communities (CCRCs) that promise comprehensive health care services—including long-term care—to all members (Chellis and Grayson 1990). CCRC customers tend to be middle- and upper-income persons who are relatively healthy when they become residents and pay a substantial entrance charge and monthly fee in return for a promise of care for life. It has been estimated that about 10% of older people could afford to join such communities (Cohen 1988). Most of the 1,000 CCRCs in the United States, however, do not provide complete benefit coverage in their contracts, and those that do have faced financial difficulties (Williams and Temkin-Greener 1996). Because most older people prefer to remain in their own homes rather than join age-segregated communities, an alternative product termed *life care at home* (LCAH) was developed in the late 1980s and marketed to middle-income customers with lower entry and monthly fees than those of CCRCs (Tell et al. 1987). There are, however, only about 500 LCAH policies in effect (Williams and Temkin-Greener 1996).

A relatively new approach for providing long-term care in residential settings is the assisted-living facility. It has been created for moderately disabled persons—including those with dementia—who are not ready for a nursing home and provides them with limited forms of personal care, supervision of medications and other daily routines, and congregate meal and housekeeping services (Kane and Wilson 1993). Assisted living has yet to be tried out with a private insurance approach. The monthly rent in a first-class nonprofit facility averages about $2,400 for a one-bedroom apartment; the rent is higher in for-profit facilities.

The Role of Medicaid

For those who cannot pay for long-term care out of pocket or through various insurance arrangements and who are not eligible for care through programs of the Department of Veterans Affairs, the available sources of payment are Medicaid and other means-tested government programs funded by the Older Americans Act, Social Service Block Grants (Title XX of the Social Security Act), and state and local governments. The bulk of such financing is through Medicaid, which paid an estimated 52% of total national nursing home expenditures in 1993, accounting for one-quarter of all Medicaid spending (Burner et al. 1992).

Medicaid, the federal-state program for the poor, finances the care—at least in part—of about three-fifths of nursing home patients (Wiener and Illston 1996). Medicaid does not pay for the full range of home care services that are needed for most clients who are functionally dependent. Most state Medicaid programs provide reimbursement only for the most "medicalized" services necessary to maintain a long-term care patient in a home environment; rarely reimbursed are essential supports such as chore services, assistance with food shopping and meal preparation, transportation, companionship, periodic monitoring, and respite programs for family and other unpaid caregivers.

Medicaid does include a special waiver program that allows states to offer a wider range of nonmedical home care services, although it is limited to those patients whose services will be less costly than Medicaid-financed nursing home care. But the volume of services in these waiver programs—which in some states combine Medicaid with funds from the Older Americans Act, the Social Services Block Grant program, and other state and local government sources—is small in relation to the overall need (Miller 1992).

Although many patients are poor enough to qualify for Medicaid when they enter a nursing home, a substantial number become poor after they are institutionalized (Adams et al. 1993). Persons in this latter group deplete their assets to meet their bills and eventually "spend down" and become poor enough to qualify for Medicaid. Still others become eligible for Medicaid by sheltering their assets—illegally or legally with the assistance of attorneys who specialize in so-called Medicaid estate planning. Because sheltered assets are not counted in Medicaid eligibility determinations, such persons are able to take advantage of a program for the poor without being poor. An analysis in Virginia estimated that the aggregate of assets sheltered through the use of legal loopholes in 1991 was equal to more than 10% of what the state spent on nursing home care through Medicaid in that year (Burwell 1993). Asset sheltering has become a source of considerable concern to the federal and state governments as Medicaid expenditures on nursing homes continue to increase rapidly; they are projected to triple between 1990 and 2000 (Burner et al. 1992).

Experimental Programs

Private Insurance and Medicaid Partnerships

The Robert Wood Johnson Foundation has undertaken an experimental program in four states intended to enable middle- and upper-income older persons to protect their assets from being spent down and yet have Medicaid pay for their long-term care (Meiners 1996). Through this Partnership for Long-Term Care Program, state governments agree to exempt spending of assets by Medicaid clients if they have previously had their long-term care paid for by a state-certified private insurance policy.

In California, Connecticut, and Indiana, the Medicaid agencies will allow a dollar of asset protection for each dollar that has been paid by insurance. In New York, after 3 years of private insurance coverage for nursing home services or 6 months of home health care, protection is granted for all assets, although the individual's income must be devoted to the cost of care along with Medicaid. This experiment is in its early stages and cannot yet be evaluated.

Financing Through Integration With Acute Care

Experimental models have also been developed in recent years for financing long-term care services by integrating them with acute care. These models are being refined through field demonstrations. Each involves mechanisms of managed care, but their differences illustrate some of the issues and challenges generated by various sources of funding and different types of older patient populations.

A model initially tested at several sites in the 1980s is the Social/Health Maintenance Organization (S/HMO), financed experimentally with waivers from the federal Health Care Financing Administration (HCFA). The S/HMO offers customers a limited package of home- and community-based long-term care benefits on a capitated basis as a supplement to Medicare HMO benefits and attempts to enroll primarily healthy older customers (Leutz et al. 1985). Results from these early experiments were equivocal with respect to the viability of financing arrangements and target populations (Newcomer et al. 1990). Consequently, Congress has called for a second round of S/HMO demonstrations to test refinements such as heavy involvement of geriatricians and geriatric nurse practitioners, standard protocols for obtaining adequate medical and social histories and for diagnosing and managing conditions frequently found in older patients, increased attention to the effects of prescription drugs on patients, and outpatient alternatives to hospitalization and nursing home placement.

Whereas the S/HMO attempts to enroll healthy older persons to demonstrate what is feasible financially with such a population, the On Lok model, developed at a San Francisco neighborhood center in the 1970s and early 1980s, is targeted to community-based older persons who are already sufficiently dependent in daily functioning to be appropriately placed in a nursing home. Most patients are eligible for both Medicare and Medicaid. Services are organized around an adult day-care program that not only serves as a social program and as a respite for caregivers but also functions much like a geriatric outpatient clinic, with substantial medical observation and supervision (Zawadski and Eng 1988).

The On Lok model, now being replicated at 10 demonstration sites as a Program for All-Inclusive Care for the Elderly (PACE), appears to have integrated acute and long-term care fairly well under its managed care approach. Whether it can be extended beyond the very frail population it has served to date—patients who are already functionally dependent and dually eligible for Medicare and Medicaid—remains to be seen. (To some extent, this issue is what is being explored in the second round of the S/HMO demonstrations.) Early evaluations of the PACE demonstrations indicate that they are experiencing problems of financial viability, high staff turnover among physicians and adult day health center directors, and obtaining the right patient mix in terms of both acuity and dementia (Kane et al. 1992).

Still another model for attempting to integrate the financing and delivery of acute and long-term care for older persons is the Minnesota Long-Term Care Options Project (LTCOP). Still in the planning stage, it is incorporating elements of both the S/HMO and On Lok models. In contrast to the S/HMO, however, LTCOP will target Medicaid-eligible enrollees and accordingly offer a benefit package that includes nursing home care as well as home- and community-based care. It will also include a less functionally dependent population than the On Lok model. Hence, it provides an opportunity to test broader approaches to integrating acute and long-term care than have been tried to date.

To the extent that any of these demonstration models seem to be effective in integrating care as they are tested in the years immediately ahead, their broader import in the American health care delivery system for older adults will still depend on further action by the federal government and the private sector. The government would need to allow the pooling of Medicare and Medicaid funds more generally for this purpose (the various demonstration models operate under special waivers from HCFA). And to make such care integration available for those older persons not covered by Medicaid for long-term care expenses, private insurance companies will need to be satisfied that such managed care arrangements are financially viable.

Health Care Reform

In the late 1980s and early 1990s, it appeared that a new federal policy that would establish public insurance for long-term care would be enacted. Today it appears far more likely that public funds for long-term care—in particular, Medicaid funds—will be scarcer than they are projected to be under current law.

Proposals to Expand Public Funds for Long-Term Care

The major initial impetus for public long-term care insurance was successful advocacy efforts on behalf of older people. Particularly noteworthy in this regard were the efforts undertaken by a political coalition concerned about Alzheimer's disease (AD) that began to form in the mid 1970s (Fox 1989). By the mid 1980s, advocates for older and younger disabled people began meeting to explore their common ground of interests (see Brody and Ruff 1986; Mahoney et al. 1986). And in 1989 a broad coalition named the Long-Term Care Campaign was formed. A Washington-based interest group claiming to represent 140 national organizations with more than 60 million members, it had as one of its key legislative goals that "Long Term Care services should be available to all who need them, regardless of age" (Long-Term Care Campaign 1990, p. 1).

A specific policy link was forged between younger and older disabled people in 1989 when Representative Claude Pepper introduced a bill to provide comprehensive long-term home care insurance coverage for persons of any age who were dependent in at least two activities of daily living (ADLs). Since then, a number of such long-term care bills have been introduced, with projected expenditures ranging from \$10 billion to \$60 billion, depending on provisions regarding the specific populations to be eligible and details regarding the timing, nature, and extent of insurance coverage.

The long-term care component in President Clinton's 1993 proposal for health care reform carried forward the principle of age irrelevance in determining eligibility for benefits. It posited that to be eligible for publicly financed services, an individual must meet one of the following conditions: 1) requires personal assistance, standby assistance, supervision, or cues to perform three or more of five ADLs—eating, dressing, bathing, toileting, and transferring in and out of bed; 2) presents evidence of severe cognitive or mental impairment as indicated by a specified score on a standard mental status protocol; 3) has severe or profound mental retardation; or 4) is a child under the age of 6 who is dependent on high technology or otherwise requires hospital or institutional care (White House Domestic Policy Council 1993, pp. 171–172).

Medicaid Block Grants

The Clinton proposal for health care reform failed in 1994, and the promise of federal long-term care insurance faded. In 1995 a Republican-dominated 104th Congress shifted legislative focus from creating a new program to curbing the costs of public expenditures for long-term care. Medicaid's expenditures on long-term care had been growing at an annualized rate of 13.2% since 1989 (U.S. General Accounting Office 1995).

As part of its overall effort to achieve a balanced budget by 2002, the 104th Congress initially proposed to curb the rate of growth in Medicaid expenditures to achieve savings of \$182 billion, to eliminate federal requirements for determining individual eligibility for Medicaid (as an entitlement), and to turn over control of the program to state governments through capped block grants. Late in the year, President Clinton vetoed a budget bill containing such changes.

The reductions and structural changes in Medicaid proposed by Congress in 1995 remain on the policy agenda, supported by the National Governors Conference. If they are enacted, state governments would have to face a number of critical issues, the resolution of which would vary, of course, from state to state. But the contour of the issues associated with a Medicaid block grant suggests that generally, throughout the states, the long-term care safety net that Medicaid provides for persons with dementia and their families (as well as other constituencies) could be substantially weakened.

One decision that states would have to face is whether to make up from their own funds the gap between the federal funds they would have received under current law and the lower amounts (after the first year of the new program) that they would receive in the form of a block grant. According to one analysis (Kassner 1995), the 1995 Congressional proposal for a Medicaid block grant would have trimmed long-term care funding by as much as 11.4% by 2000, meaning that 1.74 million Medicaid beneficiaries would have lost or been unable to secure coverage. It is unlikely that any states will provide their own funds to compensate for such a gap in federal funding. State expenditures on Medicaid are already 20% of the budget in some states and are growing fast in almost all states.

A second decision is whether to maintain the present level of expenditure, and perhaps keep up with health care cost inflation, for the state's own share of Medicaid funding. This maintenance would be politically and budgetarily difficult in most states. Most state budgets, unlike the federal budget, must be balanced each year in accordance with their constitutions. It is possible, of course, that Congress might follow the precedent it set in 1996 with legislation that turned welfare (Aid to Families with Dependent Children) into a block grant program in which it required states to maintain at least 75%–80% of their current Medicaid funding in order to receive federal grants.

The decisions of most states on these two issues—making up the federal funding gap and maintaining present state levels of funding—are likely to result in shrinking Medicaid resources for long-term care. Medicaid funding of home- and community-based care may disappear in some states and be cut back severely in others. Nursing home rates of reimbursement may, at best, be held constant, which would have the effect of ratcheting them down because of ongoing inflation in the costs of providing nursing home care.

A third issue that the states would confront is how to allocate limited and shrinking resources among the categorical groups eligible for Medicaid—the aged, disabled, and single mothers and children. This issue, unfortunately, is likely to engender heated political conflict among advocates for the respective constituents in these groups.

In tandem is a fourth set of decisions. States would have to set income and asset eligibility standards for Medicaid applications to replace the minimum federal entitlement standards that may be eliminated under a block grant program. Some states that now employ the minimum required levels may well set their criteria at lower levels, drastically reducing the number of persons eligible for Medicaid. Others, that presently have levels more generous than the federal minimum, may also be tempted to reduce the pool of Medicaid participants when faced with a cap on federal grant funds.

A fifth type of decision would be whether to maintain, through state implementation, the federal regulation standards established in 1987 for quality of care in nursing homes. It is worth noting that the 1987 federal standards were enacted because most states were not regulating quality of care in an adequate fashion. Now that the positive effects of such regulation have been empirically documented, perhaps states might do better on this front than they have previously.

Underlying these five issues that states would confront is a sixth very fundamental policy decision: How does the state intend to deal with people with dementia and other functionally disabled elders who have no place to turn—persons who cannot afford to pay for long-term care out of pocket, are not eligible for Medicaid, and do not have access to informal care from family and friends? This issue will become more and more pressing with capped block grants, especially in states that do not choose to make up for the gap in federal funding, do not maintain state funding levels at an adequate rate, curtail the portion of Medicaid funds available to the elderly (as opposed to other categories of Medicaid eligibility), lower income and asset eligibility standards, and do not wish to invest in regulation of quality of care. What is the state's social policy toward those who are not capable of taking care of themselves and have no place to turn? This issue has always been implicit, of course, but in the context of Medicaid block grants, it will need to become explicit and urgent.

What Lies Ahead?

In the years immediately ahead, it is likely that policy makers in Washington and the states will remain focused on limiting public funds for long-term care rather than expanding them. As indicated previously, federal and state outlays for Medicaid are expanding rapidly. Moreover, projections regarding spending for Medicaid when the baby boomers begin to reach the ranks of old age early in the twenty-first century are enormous, assuming current Medicaid policy stays the same (see Binstock et al. 1996).

A Coalition of Older and Younger Disabled Persons?

For the political milieu to change in favor of expanding public funds for long-term care, substantial grassroots support will be required from the constituencies who would most likely benefit from such a program. The principle of providing long-term care benefits on the basis of need for services, without regard to age, seems well established. Yet younger and older disabled persons have so far failed to find a common ground that is solid enough to develop a powerful political coalition.

Even if the fiscal costs of expanded public support for long-term care come to be perceived by policy makers as manageable, it is far from certain that older and younger disabled people—the latter including persons with spinal cord injury, cerebral palsy, mental retardation, AIDS, and other disabling conditions—will emerge as a sufficiently influential unified constituency to back such legislation. Unity will require substantial resolution of divergent outlooks and needs among the constituencies to be served.

Traditionally, advocates for the aged and for younger disabled populations have not been united in supporting long-term care initiatives and have sometimes engaged in sharp conflict (see Torres-Gil and Pynoos 1986). From the perspective of older persons, long-term care has been seen as a problem besetting elderly people, categorically, to be dealt with through a medical model of health and social services. And a major, though not exclusive, element of interest in public insurance has been generated by an economic concern. This concern is the possibility of becoming poor through spending down, that is, depleting one's assets to pay for long-term care and then becoming dependent on a welfare program, Medicaid, to pay long-term care bills. There is a distinct middle-class fear—both economic and psychological—of using savings and selling a home to finance one's own health care. This anxiety reflects a desire to preserve estates for inheritance, as well as the psychological intertwining of personal self-esteem with one's lifetime accumulation of material worth and sense of financial independence. This kind of concern has little political appeal beyond segments of the old-age constituency, of course, in the contemporary political environment structured by the generational equity paradigm (see Binstock 1994a).

In contrast to older persons, younger disabled persons and their advocates do not perceive long-term care insurance as mostly an issue of whether the government or the individual client or family pays for the care. At least as important to them is the issue of basic access to services, technologies, and environments that will make it feasible to carry forward an active life. They argue that they should have assistance to do much of what they would be able to do if they were not disabled.

The Americans with Disabilities Act of 1991 is helping to eliminate discriminatory as well as physical barriers to the participation of people with disabilities in employment, public services, public accommodations and transportation, and telecommunications. But it will not provide the elements of long-term care desired by disabled younger adults, such as paid assistance in the home and for getting in and out of the home, peer counseling, semi-independent modes of transportation, and client control or management of services.

Although the disabled have advocated for long-term care services, they have rejected a medical model that emphasizes long-term care as an essential component of health services. This stance is understandable given their strong desires for autonomy, independence, and as much normalization of daily life as possible. By the same token, disabled people have tended to eschew symbolic and political identification with elderly people because of traditional stereotypes of older people as frail, chronically ill, declining, and marginal to society.

Beyond issues of disparate philosophy lie specific divergences in service needs. As Benjamin (1996) points out, persons disabled through spinal cord injuries tend to remain in stable medical and functional condition for many years. Persons with AIDS have a trajectory of decline, punctuated by intermittent and continual episodes of acute illness. Although the trajectory for many elderly persons in long-term care—especially dementia patients—is gradual decline, on average their need for acute care is not as frequent as that of persons with AIDS.

Even among older persons in long-term care there are divergent needs. For instance, the cognitive impairments of people with dementia often require that the nature of a service be altered. A patient with dementia often fails to understand and cooperate with service providers; at the same time, many service providers are not especially knowledgeable about or skilled at working with patients who have dementia (see Office of Technology Assessment 1990).

Despite their traditional differences, advocates for the aged and the disabled worked together temporarily in the planning process for President Clinton's 1993 initiative on long-term care. This cooperation was reflected in the fact that the president's proposal incorporated many specific concerns that have been put forward by advocates for the younger disabled population over the years, for example, the principle that clients should be able at their own discretion to hire and fire service providers.

This unity eroded shortly thereafter, however, in the context of considerable reservations that the respective constituencies had regarding the overall Clinton plan for health care reform. On the one hand, advocates for the younger disabled were concerned that persons with what they term *special needs* would shortchanged in terms of attention and appropriate services within the acute care range of needs if their health care were to be provided in the context of the limited budgets of HMOs, preferred provider organizations (PPOs), and other health care provider groups that would have been assembled for the purchasing alliances. On the other hand, old-age interest groups, particularly the American Association of Retired Persons (AARP) and the National Committee to Preserve Social Security and Medicare (see McSteen 1993), were concerned with what they regarded as inequities between the insurance provided to Medicare enrollees as compared with the coverage that the president's plan proposed for most other Americans. Moreover, a provision that would have allowed states to integrate Medicare into purchasing alliances raised the specter of unofficial rationing of health care on the basis of old age—a fear paralleling that expressed by advocates for younger disabled persons (see Binstock 1994b).

The Politics of Aging

Although elements of the old-age constituency—most notably the victims of AD and their families and the Alzheimer's Association—are committed to achieving public long-term care insurance, the broader constituency of older persons does not appear to be very committed as yet. Even though many old-age interest groups support this goal, the political heterogeneity of older persons—even with respect to aging-related policy issues—makes it difficult for these organizations to develop broad, cohesive constituent support.

Media stereotypes portray some 33 million older persons as comprising a monolithic block of voters who promote and defend their self-interests successfully. In fact, however, older people are not a cohesive political constituency (Binstock and Day 1996). They distribute their votes among electoral candidates in the same proportions as do other age groups. Old-age interest groups, such as AARP, have shown no capacity to cohere or "swing" the votes of older people. And the organized demands of older persons have had little to do with the enactment and amendment of the major old-age policies such as Social Security, Medicare, and the Employee Retirement Income Security Act. Rather, such legislative actions over the years have been largely attributable to the initiatives of public officials who have focused on their own agendas for social and economic reforms.

However, extrapolation from the past and present is not always a good mode of prediction. Changing factors, especially in the lives of older persons and their families, could engender much broader and deeper popular support for long-term care legislation than has been observable to date. Some analysts have argued for years that an "age consciousness" will develop among older persons and, in turn, transform them into a cohesive political force (Bengtson and Cutler 1976; Cutler 1981; Cutler et al. 1984). Although such predictions have not been accurate in general, the development of age consciousness may be possible with respect to the issue of long-term care.

Various projections suggest that dementia and other disabling conditions will affect ever-increasing numbers of older persons and their families (see Williams and Temkin-Greener 1996). As they do, the frustrations of financing and obtaining adequate supportive services may become even more pervasive within the American population than they are now.

Of particular importance in contributing to such frustrations may be a change in the capacities and willingness of family members to care for disabled older persons—particularly when the baby boom cohort reaches old age. Family members—spouses, siblings, adult children, and broader kin networks—currently provide from 80% to 85% of all long-term care and support, through direct, unpaid services, to frail older persons who are not in nursing homes. About 74% of dependent community-based older persons receive all their care from family members or other unpaid sources; about 21% receive both formal and informal services, and only about 5% use just formal services (Liu et al. 1985). The family also plays an important role in obtaining and managing services from paid service providers, but it is possible that these roles of the family may diminish substantially during the next few decades.

The family, as a fundamental unit of social organization, has been undergoing profound transformations that will become more fully manifest over the next few decades as baby boomers reach old age. The striking growth of single-parent households, the growing participation of women in the labor force, and the high incidence of divorce and remarriage (differentially higher for men) all entail complicated changes in the structure of household and kinship roles and relationships. There will be an increasing number of blended families, reflecting multiple lines of descent through multiple marriages and the birth of children outside of wedlock through other partners. This growth in the incidence of step and half relatives will make for a dramatic new turn in family structure in the coming decades. Already such blended families constitute about half of all households with children (National Academy on Aging 1994).

As such changes begin to coincide with the growth of three- and even four-generation families, what emerges is a very complex picture that has hardly even begun to be analyzed and understood with respect to its potential ramifications. One clear implication, however, is that while kinship networks in the near future will become much more extensive than in the past, they will also become more complex, attenuated, and diffuse (Bengtson et al. 1990).

There is much room for speculation and debate about what blended families will mean for the functioning of the family as a system of social support and resource transfers among generations. Yet early research evidence of a weakened sense of filial obligation in blended families gives some cause for concern. If changes in the intensity of kinship relations significantly erode the capacity and sense of obligation to care for older family members when the baby boom cohort is in the ranks of old age and disability, there is a distinct possibility that support for public long-term care insurance will become an issue on which most older Americans and their families become united.

It is also possible that if new bills to expand long-term funding are introduced in Congress they may be more appealing to both the younger and older disabled constituencies than was the 1993 Clinton proposal. For one thing, such bills could be more carefully crafted to assure these groups that none of them will be short-changed with respect to either their share of program resources or the appropriateness of services for different types of clients and the suitability of arrangements through which they are available.

Perhaps more important, if such new initiatives are introduced without being part of an overall plan for reforming the nation's health care system, the various constituencies may embrace them far more readily than the Clinton long-term care plan. The latter was part of a broader proposal that, as noted earlier, engendered significant reservations among advocates for younger and older dis-abled persons regarding provisions affecting the acute care arena.

In the last analysis, even if substantial grassroots support for public long-term care develops, enactment of such legislation will also require strong national leadership. As indicated, none of the major policies that have comprised a welfare state for the elderly—such as Social Security, Medicare, the Employee Retirement In-come Security Act, and others—came about because of pressure from old-age interest groups or in response to broad popular de-mands for their enactment. Public long-term care insurance will need to be perceived by a president and congressional leaders as an essential response to a social issue of national importance.

However, unlike programs enacted in previous eras, grassroots support will also be needed to complement top-down leadership. The political climate—structured by deficit reduction, entitlement program reduction, and the paradigm of intergenerational equity—will undoubtedly generate a bill that requires many of the disabled beneficiaries, in accordance with their economic status, to finance substantial proportions of their services themselves. Under such circumstances, a broad base of potential beneficiaries—including those who must pay for some of the cost of their services—will need to be strong supporters of such a policy if it is to be enacted and endure. In the absence of such support, substantial reform to increase access to services and to improve their quality for persons with dementia (and their families) is unlikely to take place in the foreseeable future.

References

Adams EK, Meiners MR, Burwell BO: Asset spend-down in nursing homes: methods and insights. Med Care 31:1–23, 1993

Bengtson VL, Cutler NE: Generations and intergenerational relations: perspectives on age groups and social change, in Handbook of Aging and the Social Sciences. Edited by Binstock RH, Shanas E. New York, Van Nostrand Reinhold, 1976, pp 130–159

Bengtson VL, Rosenthal C, Burton L: Families and aging: diversity and heterogeneity, in Handbook of Aging and the Social Sciences, 3rd Edition. Edited by Binstock RH, George LK. San Diego, Academic Press, 1990, pp 263–287

Benjamin AE: Trends among younger persons with disabilities and chronic diseases, in The Future of Long-Term Care: Social and Policy Issues. Edited by Binstock RH, Cluff LE, von Mering O. Baltimore, Johns Hopkins University Press, 1996, pp 75–95

Binstock RH: Transcending intergenerational equity, in Economic Security and Intergenerational Justice: A Look at North America. Edited by Marmor TR, Smeeding TM, Greene VL. Washington, DC, The Urban Institute Press, 1994a, pp 155–185

Binstock RH: The Clinton plan, Medicare integration, and old-age-based rationing: the need for public debate. Gerontologist 34:612–613, 1994b

Binstock RH, Day CL: Aging and politics, in Handbook of Aging and the Social Sciences, 4th Edition. Edited by Binstock RH, George LK. San Diego, Academic Press, 1996, pp 362–387

Binstock RH, Cluff LE, von Mering O: Issues affecting the future of long-term care, in The Future of Long-Term Care: Social and Policy Issues. Edited by Binstock RH, Cluff LE, von Mering O. Baltimore, Johns Hopkins University Press, 1996, pp 3–18

Brody SJ, Ruff GE (eds): Aging and Rehabilitation: Advances in the State of the Art. New York, Springer, 1986

Burner ST, Waldo DR, McKusick DR: National health expenditures projections through 2030. Health Care Financing Review 14:1–29, 1992

Burwell B: State Responses to Medicaid Estate Planning. Cambridge, MA, SysteMetrics, 1993

Chellis RD, Grayson PJ: Life Care: A Long-Term Solution? Lexington, MA, Lexington Books, 1990

Cohen M: Life care: new options for financing and delivering long-term care. Health Care Financing Review, Annual Supplement 139–143, 1988

Cohen MA, Tell E, Greenberg J, Wallack SS: The financial capacity of the elderly to insure for long-term care. Gerontologist 27:494–502, 1987

Congressional Research Service, Library of Congress, Congress of the United States: Financing and Delivery of Long-Term Care Services for the Elderly. Washington, DC, U.S. Government Printing Office, 1988

Crown WH, Capitman J, Leutz WN. Economic rationality, the affordability of private long-term care insurance, and the role for public policy. Gerontologist 32:478–485, 1992

Cutler NW: Political characteristics of elderly cohorts in the twenty-first century, in Aging: Social Change. Edited by Kiesler S, Morgan JN, Oppenheimer VK. New York, Academic Press, 1981, pp 127–157

Cutler NE, Pierce R, Steckenrider J: How golden is the future? Generations 9:38–43, 1984

Eckert SK, Smyth K: A Case Study of Methods of Locating and Arranging Health and Long-Term Care for Persons With Dementia. Washington, DC, Office of Technology Assessment, Congress of the United States, 1988

Fox P: From senility to Alzheimer's disease: the rise of the Alzheimer's disease movement. Milbank Q 67:58–102, 1989

Friedland R: Facing the Costs of Long-Term Care: An EBRI-ERF Policy Study. Washington, DC, Employee Benefits Research Institute, 1990

Kane RA, Wilson KB: Assisted Living in the United States: A New Paradigm for Residential Care for Older People? Washington, DC, American Association for Retired Persons, 1993

Kane RL, Illston LH, Miller NA: Qualitative analysis of the Program of All-Inclusive Care for the Elderly (PACE). Gerontologist 32:771–780, 1992

Kassner E: Long-Term Care: Measuring the Impact of a Medicaid Cap. Washington, DC, Public Policy Institute, American Association of Retired Persons, 1995

Leutz W, Greenberg JN, Abrahams R, et al: Changing Health Care for an Aging Society: Planning for the Social/Health Maintenance Organization. Lexington, MA, Lexington Books, 1985

Liu K, Manton KM, Liu BM: Home care expenses for the disabled elderly. Health Care Financing Review 7:51–58, 1985

Long-Term Care Campaign: Pepper Commission recommendations released March 2nd. Insiders' Update, January/February 1990, p 1

Mahoney CW, Estes CL, Heumann JE (eds): Toward a Unified Agenda: Proceedings of a National Conference on Disability and Aging. San Francisco, Institute for Health and Aging, University of California, San Francisco, 1986

McSteen M: Testimony before the Subcommittee on Health, Committee on Ways and Means, U.S. House of Representatives. Washington, DC, October 21, 1993.

Meiners MR: The financing and organization of long-term care, in The Future of Long-Term Care: Social and Policy Issues. Edited by Binstock RH, Cluff LE, von Mering O. Baltimore, Johns Hopkins University Press, 1996, pp 191–214

Miller NA: Medicaid 2176 home and community-based care waivers: the first ten years. Health Aff 11:162–171, 1992

National Academy on Aging: Old Age in the 21st Century. Washington, DC, National Academy on Aging, 1994

Newcomer RJ, Harrington C, Friedlob A: Social health maintenance organizations: assessing their initial experience. Health Serv Res 25: 425–454, 1990

Office of Technology Assessment, Congress of the United States: Losing a Million Minds: Confronting the Tragedy of Alzheimer's Disease and Other Dementias. Washington, DC, U.S. Government Printing Office, 1987

Office of Technology Assessment, Congress of the United States: Confused Minds, Burdened Families: Finding Help for People with Alzheimer's and Other Dementias. Washington, DC, U.S. Government Printing Office, 1990

Rivlin AM, Wiener JM: Caring for the Disabled Elderly: Who Will Pay? Washington, DC, The Brookings Institution, 1988

Tell EJ, Cohen MA, Wallack SS: New directions in lifecare: an industry in transition. Milbank Q 65:551–574, 1987

Torres-Gil FM, Pynoos J: Long-term care policy and interest group struggles. Gerontologist 26:488–495, 1986

U.S. General Accounting Office: Long-Term Care: Current Issues and Future Directions. Washington, DC, U.S. Government Printing Office, 1995

Weissert WG: Strategies for reducing home care expenditures. Generations 14:42–44, 1990

White House Domestic Policy Council: The President's Health Security Plan. New York, Random House, 1993

Wiener JM, Illston LH: Health care financing and organization for the elderly, in Handbook of Aging and the Social Sciences, 4th Edition. Edited by Binstock RH, George LK. San Diego, Academic Press, 1996, pp 51–74

Wiener JM, Illston LH, Hanley RJ: Sharing the Burden: Strategies for Public and Private Long-Term Care Insurance. Washington, DC, The Brookings Institution, 1994

Williams TF, Temkin-Greener H: Older people, dependency, and trends in supportive care, in The Future of Long-Term Care: Social and Policy Issues. Edited by Binstock RH, Cluff LE, von Mering O. Baltimore, Johns Hopkins University Press, 1996, pp 75–95

Zawadski RT, Eng C: Case management in capitated long-term care. Health Care Financing Review, Annual Supplement 75–81, 1988

Index

Page numbers printed in **boldface** *type refer to tables or figures.*

A

Aβ-amyloid precursor protein. *See*
    β-Amyloid precursor protein
Aβ-amyloid protein. *See*
    β-Amyloid protein
Acquired genetic
    neurodegenerative disease,
    214
  HIV-1 infection, 215–216
Acquired immunodeficiency
    syndrome (AIDS)
  as acquired genetic
      neurodegenerative disease,
      215–216
  research, 213–214
Aging, politics of, 401–405
AIDS dementia complex (ADC),
    214
  brain injury in, 217–218
  cytokines, 219
  definition, 214–215
  as model for neurodegenerative
    diseases, 226
  neurotoxicity, 224–226

pathogenesis, 219–220, **221,**
    222
treatment
  immune enhancement, 227
  neurotoxicity suppression,
    227–229
  replication suppression,
    226–227
AIDS. *See* Acquired
    immunodeficiency syndrome
Alzheimer, A., 168
Alzheimer's disease
  animal models, 120–121
    nonhuman primates, 126–
      128
    transgenic mice, 128–131
  and antioxidants, 299–300, 356
  behavioral symptoms, 311–312
  compared with schizophrenia,
    313–314
  brain imaging
    brain activation, 256–260,
      257, 258, 259, 260
    computed tomography (CT),
      236, 238